REFRACTIVE SURGERY

AN INTERACTIVE CASE-BASED APPROACH

J. Bradley Randleman, MD

Editor-in-Chief, *Journal of Refractive Surgery*

Professor, Emory University Department of Ophthalmology

Director, Cornea, External Disease, and Refractive Surgery Section

Emory Eye Center, Emory University

Atlanta, Georgia

CRC Press
Taylor & Francis Group
Boca Raton London New York

CRC Press is an imprint of the
Taylor & Francis Group, an **informa** business

Dr. J. Bradley Randleman has no financial or proprietary interest in the materials presented herein.

Dr. Douglas D. Koch is a consultant for Alcon, AMO, Revision Optics, and Ziemer.

First published 2014 by SLACK Incorporated

Published 2024 by CRC Press
2385 NW Executive Center Drive, Suite 320, Boca Raton FL 33431

and by CRC Press
4 Park Square, Milton Park, Abingdon, Oxon, OX14 4RN

CRC Press is an imprint of Taylor & Francis Group, LLC

Library of Congress Cataloging-in-Publication Data

Randleman, J. Bradley (James Bradley), 1970- author.
Refractive surgery : an interactive case-based approach / J. Bradley Randleman.
p. ; cm.
Includes bibliographical references and index.
ISBN 978-1-61711-036-8 (paperback)
I. Title.
[DNLM: 1. Refractive Surgical Procedures--methods--Case Reports. WW 340]
RE925
617.7'55--dc23

2013044408

ISBN: 9781617110368 (pbk)
ISBN: 9781003526292 (ebk)

DOI: 10.1201/9781003526292

Dedication

To my darling Claudia, who loves me, supports me, amazes me, and inspires me…

To my three wonderful children, Taylor, Casey, and Mia, who enliven me and keep me young in mind and spirit…

To my father, who demonstrated teaching through coaching, and who taught me to always do my best to teach what I know to others…

…and to my mother, Patricia, whose boundless curiosity about life stimulated my scientific pursuits, and who loved a good puzzle—she would have definitely enjoyed reading this book!

Contents

Acknowledgments

This project grew out of my work over the years with cornea fellows and residents at Emory University, and I would like to thank all of them for their direct and indirect contributions to this process.

The cases may never have made it to print if not for the diligent efforts by two wonderful women who assisted me in their compilation: Cassandra Battle and Rhonda Hardaway-Brown.

Sonia Yoo, MD provided exceptional images to accompany the text in key sections, and I thank her for that help!

Of special note, the following individuals were instrumental in bringing this text to its final form through their critical review: Jenifer G. Bromley, MD; Sumitra S. Khandelwal, MD; Claudia E. Perez-Straziota, MD; Rupa D. Shah, MD; and Maria A. Woodward, MD.

About the Author

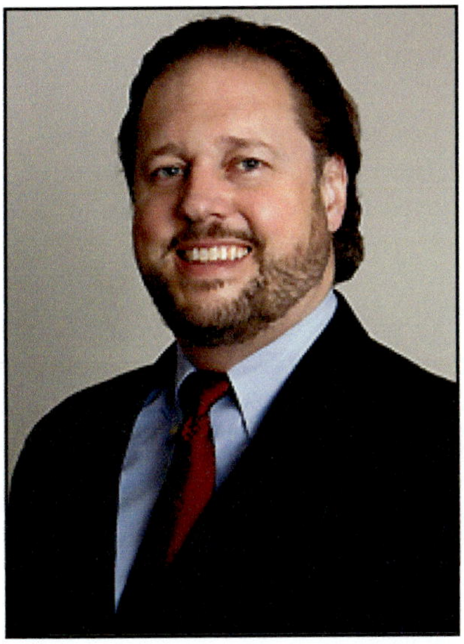

J. Bradley Randleman, MD, is a Professor in the Department of Ophthalmology at the Emory University School of Medicine and director of the Cornea, External Disease, and Refractive Surgery Section at the Emory Eye Center. A widely respected cornea specialist, his areas of expertise include corneal and intraocular refractive surgical procedures, the management of corneal and external eye diseases, corneal collagen cross-linking, corneal transplantation and cataract surgery. His primary research interests include preoperative refractive surgical screening, the avoidance, diagnosis, and management of refractive surgical complications; and diagnosis and management of corneal ectatic disorders.

Dr. Randleman received his BA degree from Columbia College at Columbia University in New York City with a joint major in biology and psychology. He earned his MD degree from Texas Tech University School of Medicine in Lubbock, Texas, where he was elected to the Alpha Omega Alpha Medical Honor Society in his junior year. He then completed his ophthalmology residency training at Emory University, where he received the Outstanding Teaching Resident award while he served as Chief Resident in his final year. Dr. Randleman joined the Emory faculty and served as Assistant Residency Director for 2 years while also completing a fellowship in cornea/external disease, and refractive surgery at Emory University. In 2004, he was awarded the prestigious Claes Dohlman Society Award, which is given annually to only one individual in the United States for academic and surgical excellence in cornea and refractive surgery training. Since practicing and teaching at Emory, he has trained more than 80 physicians in cataract surgery, refractive surgery, and corneal transplantation.

In 2007, Dr. Randleman was awarded the Secretariat Award from the American Academy of Ophthalmology (AAO) for special contributions to the field of ophthalmology. In 2010, he was presented the innagural Binkhorst Young Ophthalmologist Award from the American Society of Cataract and Refractive Surgery (ASCRS).

In 2011, Dr. Randleman was awarded the Kritzinger Memorial Award from the International Society of Refractive Surgery (ISRS). He was elected to the "135 Leading Ophthalmologists in America" listing by Becker's ASC Review (Ambulatory Surgery Centers). Dr. Randleman was also named as a "Top Ophthalmologist in America" by Castle Connolly Medical Ltd since 2010 and he is named as one of the "Best Doctors in America" by *US News & World Reports.*

Dr. Randleman has served as Editor-in-Chief for the *Journal of Refractive Surgery* since 2010. He has authored more than 90 peer-reviewed publications in leading ophthalmology journals in addition to 15 book chapters on refractive surgery evaluation and management of complications, and he co-edited the book *Corneal Collagen Cross-Linking* with Farhad Hafezi, MD, PhD.

Foreword

Every year my fellows, residents, and students ask me to recommend the best book for learning about refractive surgery. Every year I tell them that, although there are many excellent books on this topic, there isn't one go-to text. Until now.

Refractive Surgery: An Interactive Case-Based Approach by J. Bradley Randleman is that book. It has just what learners, and more experienced surgeons as well, need to grasp the basics of refractive surgery and to begin developing the clinical acumen required to care for refractive surgery patients.

Why this book?

- It is engaging. When I picked it up, I expected to read small sections at a time, but instead I read most of it at one sitting. Really? A "textbook" that one cannot put down? The case-based approach is ideal for involving the reader by stimulating inquiry and forcing one to think as a clinician. The cases are clinical puzzles that challenge (and entertain) us.
- It is comprehensive. It addresses all of the key refractive surgery procedures and remarkable array of preoperative clinical presentations and postoperative complications.
- It is beautifully illustrated. So much of what we decide in refractive surgery is based on evaluation of studies, and Dr. Randleman provides superb illustrations for each case and often supplements these with additional figures that enrich the discussion.
- It is informative. Each case is discussed in detail with clearly delineated sections and informative, pertinent references.
- It is a reference text. The initial chapters provide an excellent introduction to refractive surgery, and the appendix enables the reader to look up cases and study selected topics as needs or interests might dictate.

This book belongs in the hands of all aspiring refractive surgeons and those who simply want to know more about this field. I finally have "the" book that I will recommend to my trainees.

Douglas D. Koch, MD
Professor and Allen, Mosbacher, and Law Chair in Ophthalmology
Cullen Eye Institute
Baylor College of Medicine
Houston, Texas

Introduction

Refractive surgery has gone through extraordinary changes over the past 30 years; moving from a rogue surgical concept, with limited procedural options suitable for only the most pioneering patients and surgeons, to mainstream acceptance by surgeons and patients as a safe, effective, and reasonable choice for appropriate individuals. Although initial procedures focused primarily on altering the cornea to modify refraction for a narrow range of errors, surgeons now have a variety of corneal techniques, including corneal (incisional, laser ablative, implants) and intraocular (phakic lens implantation and refractive crystalline lens exchange) procedures. These procedures, to varying degrees, can address most refractive errors through the functional range of human vision.

Although some of these techniques have reached relative maturity in their development, even our most venerable procedures to date—excimer laser corneal ablation and cataract surgery with intraocular lens implantation—are constantly undergoing revision of surgical indications, techniques, and the technology available to reach our goals.

At the same time, refractive surgery is finally getting the academic attention it deserves! In the United States, medical residents are now required to become exposed to, and educated about, refractive surgery. For example, an entire volume of the *Basic and Clinical Science Course* from the American Academy of Othalmology is dedicated solely to the study of refractive surgery, and there are now Accreditation Council for Graduate Medical Education guidelines in place to ensure medical residents are exposed to refractive surgery didactics and surgery (www.acgme.org). This means that all eye care professionals, not just those who maintain a dedicated refractive surgical practice, must be aware of the conditions with which their patients may present before and after refractive surgery to most effectively counsel, diagnose, and treat their patient population. With the constant addition of new techniques and technologies comes the need for learning strategies to educate the novice surgeon, and keep even the seasoned veteran up to date, on the best practice patterns for the wide variety of patients who will present to our offices searching for improved vision independent from visual aids.

However, most medical residents feel they receive insufficient exposure to refractive surgical concepts and few actually perform any refractive surgery during training. Furthermore, although many conclusions have been collectively reached in numerous areas of patient evaluation, surgical technique, and avoidance and management of surgical complications, countless areas of debate and controversy remain. The goal of this book is to present where consensus exists today and to present varying elements of discussion in areas where controversy remains.

Developing the Interactive Case-Based Approach

This book has evolved from the hands-on exercises my cornea fellows and residents have gone through with me over the years. Refractive surgery patient evaluations are particularly well suited for chart review, and my trainees have walked themselves through each chart, looking for salient information contained within the notes and images. We discuss the relevant and irrelevant data in each situation, which is similar to having the medical chart accessible when these same patients are evaluated by them or you. Some cases were easily navigated, while others proved puzzling over and over again. These puzzling cases made it into the "interesting case file" folder, which finally outgrew its confines and became this text.

How to Use This Book

Regular textbooks and peer-reviewed publications are an invaluable source of knowledge. However, knowledge acquisition through simple reading is a passive process; the information is presented and you, the reader, absorb it. In contrast, many studies have shown that most "learners" learn best when the process is active and engaging, forcing them to think rather than merely absorb. Consider the information that came to you by way of a question with which you were charged to answer, or a specific clinical dilemma you had to solve, or a specific patient you had to treat. When one is forced to find information rather than remember it, to think instead of absorb, and to become an active participant in the learning process, the knowledge acquired in this manner has the veracity to last a lifetime. That is the intent of this text—acquisition of knowledge that will last a lifetime.

After laying a foundation and defining key concepts through the first few concise chapters, each "chapter" in Section II of this book is a single case that will present similar to a patient who seeks your care in clinic. All of the necessary information will be offered so that you can make an informed decision regarding diagnosis and management plans; however, no information will be highlighted or accentuated but rather left for you to sift through for each case. The critical question for each case is simply, "What data in this chart are the most critical for me to consider when evaluating this patient for surgery?"

Instead of neatly arranged chapter headings taking you through the refractive surgery in a predictable, logical, and fully organized way, this book will challenge you to formulate your own answers first. You will sift through the available information, determine what is relevant and what is not, and make decisions in the best interest of your patient. Only after this active process should you "turn the page" to obtain the rest of the story and understand the specific relevance of the clinical scenario, including much of what is known and what is left to be determined for each scenario.

The layout of the case scenario text will necessarily be different than most other textbooks that you will encounter. Don't turn the page until you have processed the information presented and have formulated your answers! The text will also be laid out to function effectively "forwards" or "backwards" depending on the situation—meaning, as a learning tool moving "forward" or as a reference tool, moving from back to front. After the introductory chapters the remainder of the text will be organized by case scenario. A case will be presented, and pointed questions will first guide you through the scenario; second, move you onto the discussion points; and then finally direct you to the literature, which is listed in each section in alphabetical order by author, for further reading. The cases in this book cover a variety of topics that present to the refractive surgeon and anyone else who manages refractive surgical patients on a daily basis.

This approach will, by definition, result in a compilation of the most important clinical scenarios presenting to refractive surgeons today. To add further value to the case presentations, the topics will be organized, referenced, and available to the reader by approaching the book "backwards" so that if one is looking for a concise review on a particular topic, he or she can simply go to the index, find the relevant discussion pages, and use the text accordingly. My hope is that most will attack the book and its available teaching points from a forward direction first and then rely on it as a reference guide later.

The Companion Website

In addition to the material contained in this text, a variety of learning modules are contained online at the accompanying website: www.routledge.com/9781617110368

This material includes the following:

- Surgical videos (with voice overlay) highlighting and explaining the basic steps for refractive surgical procedures, including photorefractive keratectomy (PRK), LASIK, and phakic intraocular lens (IOL) implantation
- Additional cases for evaluation, specifically regarding intraoperative decision making

It is my sincere hope that the combination of text and video-based learning modules will guide you through the decision-making process for a broad range of issues that can arise when performing refractive surgical procedures.

Bibliography

McDonnell PJ, Kirwan TJ, Brinton GS, et al. Perceptions of recent ophthalmology residency graduates regarding preparation for practice. *Ophthalmology.* 2007;114(2):387-391.

Randleman JB, Stulting, RD. Refractive surgical education: what's the best time, and what's the best place? *Am J Ophthalmol.* 2006;141(1):143-144.

Yeu E, Reeves SW, Wang L, Randleman JB; ASCRS Young Physicians and Residents Clinical Committee. Resident surgical experience with lens and corneal refractive surgery: survey of the ASCRS Young Physicians and Residents Membership. *J Cataract Refract Surg.* 2013;39(2):279-284.

Section I

Refractive Surgery: An Interactive Case-Based Approach

1

Fundamentals of Refractive Surgery

Chapter Highlights

- Refractive error
- Refractive surgery terminology
- Overview of refractive surgeries
- Biological and biomechanical impact of refractive surgery

A basic understanding of the techniques, concepts, and terminology unique to refractive surgery is necessary before any relevant case discussion can begin. This chapter will focus on the fundamentals of refractive error (ametropia), available refractive surgical techniques, and the primary biological and biomechanical considerations that are critical for understanding the mechanisms by which surgical procedures induce refractive change, as well as their potential to induce complications.

Refractive Error

Refractive Errors

- Myopia
- Hyperopia
- Astigmatism
    - ◊ Regular
    - ◊ Irregular
- Presbyopia
- Higher-order aberrations

Refractive error can be subdivided into 2 primary categories: lower-order aberrations (error) and higher-order aberrations (HOA).

Lower-Order Aberrations

Lower-order aberrations include myopia, hyperopia, and astigmatism, and result from a mismatch between combined corneal and lenticular power and axial length in healthy eyes. Lower-order aberrations cause increased blur relative to the amount of error, have the greatest impact on visual function, and are the target of most

Randleman JB.
Refractive Surgery: An Interactive Case-Based Approach (pp. 3-14).

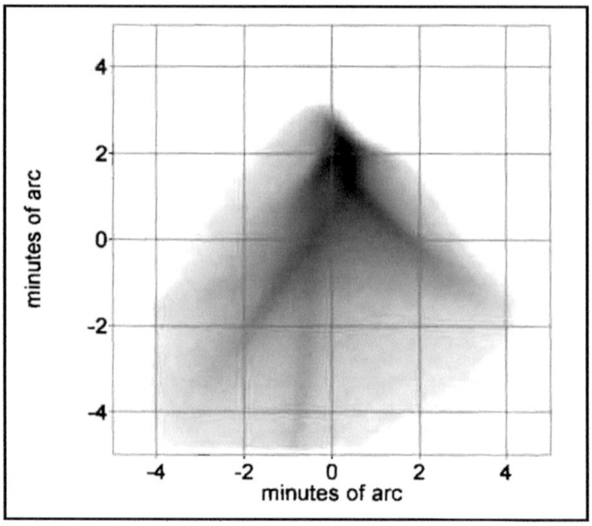

Figure 1-1. Point spread function (PSF) demonstrating relative blur generated by a point source of light in a patient with myopia. Higher refractive errors generate larger PSF.

refractive surgical procedures (Figure 1-1). Myopia induces blur at distance, whereas near objects at the patient's focal plane are clear. Hyperopia induces blur relatively greater at near than at distance focus, although in reality, distant objects also become blurred when the patient's ability to accommodate for clarity is insufficient. Regular astigmatism occurs when the eye has more than one focal plane, which can be induced by a nonspherical corneal or lenticular curvature; thus, all objects are blurred to some extent with astigmatism, regardless of their distance from the eye.

Higher-Order Aberrations

HOA are numerous and complex (Figure 1-2), and our understanding of their effects on visual quality are expanding rapidly. Among the multitude of HOA, the most significant appear to be spherical aberration, coma, and trefoil, all of which can potentially induce glare and halo and degrade contrast sensitivity. These aberrations can occur in combination with any degree of lower-order aberration, even in individuals without "regular" refractive error (lower-order aberrations).

Spherical aberration occurs when peripheral light rays reach the retina out of sync with central light rays, either reaching the retina before (positive spherical aberration) or after (negative spherical aberration) central rays. Spherical aberration is a common cause of halos around point light sources and frequently manifests as night vision complaints.

Coma causes light rays at one side of the pupil to come into focus before rays from the opposite edge and can occur horizontally or vertically, inducing relative blur, with the resulting image shaped like a comet with a blurred tail image.

Lower-order aberrations (hereafter referred to as *refractive errors* or *ametropia*) can be considered as a measure of vision quantity, as these errors determine an individual's reliance on visual aids, which increase directly proportionate to the amount of lower-order aberrations present. In contrast, HOA are associated with vision quality, with significant HOA inducing glare, halos, and blur in low contrast situations.

Presbyopia is not a true refractive error but rather an age-related phenomenon by which the process of accommodation (the ability to increase lenticular curvature and power) gradually decreases over time, making near objects blurred. The precise mechanism for presbyopia remains under debate; nevertheless, the process generally becomes clinically relevant around the age of 40 years and progressively worsens until about age 65 years. As opposed to other refractive errors, presbyopia affects all individuals, and because so many of our daily tasks are viewed at close range,

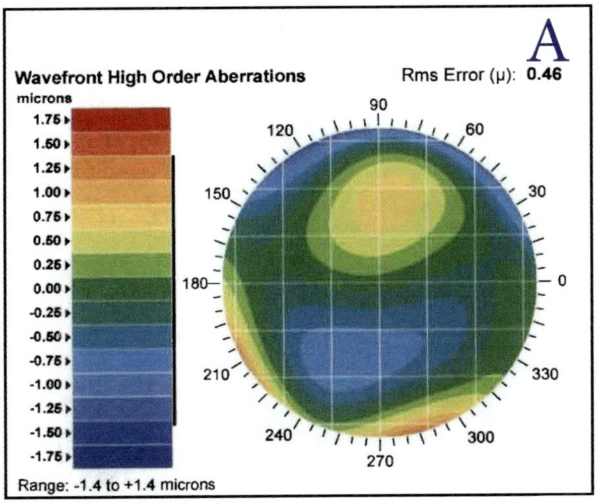

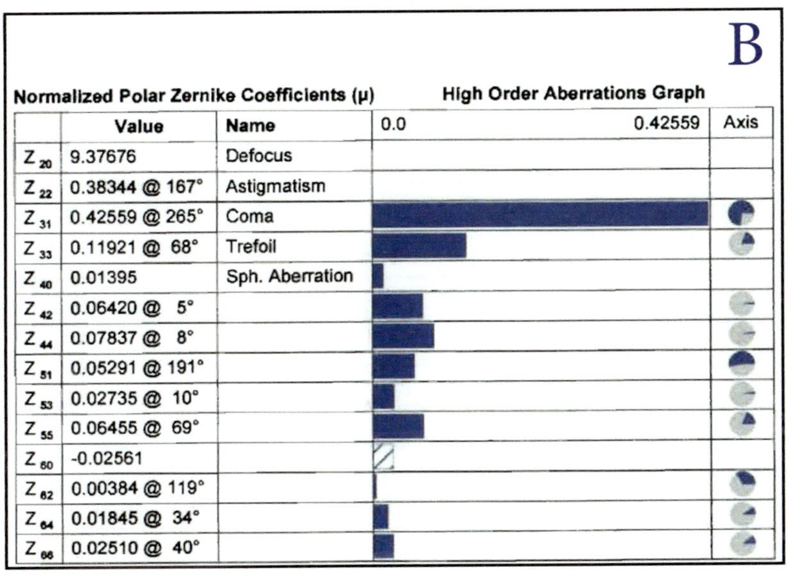

	Value	Name	0.0 — 0.42559	Axis
Z 20	9.37676	Defocus		
Z 22	0.38344 @ 167°	Astigmatism		
Z 31	0.42559 @ 265°	Coma		
Z 33	0.11921 @ 68°	Trefoil		
Z 40	0.01395	Sph. Aberration		
Z 42	0.06420 @ 5°			
Z 44	0.07837 @ 8°			
Z 51	0.05291 @ 191°			
Z 53	0.02735 @ 10°			
Z 55	0.06455 @ 69°			
Z 60	-0.02561			
Z 62	0.00384 @ 119°			
Z 64	0.01845 @ 34°			
Z 66	0.02510 @ 40°			

Figure 1-2. HOA profile demonstrating (A) the HOA pattern and overall HOA error reported as root mean square (RMS) error (in microns) and (B) specific Zernike polynomial coefficients. The most clinically significant values appear to be spherical aberration, coma, and trefoil.

presbyopia correction is of utmost importance to all individuals. Currently, accommodation cannot be restored directly; therefore, all refractive procedures aimed at improving near acuity do so by modifying the way the eye functions to provide near focus.

Irregular astigmatism occurs in eyes with abnormal corneal curvature, including those with an ectatic corneal disorder (eg, keratoconus), irregularity caused by corneal scars or opacities, or previous ocular surgery with irregular corneal healing (Figure 1-3). Irregular astigmatism is not amenable to correction with current corneal refractive surgical procedures but is the focus of many new technologies, including topography-guided laser ablations and corneal collagen cross-linking (CXL). Refer to Chapter 3 for a more complete discussion of corneal topographic analysis.

Overview of Refractive Surgeries

A wide range of surgical procedures exists to treat refractive error, which is broadly categorized as corneal or intraocular procedures. Most refractive surgical techniques are better known by their abbreviations than their full names. Table 1-1 lists the most common procedures and

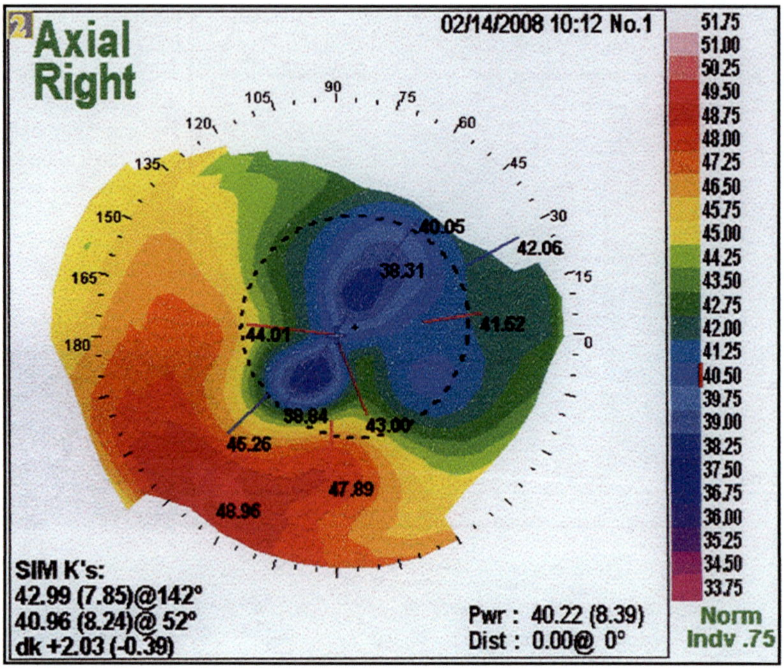

Figure 1-3. Corneal topography exhibiting significant irregular astigmatism, as seen by the multitude of color patterns with irregular orientation, in an eye after previous corneal refractive surgery that developed postoperative ectasia.

Table 1-1. Common Refractive Surgical Procedures and Their Abbreviations	
SPECIFIC PROCEDURES	COMMON ABBREVIATIONS
Incisional surgeries	
Radial keratotomy	RK
Astigmatic keratotomy	AK
Limbal relaxing incisions	LRI
Laser vision correction	LVC
Surface ablation	ASA or SA
Photorefractive keratectomy	PRK
Laser-assisted subepithelial keratomileusis	LASEK
Epipolis laser in situ keratomileusis	Epi-LASIK
Laser in situ keratomileusis	LASIK
Intracorneal ring segments	ICRS
Conductive keratoplasty	CK
Corneal collagen cross-linking	CXL
Phakic intraocular lens	PIOL
Refractive lens exchange	RLE
Multifocal IOL	MFIOL
Toric IOL	Toric IOL

Table 1-2. Overview of Corneal Refractive Surgical Procedures

PROCEDURE TYPE	SPECIFIC PROCEDURES	APPROVED REFRACTIVE ERROR TREATMENT RANGE	COMMON REFRACTIVE ERROR RANGE TREATED*
Incisional	AK, LRI	N/A	Astigmatism up to 2.00 diopters (D)
Excimer laser	Surface ablation (PRK, LASEK, Epi-LASIK)	+6.00 to -14.00 D spherical, up to 6.00 D astigmatism	+3.00 to -8.00 D
	LASIK	+6.00 to -14.00 D, up to 6.00 D astigmatism	+3.00 to -12.00 D
Corneal inlays	Intracorneal ring segments	Myopia (-1.00 to -3.00 D), keratoconus	Keratoconus
Collagen shrinkage	Conductive keratoplasty	Hyperopia, astigmatism +0.75 to +3.25 D	Not commonly used
Collagen cross-linking		Not yet approved in the United States	Keratoconus and postoperative ectasia

*The common range treated is the author's opinion and does not signify absolute practice patterns in the United States or abroad.

Abbreviation: N/A, no treatment ranges specified.

The Most Common Refractive Surgical Procedures

- LASIK
- Surface ablation
- Phakic IOL
- Refractive lens exchange

their abbreviations. Unfortunately, some abbreviations look quite similar (eg, radial keratotomy [RK] and photorefractive keratectomy [PRK]), despite the procedures being completely unrelated, whereas other related procedures (eg, laser in situ keratomileusis [LASIK] and PRK) look nothing alike. This causes great confusion among patients, especially when a procedure other than LASIK is being recommended to them.

Corneal refractive surgical procedures are by far the most widely utilized techniques specifically for refractive error. The most common types and treatment ranges are shown in Table 1-2. All corneal refractive procedures selectively alter corneal curvature to reduce specific refractive errors. Central flattening reduces myopia, whereas central steepening reduces hyperopia or induces myopia for improved near vision if the eye is targeted for this. The cornea's natural prolate shape, steeper centrally than peripherally, produces an aspheric optical system that minimizes spherical aberrations and modern treatments aim to reduce refractive error, while maintaining this prolate shape, to minimize visual aberrations such as glare and halos.

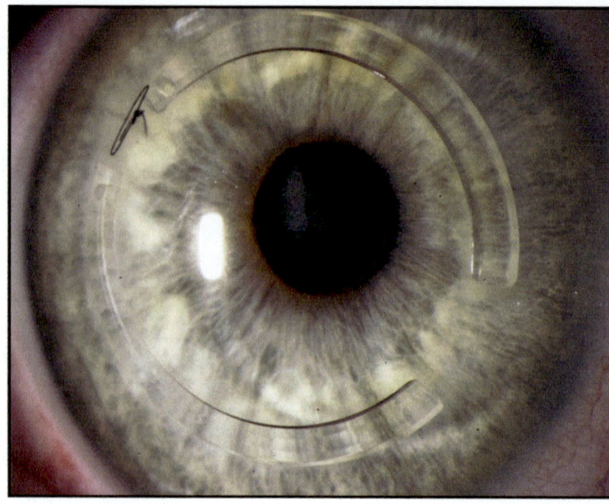

Figure 1-4. Slit-lamp image of Intacs segments within the corneal stroma (Addition Technology).

Among corneal refractive procedures, excimer laser ablation is the most utilized technique, either through surface ablation or LASIK. Excimer laser procedures, also generically termed *laser vision correction* (LVC), alter corneal curvature, thereby reducing refractive error, depending on the amount and location of the applied laser energy. Excimer laser energy and treatment patterns are identical for surface ablation and LASIK procedures. The differences in procedures derive from the location of laser application. Surface ablation procedures occur on a denuded Bowman's layer and anterior stroma, whereas LASIK occurs in the midstroma by making an anterior corneal stromal flap created with a mechanical microkeratome or femtosecond laser. The history of excimer laser refractive surgical techniques is fascinating and enlightening; however, it is also beyond the scope of this book. Please see references at the end of this chapter for further reading on these topics.

Other less common corneal refractive procedures include intracorneal ring segments (ICRS) for myopia or keratoconus (Figure 1-4), and presbyopia-correcting corneal inlays, which are not yet approved in the United States. Intracorneal ring segments are designed to reduce myopia through an arc-shortening biomechanical effect, whereby the peripheral cornea is steepened by the space-occupying ring segment, resulting in central corneal flattening. Presbyopic inlays function through a variety of mechanisms, including increased depth of focus or additional plus power, both of which may improve unaided near acuity.

Although not directly or specifically a refractive procedure, CXL is an important adjunctive technique by which corneal biomechanical strength is increased. This procedure is utilized currently for keratoconus and other naturally occurring ectatic diseases, as well as postoperative corneal ectasia. In the future, CXL may be utilized in combination with other refractive procedures to induce a positive refractive effect in previously untreatable corneas.

Other surgical techniques are less utilized presently, including incisional techniques (ie, radial keratotomy) to correct myopia and collagen thermal techniques (ie, laser thermal keratoplasty and conductive keratoplasty) to correct hyperopia or induce myopia for intended near vision improvement. However, these techniques are indirectly relevant in that many patients who had previously undergone these procedures continue to present for further refractive surgical options and for cataract surgery.

Intraocular surgical techniques (Table 1-3) include phakic intraocular lens (PIOL) implantation, where the natural crystalline lens is maintained and an intraocular lens (IOL) is implanted anterior to it, either iris-fixated (Figure 1-5) or in the sulcus. Another technique is refractive

Table 1-3. Overview of Intraocular Refractive Surgical Procedures

PROCEDURE TYPE	SPECIFIC PROCEDURES	APPROVED REFRACTIVE ERROR TREATMENT RANGE	COMMON REFRACTIVE ERROR RANGE TREATED*
Phakic	Phakic IOL		
	Iris-fixated	-5.00 to -20.00 D	-6.00 to -20.00 D (and higher)
	Posterior chamber	-3.00 to -20.00 D	-6.00 to -20.00 D
	Toric PIOL	Investigational in the United States	
Pseudophakic	Refractive lens exchange	Myopia, hyperopia, astigmatism up to 4.00 D, presbyopia	Myopia, hyperopia, astigmatism up to 4.00 D, presbyopia

*The common range treated is the author's opinion and does not signify absolute practice patterns in the United States or abroad

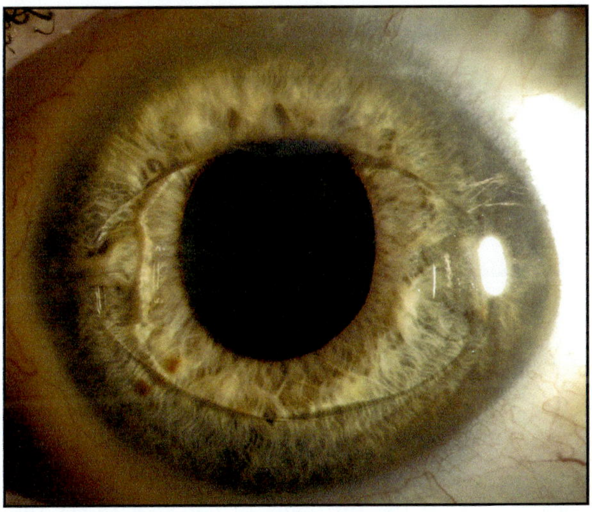

Figure 1-5. Slit-lamp image of an eye after phakic IOL implantation with an iris-claw IOL. Note the iris fixation with the IOL haptic attached to the midperipheral iris in the 3- and 9-o'clock regions. The IOL was implanted through a superior clear corneal incision.

lens exchange (RLE) (Figure 1-6), which is surgically equivalent to cataract surgery, whereby the crystalline lens is replaced with an artificial IOL intended to correct refractive error and potentially presbyopia, depending on the IOL design.

Biological and Biomechanical Impact of Refractive Surgical Procedures

Detailed explanation of laser biophysics is beyond the scope of this book. However, there are a few fundamental concepts worth digesting. All refractive procedures have both biomechanical and biological (wound healing) effects on the eye, and these factors are important to consider in each patient to best match patient and procedure to maximize safety and efficacy.

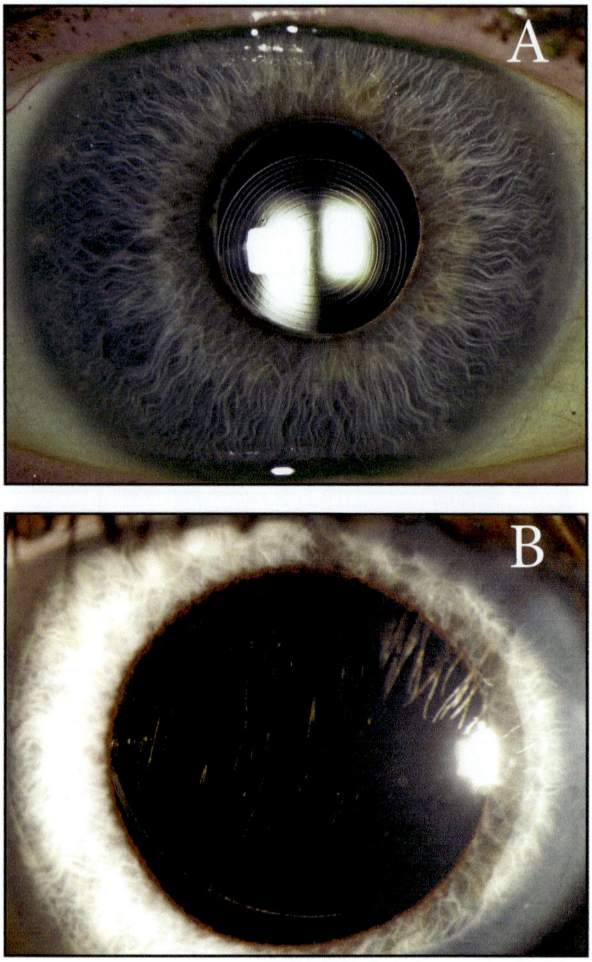

Figure 1-6. (A) Multifocal pseudophakic IOL, with multiple concentric rings visible in the pupillary margin. (B) Toric pseudophakic IOL, with the toric orientation marks (3 aligned dots on the IOL haptic) visible on the 9-o'clock region.

Laser Biophysics: Excimer and Femtosecond Lasers

Two unique lasers are utilized for laser vision correction surgeries—the femtosecond laser for LASIK flap creation and the excimer laser for ablation to induce corneal power change in all procedures.

Femtosecond laser energy is photodisruptive, causing the breakage of collagen fibers that allows for tissue plane creation sufficient to create corneal flaps or stromal channels for ICRS implantation. The femtosecond laser utilizes a 1053-nm beam in the infrared range that transforms tissue focally into plasma, resulting in microcavities within the corneal stroma at a predetermined depth that, when placed close enough together, functionally cleaves corneal tissue. The femtosecond laser's mechanism of action can also give rise to potential complications through excessive interface gas build up, resulting in anterior chamber bubbles, vertical gas breakthrough (similar to a microkeratome buttonhole flap), or an opaque bubble layer in the interface.

Excimer laser energy is photoablative, causing a relative dissolution of corneal tissue at the submicron level. The excimer laser derives its name from a combination of the words *excited dimer*, signifying the use of energized argon and fluoride gasses to create dimers, generating particles with a wavelength of 193 nm in the ultraviolet range with energy sufficient to break carbon–carbon and carbon–nitrogen bonds. A single excimer laser pulse removes a depth of approximately 0.25 μm, thus allowing for precise tissue removal. Further, at 193 nm, the laser

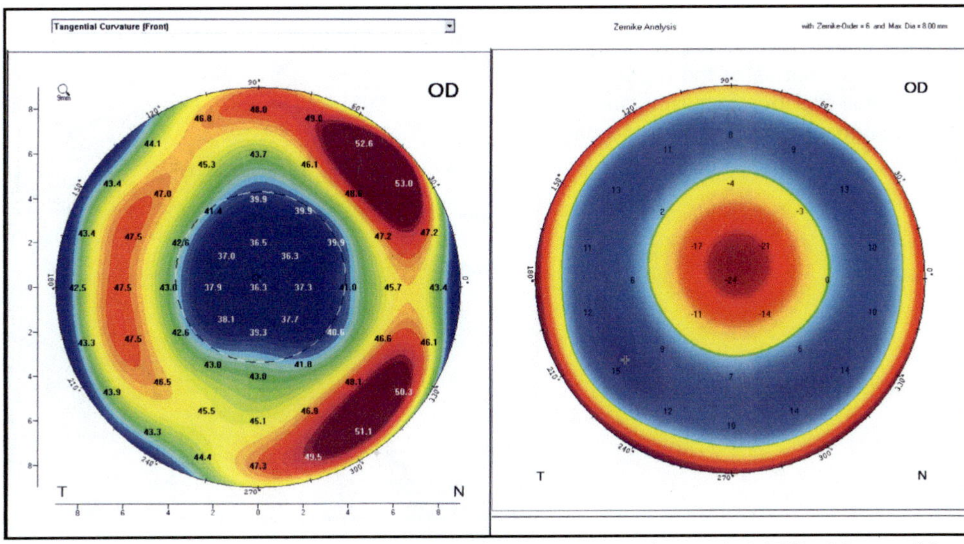

Figure 1-7. Topography (left) and HOA (right) after conventional myopic LASIK without a blend zone. Note the abrupt change in corneal power at an approximate 6-mm diameter at the edge of the ablation without a blend zone, with significant positive aberrations outside the treatment zone.

is nonmutagenic and functionally nonthermal; therefore, minimal damage to adjacent corneal tissue occurs. Excimer laser ablation occurs centrally for myopic treatments to induce central corneal flattening and peripherally for hyperopic treatments to induce central corneal steepening. Corneal tissue removal necessary to correct specific refractive errors can be approximated by the following Munnerlyn formula:

Ablation depth in microns (μm) ≈ [diopters (D) of myopia x OZ2 (mm)]/3 OZ = optical zone.

Thus, increasing the ablation zone size can dramatically increase tissue removal required for the treatment of higher myopic errors. Although smaller optical zones were utilized in the past, currently most clinicians use 6.5 to 7.0 mm OZ for standard treatments, with a "blend zone" well beyond the OZ to minimize induced spherical aberrations.

Each excimer laser platform generates a unique ablation pattern and ablation depth. These data can be entered into the laser settings prior to surgery to facilitate surgical planning by allowing for an estimation of residual stromal bed (RSB) thickness through the following formula:

RSB thickness (μm) = Central corneal thickness – flap thickness – ablation depth

There is no definitive cutoff value for RSB thickness; however, most surgeons try to leave a RSB thickness of 250 to 300 μm for all eyes to prevent biomechanical instability and progressive postoperative ectasia.

Conventional, Wavefront-Optimized, and Wavefront-Guided Ablations

Conventional laser ablations, available on some excimer lasers, essentially have no blend zone and are more likely to induce HOA, especially spherical aberration (Figure 1-7). Wavefront-optimized ablation profiles are designed to minimize spherical aberration induction by using a

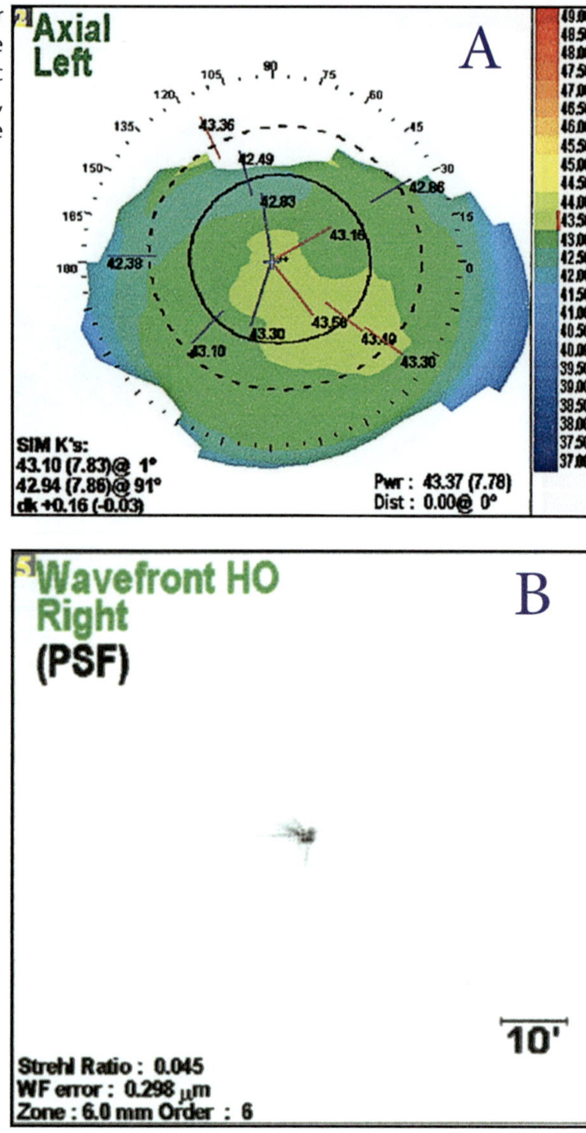

Figure 1-8. (A) Topography and (B) PSF after wavefront-optimized myopic LASIK. Note the retained prolate curvature of the topographic image and small PSF on wavefront analysis, indicating minimal residual error or image distortion.

population-based peripheral ablation pattern that adds energy to pulses directed to the periphery to account for the angle of approach for these pulses (Figure 1-8). Wavefront-guided ablations theoretically provide the most customized ablation profile by measuring specific wavefront HOA preoperatively, using specific aberrometers for each laser platform and applying selective laser ablation to account for these. However, multiple studies have found minimal differences between wavefront-optimized and wavefront-guided ablations in patients with relatively normal preoperative HOA profiles (approximately 85% to 90% of the population), and that measurement error can minimize the efficacy of wavefront-guided ablations. Both wavefront-optimized and wavefront-guided profiles are superior to conventional ablations for the majority of patients, providing superior vision in low-lighting conditions, especially at night, and, along with increased optical and blend zones, minimizing the induction of glare and halos postoperatively.

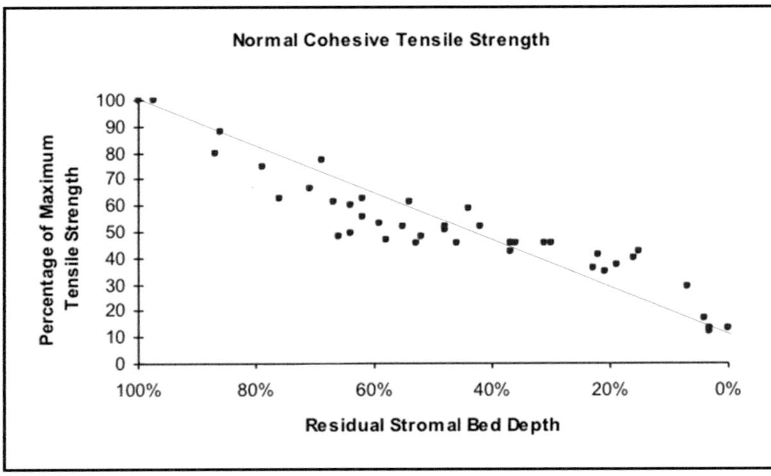

Figure 1-9. Depiction of the relative depth-dependent corneal tensile strength. Tensile strength is not uniform throughout but decreases with increasing depth in the cornea. (Adapted from Randleman JB, Dawson DG, Grossniklaus HE, McCarey BE, Edelhauser HF. Depth-dependent cohesive tensile strength in human donor corneas: implications for refractive surgery. *J Refract Surg.* 2008;24(1):S85-S89.)

Corneal Wound Healing

The mechanisms for and degree of corneal healing directly affects refractive outcomes for surface ablation and LASIK procedures. Following surface ablation, a complex cascade of events occurs, including keratocyte migration and apoptosis in response to removal of epithelium and Bowman's layer, with accompanying cytokine release. Clinically, this response can manifest as corneal haze, although in practice, significant haze occurs rarely (see Chapter 5, Figure 5-4).

Prophylactic use of mitomycin C (MMC), a chemotherapeutic agent, has significantly reduced the occurrence of clinically significant haze after surface ablation. Clinicians routinely use topical steroids after both surface ablation and LASIK to minimize inflammation and corneal haze, although the efficacy of this remains to be determined.

In contrast to surface ablation, a minimal wound healing response occurs after LASIK. With epithelial disruption only at the flap edge, minimal cytokine release occurs, minimizing the potential for corneal haze, and limited wound healing occurs between the anterior corneal flap and residual stromal bed, which is isolated to the peripheral wound region. This allows for functional corneal transparency centrally and the future ability to relift the flaps surgically for enhancement retreatment (termed *enhancements*), perhaps indefinitely, but it also significantly reduces corneal biomechanical strength.

Corneal Biomechanical Alterations After Excimer Laser Surgery

In the normal, unoperated cornea, physiologic stress is borne uniformly throughout the corneal stroma. However, corneal tensile strength does not appear uniform through the cornea in superior–inferior or anterior–posterior directions. Rather, the inferior cornea appears biomechanically weaker than its superior counterpart, and the anterior 40% of the corneal stroma has significantly greater tensile strength than the remaining 60% (Figure 1-9).

This biomechanical gradient has significant implications for excimer laser corneal refractive surgical procedures, with corneal biomechanical alterations being more significant after LASIK than after comparable surface ablation. Due to the relative increased weakness of the posterior stroma, LASIK performed with thicker corneal flaps results in deeper ablations into functionally weaker tissues, thus having an additive biomechanical effect. Thinner corneal flaps mitigate this difference; however, LASIK still appears to have a greater effect on postoperative corneal biomechanics than does surface ablation. This impacts surgical decision making in eyes where preoperative corneal thickness is low, where greater ablations are needed for higher refractive errors, or in corneas with suspicious signs for biomechanical weakness. This will be discussed in greater detail in Chapter 3.

Summary and Take Home Points

A variety of refractive surgical procedures are available to treat refractive error (ametropia). All treatments are primarily directed toward lower-order aberrations (myopia, hyperopia, and astigmatism); however, attention must be paid to minimizing the induction of HOA.

The most common refractive surgical procedures are corneal excimer laser ablation (LASIK and surface ablation) and IOL-based procedures (phakic IOL implantation and refractive lens exchange). Principles of laser biophysics determine laser accuracy and predictability, whereas wound healing and biomechanical considerations help to direct surgical decision making.

Bibliography

Dupps WJ Jr, Wilson SE. Biomechanics and wound healing in the cornea. *Exp Eye Res.* 2006;83(4):709-720.

Hafezi F, Randleman JB, eds. Corneal Collagen Cross-Linking. Thorofare, NJ: SLACK Incorporated; 2013.

Holzer MP, Rabsilber TM, Auffarth GU. Femtosecond laser-assisted corneal flap cuts: morphology, accuracy, and histopathology. *Invest Ophthalmol Vis Sci.* 2006;47(7):2828-2831.

Myrowitz EH, Chuck RS. A comparison of wavefront-optimized and wavefront-guided ablations. *Curr Opin Ophthalmol.* 2009;20(4):247-250.

Netto MV, Mohan RR, Sinha S, Sharma A, Dupps W, Wilson SE. Stromal haze, myofibroblasts, and surface irregularity after PRK. *Exp Eye Res.* 2006;82(5):788-797.

Perez-Straziota CE, Randleman JB, Stulting RD. Visual acuity and higher-order aberrations with wavefront-guided and wavefront-optimized laser in situ keratomileusis. *J Cataract Refract Surg.* 2010;36(3):437-441.

Randleman JB, Dawson DG, Grossniklaus HE, McCarey BE, Edelhauser HF. Depth dependent cohesive tensile strength in human donor corneas: implications for refractive surgery. *J Refract Surg.* 2008;24(1):S85-S89.

Schallhorn SC, Farjo AA, Huang D, et al; American Academy of Ophthalmology. Wavefront-guided LASIK for the correction of primary myopia and astigmatism a report by the American Academy of Ophthalmology. *Ophthalmology.* 2008;115(7):1249-1261.

Schallhorn SC, Tanzer DJ, Kaupp SE, Brown M, Malady SE. Comparison of night driving performance after wavefront-guided and conventional LASIK for moderate myopia. *Ophthalmology.* 2009;116(4):702-709.

Schmack I, Dawson DG, McCarey BE, Waring GO III, Grossniklaus HE, Edelhauser HF. Cohesive tensile strength of human LASIK wounds with histologic, ultrastructural, and clinical correlations. *J Refract Surg.* 2005;21(5):433-445.

Slade SG, Durrie DS, Binder PS. A prospective, contralateral eye study comparing thin-flap LASIK (sub-Bowman keratomileusis) with photorefractive keratectomy. *Ophthalmology.* 2009;116(6):1075-1082.

Solomon KD, Fernández de Castro LE, Sandoval HP, et al; Joint LASIK Study Task Force. LASIK world literature review: quality of life and patient satisfaction. *Ophthalmology.* 2009;116(4):691-701.

Stonecipher KG, Kezirian GM. Wavefront-optimized versus wavefront-guided LASIK for myopic astigmatism with the ALLEGRETTO WAVE: three-month results of a prospective FDA trial. *J Refract Surg.* 2008;24(4):S424-430.

Trokel SL, Srinivasan R, Braren B. Excimer laser surgery of the cornea. *Am J Ophthalmol.* 1983;96(6):710-715.

Virasch VV, Majmudar PA, Epstein RJ, Vaidya NS, Dennis RF. Reduced application time for prophylactic mitomycin C in photorefractive keratectomy. *Ophthalmology.* 2010;117(5):885-889.

Please visit www.routledge.com/ 9781617110368 to access additional material.

2

Preoperative Patient Evaluation

Chapter Highlights

- Evaluating patient goals and expectations
- Comparing refractive surgery to other forms of optical correction
- Patient history for refractive surgical candidates
- Physical examination for refractive surgical candidates
- Special testing for refractive surgical candidates

The goal of refractive surgery is simple—maximize potential outcomes and minimize potential complications. Corneal and lens-based approaches enjoy tremendous success rates because significant complications are rare and because the majority of patients attain the visual acuity they anticipated before surgery. The small percentage of unsatisfied patients after surgery comprises a combination of individuals. Reasons for patient dissatisfaction after refractive surgery include the following:

- Individuals who had a good objective outcome but are not satisfied because their expectations from surgery were not met.
- Individuals who developed complications because they were not good surgical candidates.
- Individuals who achieved good objective visual acuity but have postoperative symptoms that are unwanted and excessively bothersome.
- Individuals who were good surgical candidates but nevertheless developed significant complications, limiting their final visual acuity.

A thorough physical examination, including many ancillary evaluations that are relatively unique to refractive surgical preoperative screening, must be undertaken to identify individuals at higher risk for postoperative complications. These tests will be discussed in this chapter and Chapter 3, which is devoted specifically to corneal biomechanical evaluation.

Determining patient expectations can prove more challenging. Because all refractive surgery is by definition elective and serves as an alternative to other nonsurgical forms of visual aids, it

Randleman JB.
Refractive Surgery: An Interactive Case-Based Approach (pp. 15-22).

is imperative that each physician and patient accurately determines the specific patient's goals and desires for his or her surgical outcome, which should include an in-depth discussion about whether those goals are realistic and achievable. All individuals should be diligently screened preoperatively and counseled so they will have a full understanding of what surgery can and cannot accomplish in their particular situations.

Evaluating Patient Goals and Expectations

Patients with ametropias can vary in many respects, including their degree of visual disability when uncorrected, their symptoms from current visual aids, the possible benefits, potentially unrealized, that their ametropia and/or visual aids provides to their daily life, and their specific motivations for pursuing refractive surgery. All of these factors must be evaluated for patients and doctors to make sound decisions about surgical candidacy.

As brief examples, a 25-year-old moderate myope likely does not derive much functional benefit from his or her uncorrected refractive error, nor does a 45-year-old mild hyperope. However, a 45-year-old mild myope may unconsciously spend a great part of his or her day without correction, relying on his or her natural myopia to see at the office. This individual must realize what he or she will gain, as well as lose, through surgery.

For all of these reasons, it is imperative to fully counsel patients about their current and expected future visual function before they undergo surgery, comparing the visual function they may achieve with surgery to their current vision with and without correction.

How Does Surgery Compare Optically With Other Visual Aids?

Fundamentals of Patient Evaluation

- Determine surgical candidacy, both physical and psychological
- Match each patient with the most appropriate surgical procedure
- Identify any important unique aspects of the patient's status to include in informed consent discussion
- Refractive error

As a basic concept, laser vision correction (LVC) optically performs in a manner similar to soft contact lenses. Certainly, there are exceptions to this due to the inherent variability and subjectivity among individuals, with some patients reporting a subjective improvement in visual quality after surgery and some reporting slight worsening. Soft contact lenses can have a slight surface smoothing effect, which may mask subtle irregularity that surgery cannot. Laser vision correction often outperforms toric contact lenses due to the potential for shift in the lens position with blinking.

Laser vision correction outperforms spectacles in many respects, especially for peripheral vision. Spectacles can contribute to the control of strabismus in ways that surgery cannot (using a slight over-minus to control exotropia and a slight over-plus to control esotropia); therefore, in any patient with a history of amblyopia or strabismus treatment, it is critical to ascertain that individual's functional status in soft contacts. This is particularly important with monovision or in patients with active diplopia or strabismus as adults.

Surgery generally cannot recreate the same quality of vision attainable through successful rigid gas permeable (RGP) contact lens wear; therefore, all RGP contact lens wearers should be extensively counseled on this issue.

Multiple studies have found that subjective acuity is better after phakic intraocular lens (PIOL) implantation compared with LVC for patients with high myopia.

Important Aspects of Patient History

Important aspects of a patient's history include occupational issues and hobbies, family history, past medical history, and past ocular history.

Occupational Issues and Hobbies

It is critical to evaluate how a person individually uses his or her vision on a daily basis to determine the optimal surgical strategy. Although an individual may feel that distance vision for driving is most important, he or she may spend only 30 minutes each day driving but may spend 9 hours in front of a computer. Some patients desiring monovision may have extremely high near vision demands, such as small craftwork or extensive reading of exceptionally small print. Patients ultimately choose the surgical outcome they desire but in these and many other examples, it is the surgeons' responsibility to provide balanced education to facilitate that informed choice.

Finally, the risk of future ocular trauma warrants discussion about some individuals. Although most individuals have a low risk for ocular trauma in their lifetime, those involved in combat or hand-to-hand sports, such as martial arts or boxing, may carry an increased risk of flap dislocation after LASIK. These individuals may be better suited for surface ablation procedures.

Hobbies and Activities Usually Requiring Good Bilateral Distance Acuity

- Golf
- Tennis
- Night driving
- Airplane piloting
- Commercial driving license

Hobbies and Activities Usually Requiring Good Bilateral Near Acuity

- Craftwork
- Reading small print (eg, legal documents, payroll spreadsheets)
- Pleasure reading for extended periods

Family History

A family history of certain inherited corneal stromal dystrophies should exclude patients from LVC (Table 2-1). Although there are no definitive criteria for using a family history of keratoconus in screening, patients with a strong family history likely have a greater risk of ectatic disease. A family history of cataracts, glaucoma, Fuchs' dystrophy, or macular degeneration does not preclude surgery in an otherwise qualified candidate.

Past Medical History

There is limited consensus on general medical conditions that definitively predispose patients to higher complication rates after refractive surgery. Severe immunocompromised conditions, such as HIV or hematologic disorders and rheumatologic disorders, have been considered as relative contraindications for surgery. However, in most of these individuals with medically controlled disease, the risk is small and surgery may be undertaken with appropriate informed consent.

Table 2-1. Summary of Laser Vision Correction in Corneal Dystrophies
DYSTROPHIES THAT ARE APPROPRIATE FOR LASER VISION CORRECTION
EBMD (surface ablation)
Fleck corneal dystrophy
Posterior crocodile shagreen
Posterior polymorphous corneal dystrophy (PPMD)
DYSTROPHIES THAT ARE NOT APPROPRIATE FOR LASER VISION CORRECTION
BIGH3-related dystrophies
Reis-Bucklers
Avellino and variants
Granular and variants
Macular
Fuchs'
DYSTROPHIES UNDETERMINED FOR LASER VISION CORRECTION
Meesmann
Lisch

Some speculation but no concrete evidence exists of any systemic medication directly causing poor surgical outcomes. However, any and all medications with dryness as a side effect should be evaluated preoperatively and, when possible, discontinued for the early postoperative period.

Past Ocular History

Relevant ocular history issues include significant dry eye symptoms, extensive contact lens wear, past eye infections, and any history of amblyopia, strabismus, or diplopia that was treated as a child or an adult. In addition, significant changes in spectacles or contact lens over the past 1 to 2 years may be cause for concern. Finally, ocular plastic surgery for eyelids may predispose individuals to worsened dry eye symptoms, even corneal exposure, and should be discussed preoperatively. Ocular surface symptoms are generally easy to elicit; however, childhood issues related to patching, therapeutic spectacle wear, or eye muscle surgery may prove more challenging.

A history of "pink eye" should be explored in greater detail. Although most episodes of conjunctivitis are self-limited and pose no risk to future LVC, a history or findings suggestive of adenovirus with residual subepithelial infiltrates or past episodes of herpes virus with corneal involvement are relative contraindications for LVC.

Physical Examination for Refractive Surgical Candidates

In addition to a full basic eye examination, including a dilated fundus examination, there are specific aspects of the examination that should receive greater attention, and a variety of ancillary testing must be performed.

Refractive Evaluation

Both manifest and cycloplegic refraction should be performed on all refractive surgery candidates. In addition to obtaining an accurate refraction on which to base treatment, manifest refraction should match up well with the patient's current spectacles or contact lenses to assure refractive stability.

It is important to perform cycloplegic refraction to identify latent hyperopia and over-minus manifest refractions, especially in younger patients. If significant latent hyperopia is present, it may affect surgical candidacy (if outside reasonable treatment range) or surgical planning, with some target between manifest and cycloplegic refraction planned.

External Evaluation

Lid or Lash Position Abnormalities

Entropion, ectropion, trichiasis, and other eyelid/eyelash disorders may all contribute to surface symptoms of the eye and postoperative healing issues and should be addressed before any refractive surgery is considered.

Blepharitis

Blepharitis can contribute to contact lens intolerance and nonabatement of symptoms after LVC. Blepharitis can affect preoperative topography, thereby complicating surgical screening. Patients with significant lid disease may benefit from pretreatment with lid hygiene instruction and a short course of topical azithromycin or oral tetracycline antibiotics. Blepharitis increases the risk of infection and sterile infiltrates after surface ablation and LASIK, as well as LASIK interface inflammation.

Corneal Evaluation

Epithelium

Epithelial basement membrane dystrophy (EBMD) predisposes patients to epithelial defect formation with LASIK. Surface ablation is preferred and may have therapeutic as well as refractive benefits.

Subepithelial haze or scarring could be suggestive of past adenovirus or herpes simplex virus (HSV) infections. Both are relative contraindications for LVC, as both may recur after excimer laser ablation.

Stroma

"Spots and dots" may be suggestive of certain corneal stromal dystrophies, which are contraindications to LVC, as the conditions may exacerbate with excimer laser treatment (see Table 2-1).

Endothelium

The surgeon should evaluate for the presence of corneal guttae, which is a relative contraindication for LASIK due to potential problems with flap adherence. Guttae are also important for PIOL evaluation, as they may signify compromised endothelial cell function, thus excluding PIOL implantation, and indicate a relative contraindication for refractive lens exchange as well as the use of multifocal IOLs at the time of cataract surgery.

Anterior Segment Evaluation

The surgeon should evaluate for any evidence of anterior segment dysgenesis, which is more important for PIOL evaluation than LVC. Any lens opacity could be relevant for older patients desiring LVC or for patients evaluated for PIOL implantation.

Retinal Evaluation

Peripheral retinal evaluation is most important for patients with high myopia. Although neither LVC nor PIOL implantation have been found to increase the risk of retinal detachment, high myopia patients are at increased risk at baseline, and significant peripheral retinal pathology should be ruled out before surgery. Macular function evaluation with ocular coherence tomography has been advocated by some for multifocal intraocular lenses (MFIOL) evaluation.

Special Testing

Pupils

Pupil size should be formally measured in room light and dim conditions. Although pupil size has not been found to correlate with postoperative glare, halo, or night driving issues, generically termed night vision complaints, these measurements should be undertaken during LVC screening for all patients. Some adjustments to the optical zone may be beneficial for patients with large pupils (>7.5 mm). Pupil size is directly relevant for PIOL screening, as patients with pupils larger than the IOL optic will experience increased symptoms in dim light.

Tear Film

Multiple testing strategies for tear film evaluation are available, including vital dye staining, tear production testing (Schirmer's test), and tear break-up time, as well as newer tear osmolarity testing devices. Tear film should be evaluated in any patient who has preoperative dry eye symptoms and in those individuals at greater risk for decreased tear production, including older patients and women. Pretreatment may be advisable for certain patients, and some patients should be excluded from LVC due to insufficient tear production.

Pachymetry

Average central corneal thickness (pachymetry) is approximately 540 ± 30 μm, providing a normal range of 480 to 600 μm, although patients outside of this range may still have normal corneas and be surgical candidates. Central corneal thickness measurements are critical to determine surgical candidacy based on both absolute thickness and screening for biomechanical weakness. Ultrasound pachymetry measurements remain the gold standard; however, multiple technologies now provide accurate and reproducible measurements, including Scheimpflug tomography and optical coherence tomography (OCT) of the anterior segment. These technologies will be discussed more fully in Chapter 3.

Endothelial Cell Count

Patients considering PIOL implantation must have a formal endothelial cell count performed with either specular or confocal microscopy, as there are specific minimum values designated for each PIOL, stratified by patient age.

Keratometry

Keratometry should be measured using manual or reliable automated devices. This measurement information is used for laser treatment programming for most ablations, and may be important for planning flap creation if a mechanical microkeratome is utilized, as steep corneas (> 48.00 diopters [D]) are at increased risk of buttonhole formation, and flat corneas (< 40.00 D) are at increased risk for free cap formation.

Ocular Dominance

For patients considering monovision (or blended vision), ocular dominance may be relevant. Most practitioners advocate targeting the dominant eye for distance when patients have a strong dominance preference, although this is not absolute. Various ways to determine ocular dominance are available; however, the simplest and easiest method is performed by having the patient extend both hands to create a small viewing "window" or hole, through which they site a distant object. The patient is asked to close one eye at a time to determine which eye is being used to fixate through the small hole; whichever eye has the object aligned through their target is his or her dominant eye.

Topography

Topography and biomechanical evaluation is the subject of Chapter 3. Please refer to that chapter for detailed discussion.

Summary and Take Home Points

A variety of unique factors comprise patient screening and evaluation for refractive surgery. These include the patient's desires and expectations, with specific focus on the patient's hobbies and work tasks, with a focus on activities that might require optimal distance acuity. In addition to a complete routine eye examination, special attention must be paid to the ocular surface and to subtle findings that might otherwise be overlooked in a routine eye examination. Special testing for pupil size, corneal pachymetry, and endothelial cell count where indicated are important parts of every refractive surgical patient evaluation.

Bibliography

Ambrósio R Jr, Tervo T, Wilson SE. LASIK-associated dry eye and neurotrophic epitheliopathy: pathophysiology and strategies for prevention and treatment. *J Refract Surg.* 2008;24(4):396-407.

Chan A, Manche EE. Effect of preoperative pupil size on quality of vision after wavefront-guided LASIK. *Ophthalmology.* 2011;118(4):736-741.

Lee ES, Kim EK. Surgical do's and don'ts of corneal dystrophies. *Curr Opin Ophthalmol.* 2003;14(4):186-191.

Mathers WD, Fraunfelder FW, Rich LF. Risk of LASIK surgery vs contact lenses. *Arch Ophthalmol.* 2006;124(10):1510-1511.

McGee HT, Mathers WD. Laser in situ keratomileusis versus long-term contact lens wear: decision analysis. *J Cataract Refract Surg.* 2009;35(11):1860-1867.

Pollard ZF, Greenberg MF, Bordenca M, Elliott J, Hsu V. Strabismus precipitated by monovision. *Am J Ophthalmol.* 2011;152(3):479-482.

Sedaghat MR, Daneshvar R, Kargozar A, Derakhshan A, Daraei M. Comparison of central corneal thickness measurement using ultrasonic pachymetry, rotating Scheimpflug camera, and scanning-slit topography. *Am J Ophthalmol.* 2010;150(6):780-789.

Smith RJ, Maloney RK. Laser in situ keratomileusis in patients with autoimmune diseases. *J Cataract Refract Surg.* 2006;32(8):1292-1295.

Please visit www.routledge.com/ 9781617110368 to access additional material.

3

Corneal Topography and Biomechanical Evaluation

Chapter Highlights

- Corneal topographic evaluation
- Corneal tomographic evaluation
- Additional biomechanical evaluation considerations
  - ◊ Ocular coherence tomography
  - ◊ Corneal hysteresis
- Topography versus tomography

This is the single most important chapter in this book; yet, you may still feel less than completely prepared to evaluate the biomechanics of the cornea after reading it. Corneal biomechanical evaluation is the most critical, and controversial, aspect of preoperative patient evaluation. All corneal refractive surgical procedures reduce corneal strength to varying degrees, and excessive corneal weakening can result in nonprogressive irregular astigmatism or progressive corneal ectasia postoperatively. That concern underlies many surgucal decisions, including whether or not to offer LASK or declining to operate altogether for some patients. Unfortunately, biomechanical concerns may overshadow other important issues, such as the comparative risk of other surgical approaches and the long-term effects of contact lens wear.

To date, the majority of corneas that have developed postoperative corneal ectasia have, in hindsight, had indicators of increased risk; thus, a variety of screening algorithms have been developed to appropriately evaluate refractive surgical candidates. Subtle corneal irregularities in curvature, thickness, elevation, and other corneal parameters are the initial indicators of biomechanical instability and increased risk for worse surgical outcomes. Therefore, learning to identify risk factors is key.

Randleman JB.
Refractive Surgery: An Interactive Case-Based Approach (pp. 23-38).

A few years ago this chapter would have been appropriately titled "Topographic Analysis." However, advances in corneal biomechanical evaluation have moved our field beyond (but not away from) relying on anterior corneal curvature (topography) toward a more comprehensive approach, including regional corneal thickness (tomography), anterior and posterior corneal elevation mapping (available through scanning slit-beam and Scheimpflug imaging), and corneal hysteresis measurements.

Although corneal topographic analysis has evolved through multiple generations of technology and has matured as a corneal evaluation method, the other aforementioned evaluations are earlier in their developmental phases. Therefore, the bulk of this chapter will focus on topographic pattern analysis and interpretation. Note that entire texts have been written on this topic alone; what follows is a basic overview of corneal biomechanical analysis, which is a primer to allow you to work through the cases that follow. Among all topics covered in this text, you are strongly encouraged to spend the time and energy necessary to seek out additional information on corneal evaluation through texts, peer-reviewed publications, and courses provided at all national meetings, as this field is evolving rapidly.

Corneal Topographic Evaluation

Color corneal topography allows for rapid evaluation of corneal surface curvature by assigning a color code to curvature values derived by measuring the distance between individual Placido rings (Figure 3-1). By using this system, changes in corneal curvature, especially focal changes, become readily apparent. Accurate topographic evaluation requires a systematic, consistent approach to the evaluation of these scans.

Fundamental Elements of Topographic Evaluation

- Identify color scale
- Confirm adequate scan
- Evaluate for artifacts
- Identify topographic pattern

Color Scale

The first step in topographic analysis is the determination of the color steps being utilized in the topography. Most topography machines are programmable to output in 0.25- to 2.00-diopter (D) scales; however, most refractive surgeons utilize 0.50- or 1.00-D scales. Smaller scales (0.25 D) add "noise" to the analysis by including multiple colors to any pattern, whereas large scales (2.00 D) miss all but major curvature changes. Because refractive surgeons are looking for subtle curvature differences, most advocate using the 0.50-D scale. Color-step identification is critical because identical topographies can look significantly different based on the color step used (Figure 3-2).

Topographic Pattern Analysis

When the color steps are identified, specific topographic patterns can be evaluated. Although a variety of subtle differences exist between many specific topographies, the patterns can be divided into 4 major categories (Table 3-1).

A spectrum of topographic patterns from normal to suspicious is demonstrated in Figure 3-3. Abnormal patterns include any significant steepening that meets the criteria for forme fruste keratoconus, as studies have shown more advanced focal steepening qualifying as early keratoconus (Figure 3-4); or pellucid marginal corneal degeneration (PMCD) patterns (Figure 3-5), which typically demonstrate a "crab-claw" pattern, with steepening in the far inferior periphery between the 4- and 8-o'clock meridians. Although the crab-claw pattern has been traditionally associated

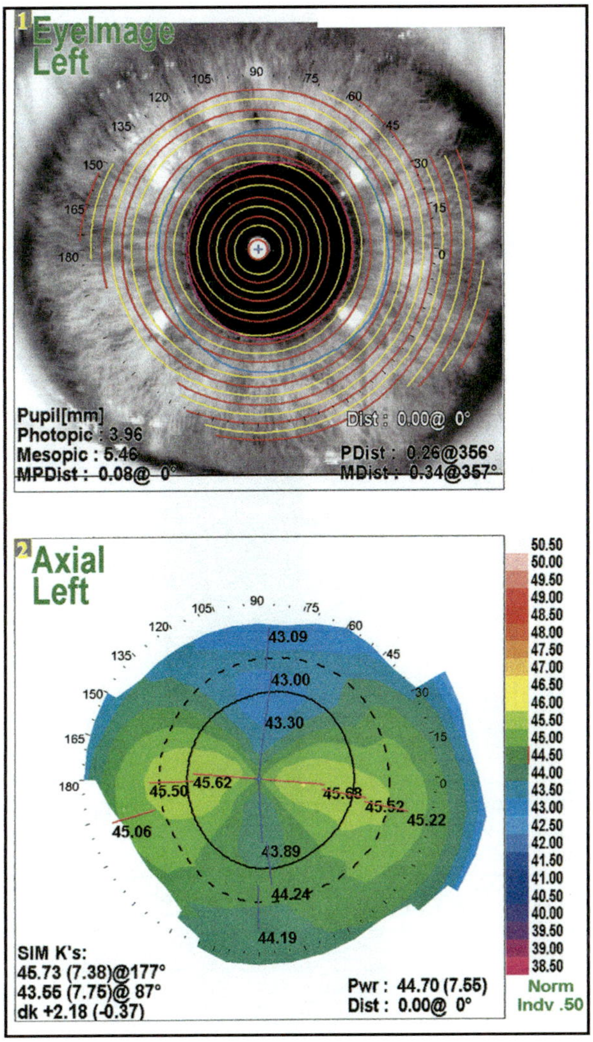

Figure 3-1. Placido image showing actual reflected Placido rings (top) that are subsequently converted into color scale patterns (bottom).

with PMCD, it can also be found in keratoconus eyes. However, the difference is of minimal significance in refractive surgical evaluation, as both conditions are general contraindications for corneal refractive surgery.

Although most practitioners feel comfortable identifying grossly normal and grossly abnormal topographies, the patterns that fall in between these extremes can prove challenging, especially considering that up to one third of all patients presenting for refractive surgical evaluation have at least mild topographic asymmetry. Among these asymmetric patterns, certain specific patterns warrant special attention. These patterns include the following:

- Between-eye asymmetry (Figure 3-6), where the pattern found in one eye deviates significantly from that of the fellow eye, even if neither pattern in itself is abnormal.
- Against-the-rule steepening (Figure 3-7), which is an unusual topographic pattern for patients aged 40 years or less.
- Focal steepening in atypical meridians (other than the traditional inferior location) (Figure 3-8).

For the purposes of refractive surgical evaluation, the most suspicious topographic pattern between the patient's two eyes should be given the most weight, as keratoconus is a bilateral

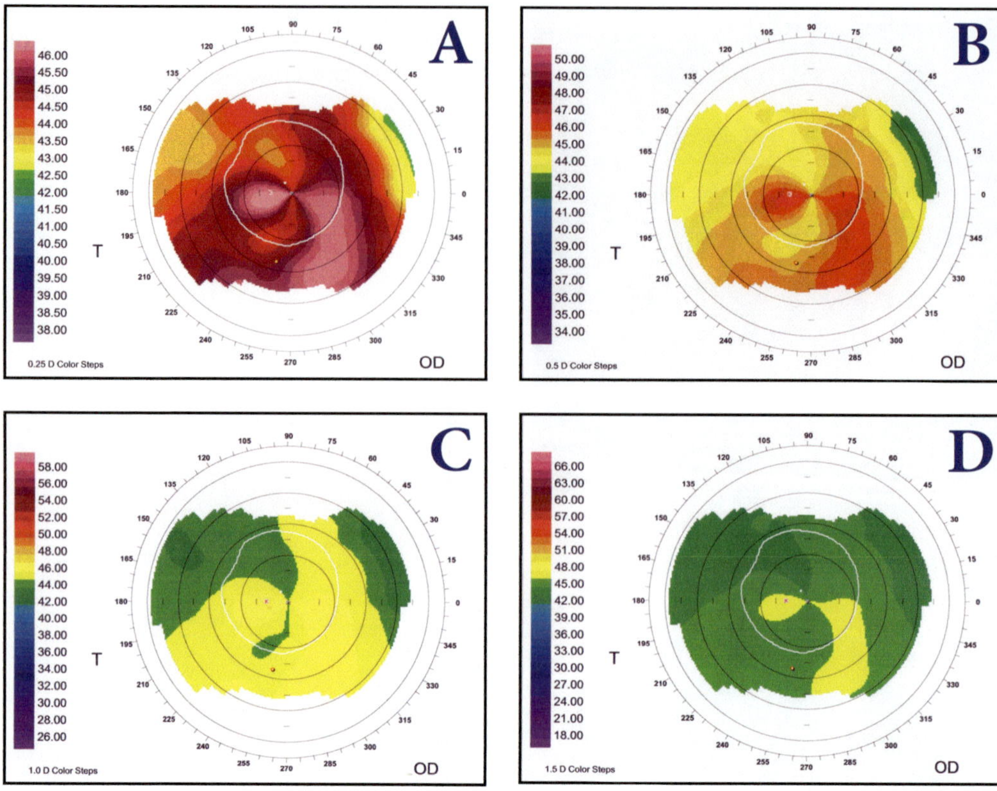

Figure 3-2. Placido image demonstrating the importance of color steps: The same topography is displayed in (A) 0.25-D, (B) 0.50-D, (C) 1.00-D, and (D) 1.50-D color steps.

Table 3-1. Topographic Pattern Categories

Normal (including round, oval, or regular bowtie patterns)
Asymmetric (Mild) • Asymmetric bowtie patterns with irregularity of 0.50 D or less • Mild skewing of the axis (less than 25 degrees)
Asymmetric (Significant) • Focal steepening of 1.00 D or more in any meridian • Skewed radial axis patterns (25 degrees or more of skewing)
Abnormal patterns • Keratoconus suspect patterns (also called forme fruste keratoconus or keratoconus suspect) • Keratoconus • Pellucid marginal corneal degeneration

disease process. In against-the-rule astigmatic patterns, special attention should be paid to the far periphery of the image to make sure that the pattern does not begin to "droop" downwards, indicating the early stages of a crab-claw type pattern.

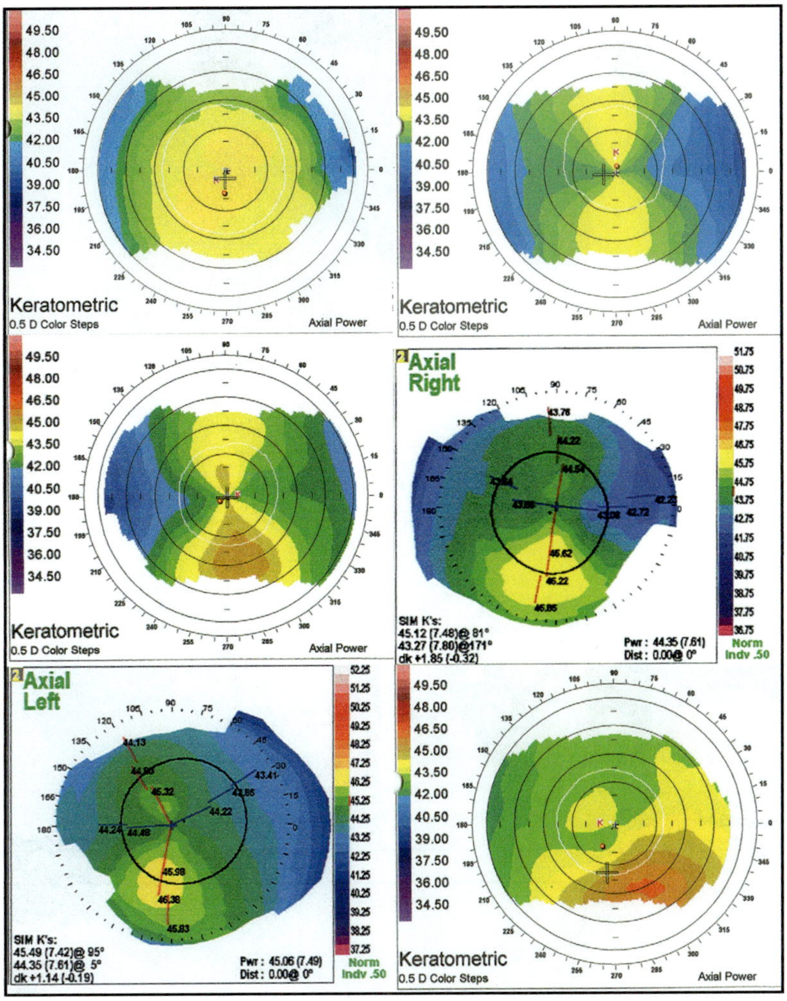

Figure 3-3. Composite images of preoperative topographic patterns, ranging from (A) normal to (F) abnormal. Note the increasing degree of asymmetry in the images. (Adapted from Randleman JB. Pre-refractive surgery topographic evaluation. In Wang M, ed. *Corneal Topography: A Guide for Clinical Application in the Wavefront Era, Second Edition*. Thorofare, NJ: SLACK Incorporated; 2011: 231-242.)

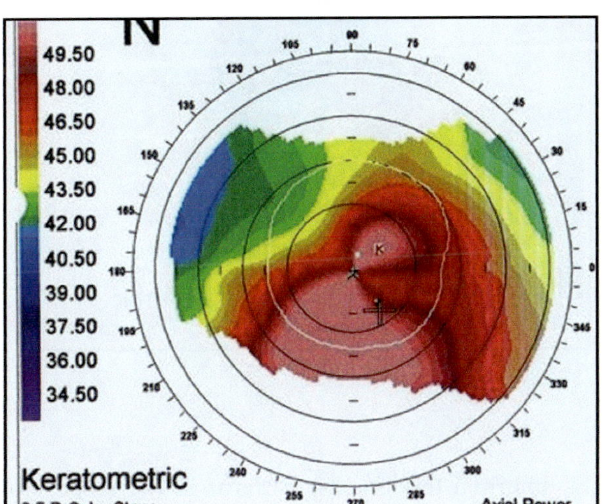

Figure 3-4. Placido image in 0.50-D color-scale steps with dramatic pattern irregularity, including a skewed radial axis and pronounced inferior steepening.

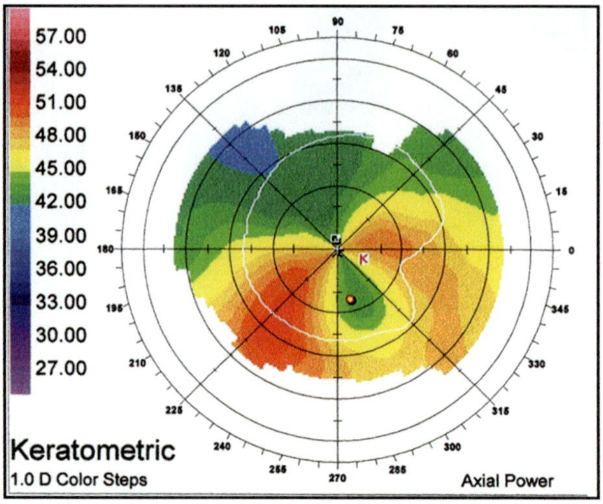

Figure 3-5. Placido image demonstrating a typical crab-claw pattern, with the steepest regions coming together centrally, mimicking a crab's claw, and similar steepening in the far periphery inferiorly.

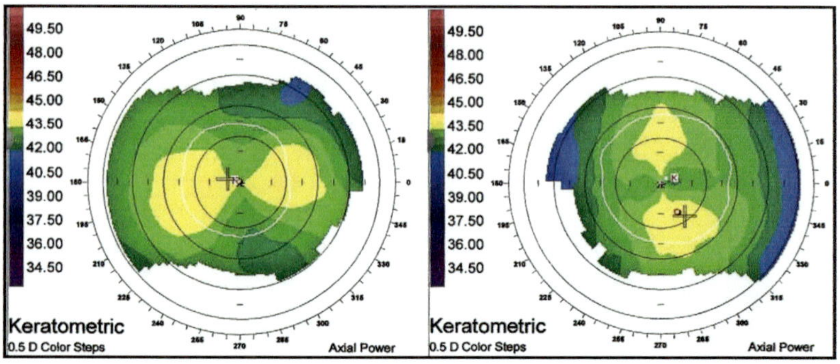

Figure 3-6. Placido image of the right and left eyes demonstrating between-eye asymmetry, with against-the-rule astigmatism in the right eye and with-the-rule in the left eye.

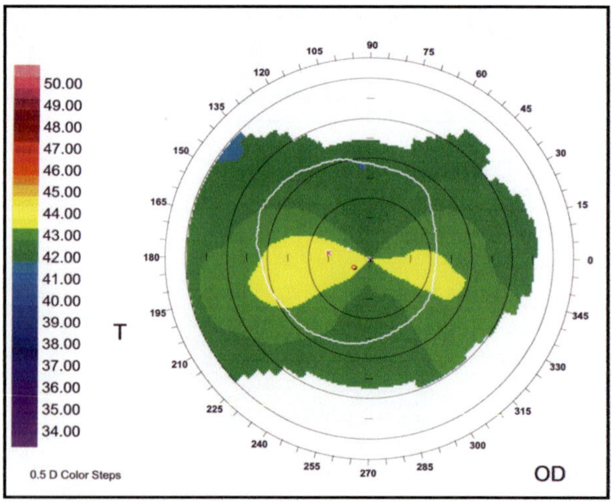

Figure 3-7. Placido image demonstrating against-the-rule steepening, with inferior sagging in the far periphery, indicating potential abnormality.

Topographic Artifacts

Other conditions may generate seemingly abnormal topographic patterns in the absence of true corneal biomechanical weakening. The most common ocular surface issues affecting the tear film include dry eye and blepharitis, corneal scars, and epithelial abnormalities, such as epithelial basement membrane dystrophy (EBMD). Although in the aforementioned situations it is usually reasonable to proceed with corneal refractive surgery, it is important to identify each

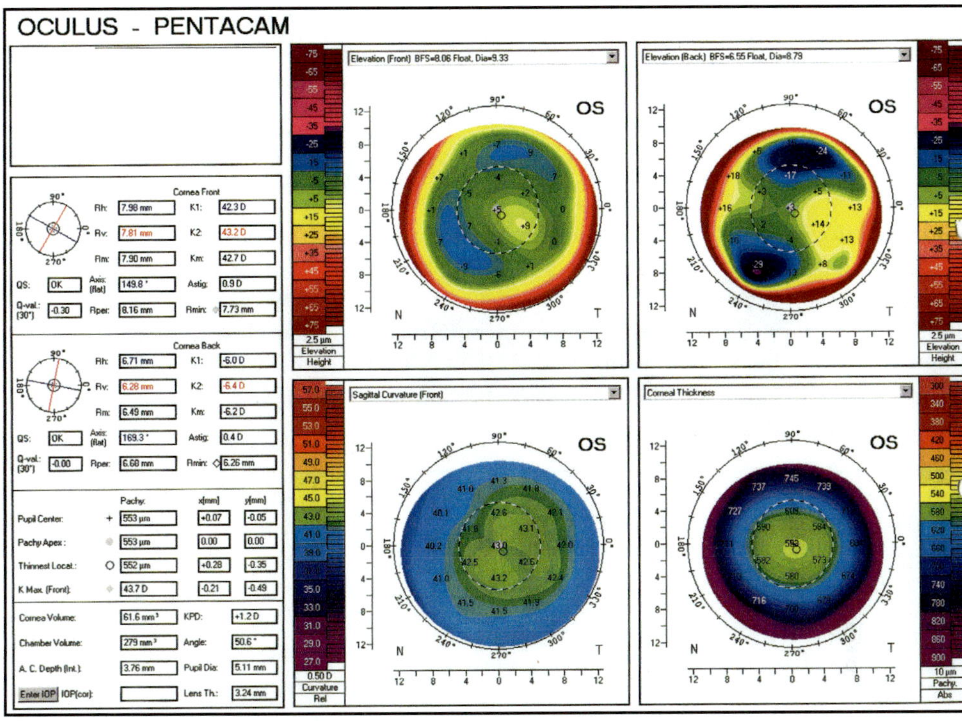

Figure 3-8. Scheimpflug image demonstrating focal steepening in the 3-o'clock meridian, as evidenced in the sagittal curvature map (lower left). The front (top left) and back (top right) elevations are both displaced in the same direction.

of these conditions preoperatively because some, such as dry eye or blepharitis, may require treatment prior to surgery to maximize ocular surface health and promote rapid visual recovery postoperatively. However, other conditions, such as mild anterior corneal scars and EBMD, may be better suited for surface ablation, which may be therapeutic as well as refractive, rather than LASIK, where epithelial defects may result. Extensive contact lens wear may also generate seemingly abnormal topographic patterns. In such cases, extended periods without contact lens wear preoperatively may be necessary to obtain a true evaluation of corneal curvature.

Finally, because accurate topographic analysis completely depends on the quality of the scan, the importance of training staff to produce high quality, reproducible scans cannot be overemphasized. If any question exists about the topographic quality, repeating the scan is always warranted. The most common causes of poor quality scans include patient–topographer misalignment; small images, with inferior and superior data loss generated from poor corneal exposure; drop-out of data due to debris in the tear film or eye lashes; and tear lake irregularities.

The Role of Patient Age in Topographic Pattern Analysis

Among all other mitigating factors, the most significant factor to include in one's thought process when analyzing topographic patterns is patient age. Young patient age is a defined risk factor for ectasia development, and naturally occurring ectatic corneal disorders (eg, keratoconus and PMCD) are progressive in nature, usually becoming manifest around the age of 20 years in keratoconus and age 40 years in PMCD. Therefore, it is logical that more subtle forms of ectatic corneal disorders, so-called suspect or forme fruste patterns, also develop in a progressive, albeit abortive, fashion. Thus, younger patients may display milder topographic asymmetry than their older counterparts. For this reason, any degree of topographic asymmetry in very young patients (less than age 25 years) should be considered potential markers of abnormality until proven otherwise, whereas the same pattern in a 45 year old would not cause concern.

Corneal Tomographic Evaluation

In addition to anterior corneal curvature data available from corneal topographic images, corneal tomography can generate regional corneal thickness profiles and create anterior and posterior corneal elevation profiles. A variety of different specific tomographic units are available, but these can be categorized as scanning slit-beam (Orbscan II; Bausch & Lomb), or Scheimpflug imaging devices (including the Pentacam; OCULUS Optikgerate GmbH and Galilei; Zeimer Ophthalmic Systems AG). Ocular coherence tomography (OCT) can also generate regional corneal thickness profiles and will be discussed in this chapter.

Basics of Tomographic Evaluation

- Identify color scales and units of measurement
- Assess image quality
- Evaluate regional corneal thickness profiles
- Evaluate focal anterior and posterior elevation changes

When evaluating corneal tomographic images, one must first establish the color-step pattern in use and the quality of the image. The Orbscan II device incorporates both Placido imaging and scanning slit beam–based imaging to generate both standard topographic and tomographic data. Overall corneal thickness profiles are measured, and from these, anterior and posterior elevation data are generated, which are then measured against a *best-fit sphere* to give an overall impression of focal elevations (Figure 3-9A). Some reports have discussed the value of these individual elevation parameters, especially posterior float metrics; however, they remain to be validated clinically. Scheimpflug imaging systems also generate analogous scans, but they do so through different optical mechanisms (Figure 3-9B). The specific relevance and validity of anterior and posterior elevation measurements and screening values also remains to be accurately determined, although focal areas of elevation are suspicious for biomechanical insufficiency (Figure 3-9C).

Corneal thickness relational profiles may prove the most useful metric in evaluating corneal biomechanics (Figure 3-10). The normal cornea becomes progressively thicker as measured from the center to the periphery, and although no absolute ratio has been definitively established, studies have reported significant differences in corneal thickness spatial profiles and corneal volume distribution between keratoconic and normal corneas, and these metrics may be useful in screening, especially in eyes with borderline topographic patterns.

Additional Biomechanical Evaluation Considerations

Ocular Coherence Tomography

Corneal thickness profiles can also be generated by high-resolution ultrasound and OCT (Figure 3-11). Subtle changes in epithelial and stromal thickness may have implications for screening, as compensatory epithelial thinning overlying an ectatic region may be an early sign

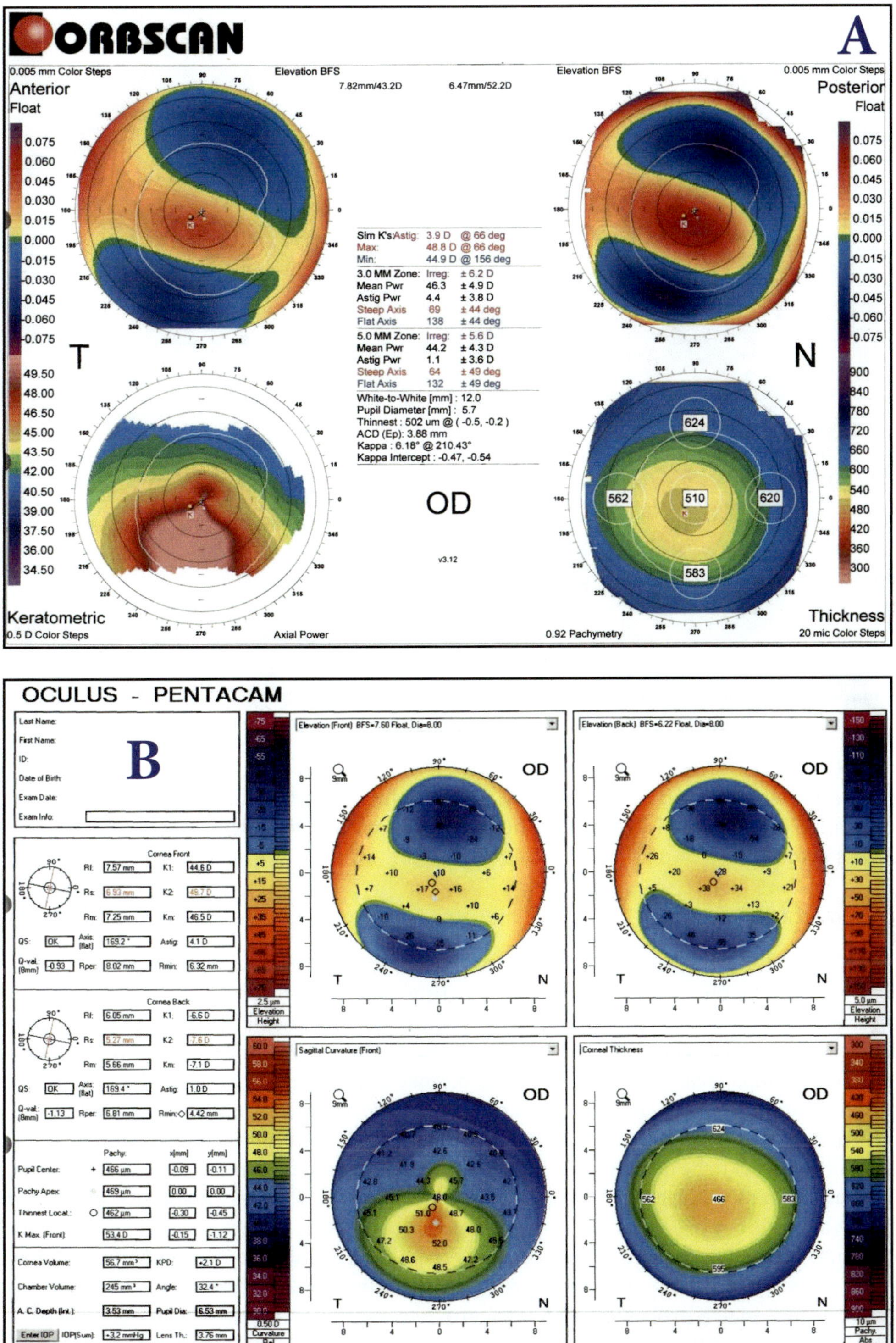

Figure 3-9. Corneal tomography analysis with the (A)Orbscan scanning-slit and (B, C) Pentacam Scheimpflug technologies. Note the Placido-based keratometric map (A, lower left image) and the analogous sagittal curvature map (B, lower left image) in the same eye demonstrates inferior steepening with keratoconus. Corneal thickness is thin centrally in both maps (A, B, lower right), and elevation/float maps (upper right and upper left images in A and B, respectively) are increased over normal. *(continued)*

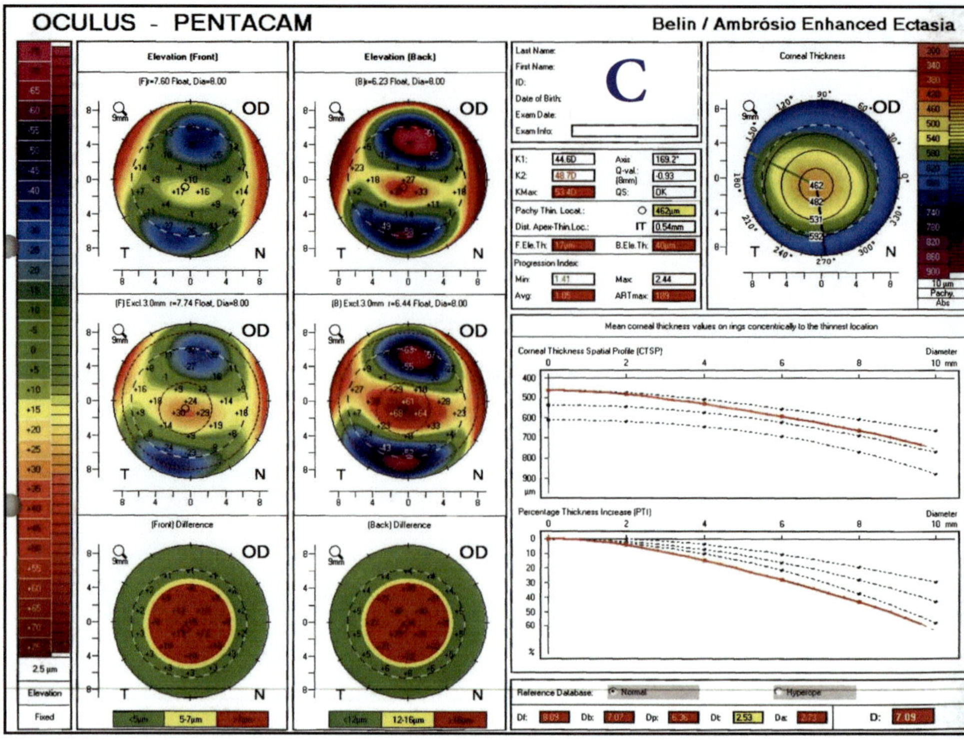

Figure 3-9 (continued). (C) In the Pentacam's Belin/Ambrosio display, the posterior elevation is marked abnormal, as evidenced by the large red circles at the bottom left and right map images.

of a corneal ectatic disorder. Unfortunately, high-resolution ultrasound is not yet widely commercially available for corneal evaluation; however, numerous OCT devices can evaluate corneal thickness profiles.

Corneal Hysteresis

All of the aforementioned techniques for evaluating corneal biomechanical integrity are, in reality, indirect measures, relying on detecting changes in curvature, thickness, or shape to indicate structural weakening. In theory, direct biomechanical measurements would be of greatest value, as these could determine the strength of a cornea prior to any of the mentioned changes occurring. Measurement of corneal biomechanics, currently clinically available as the Ocular Response Analyzer (Reichert Technologies), theoretically provides these data in the form of corneal hysteresis (CH) and corneal resistance factor (CRF) (Figure 3-12); however, the clinical applicability has yet to be determined. Lower CH and CRF values (generally lower than 10 mm Hg for both measurements) signify a weaker cornea (ie, a cornea with less resistance to deformation forces). Although corneal hysteresis measurements can detect differences between normal and keratoconus populations, there is significant overlap in individual eyes, making this technology of questionable value currently. Newer algorithms, including the keratoconus match indices (KMI) and keratoconus match probabilities (KMP), provide additional information based on a variety of novel parameters, and these may provide better sensitivity and specificity in the screening process (see Figure 3-12). However, for now, ocular hysteresis is not a primary method of patient screening in most clinical settings.

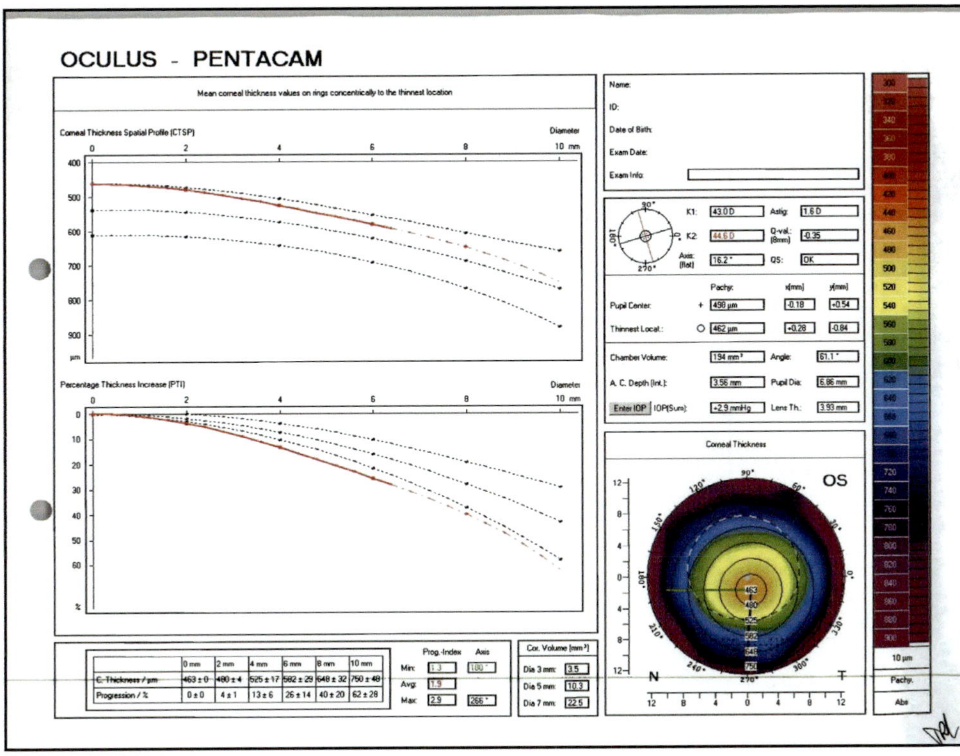

Figure 3-10. Scheimpflug regional corneal thickness map demonstrating an abnormal corneal thickness spatial profile (CSTP, top left) and percentage thickness increase (PTI, bottom left), evidenced by the line trailing off inferiorly as viewed from left to right, indicating relative thinning centrally compared with peripheral thickness values.

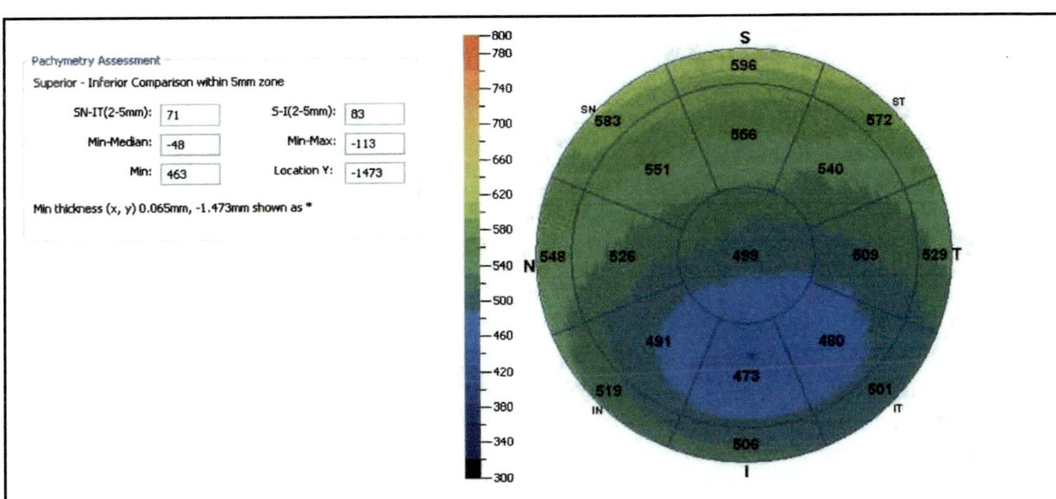

Figure 3-11. Anterior segment OCT (RTVue, Optovue Inc) of the same eye as shown in Figure 3-10, indicating a displaced thinnest point inferiorly, with an abnormally low peripheral corneal thickness inferiorly.

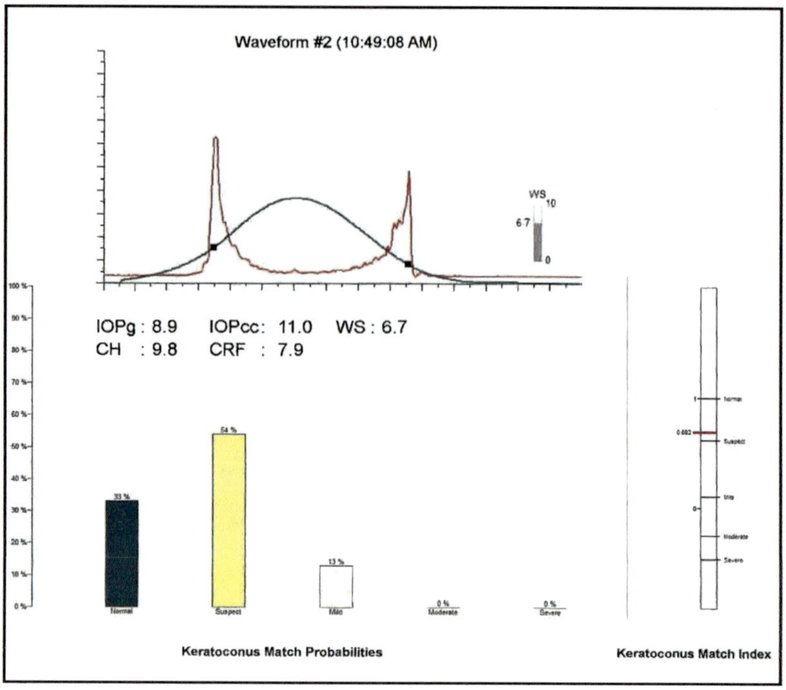

Figure 3-12. Composite image from the Ocular Response Analyzer demonstrating low corneal hysteresis (9.8 mm Hg) and CRF (7.9 mm Hg) and abnormal keratoconus match probabilities and keratoconus match index scores.

Topography Versus Tomography

The relative weight given to tomographic data versus topographic data is currently hotly debated; however, the two technologies are likely additive, rather than superior or inferior to one another. Anterior curvature changes with concomitant elevation abnormalities and abnormal corneal thickness profiles increase the odds that a cornea is biomechanically weaker and should be excluded for corneal refractive surgery.

Other Screening Factors: Age, Corneal Thickness, and Residual Stromal Bed Thickness

Patient Age

Young patient age also is a significant risk factor. As mentioned previously, younger patients may have only subtle topographic abnormalities, which may not be deemed as being suspicious in an older patient, or they may be destined to develop keratoconus with or without corneal refractive surgery but have undergone LASIK prior to having the keratoconus fully manifest. In addition, natural corneal collagen cross-linking occurs with age, resulting in increased corneal tensile strength. Young patients are still potential candidates for corneal refractive surgery; however, added diligence is warranted, especially in the topographic analysis in these individuals.

Preoperative Central Corneal Thickness

Low preoperative central corneal thickness (CCT) also increases the risk of developing ectasia, which is confirmed in every published analysis of CCT. Thinner corneas may be indicative of an abnormal cornea (predisposed to keratoconus or ectasia), or thinner corneas may be at risk because there is a higher probability of low residual stromal bed (RSB) thickness resulting from a combination of subtly thicker-than-intended flaps and deeper-than-anticipated ablations. However, many patients with thin corneas have had successful LASIK outcomes, and similar to other variables, no predictive cut-off value exists. Rather, corneal thickness values should be assessed within the context of other screening parameters.

Residual Stromal Bed Thickness

Low RSB thickness is a known risk factor for the development of ectasia. Low RSB thickness can result from large ablations compared with baseline corneal thickness, excessive flap thickness, and/or deeper-than-expected stromal ablations.

RSB thickness is derived by subtracting the flap thickness and ablation depth from the preoperative CCT. Because variations in flap thickness can exist, intraoperative pachymetry should be done to exclude the presence of an excessively thick flap before ablation is performed. To calculate estimated RSB thickness preoperatively, it is best to use the mean flap thickness + 2 standard deviations formula in the device used for flap creation for your estimated flap thickness to increase the safety index:

RSB = Central corneal thickness – flap thickness (+2 SD) – ablation depth

For all eyes undergoing surgery, biomechanical strength will be greater after photorefractive keratectomy (PRK) than after LASIK because less stroma is surgically altered and because tensile strength is not uniform throughout the cornea but higher in the anterior third of the cornea. For purposes of RSB thickness calculations, epithelial thickness is assumed to be 50 µm and should be subtracted from estimated flap thickness when comparing functional RSB thickness between PRK and LASIK.

Ectasia Risk Score System

The aforementioned factors, along with topographic patterns, have been used for screening in a weighted system the Ectasia Risk Score System (Table 3-2). This system is far from perfect, but it does provide users with a logical approach to considering various risk factors, and it has demonstrated its utility in case-control studies.

Evaluate Topographic and Tomographic Data Independently From Other Patient Factors First!

Although a complete surgical evaluation requires the clinician to evaluate and consider a variety of information in addition to topographic pattern, including refraction, corneal thickness, overall ocular health, and patient age, it is critical that topographic pattern evaluation be done independently initially. That is, you should first evaluate topographic and tomographic patterns independent of other patient information. This is critical for accurate evaluations, as abnormal topographic patterns can occur in any age group, with any refraction or corrected visual acuity, and with any corneal thickness. Some clinicians may be tempted to "overlook" subtle abnormalities if the patient has a low myopic or hyperopic refraction, if their correctable acuity is "excellent," or if the cornea is "thick enough"; however, abnormal topography can occur in any eye

Table 3-2. Ectasia Rick Score System					
PARAMETER	**POINTS**				
	4	3	2	1	0
TOPOGRAPHY PATTERN	Abnormal	Inf. Steep/ SRA		ABT	Normal/SBT
RSB	<240 µm	240-259 µm	260-279 µm	280-299 µm	>300 µm
AGE		18-21 yrs	22-25 yrs	26-29 yrs	>30 yrs
CORNEAL THICKNESS	<450 µm	451-480 µm	481-510 µm		>510 µm
MRSE	>-14 D	>-12 to -14 D	>-10 to -12 D	>-8 to -10 D	-8 D or less
Low: (0,1,2) OK to proceed with LASIK					
Moderate: (3) discussed at length with patient potential increased rick of ectasia. Alternatives discussed.					
High: (≧4) Recommend no LASIK. Discussed alternatives with patient including ASA. Unknown ectasia risk with this procedure.					

and is an independent risk factor for ectasia. Ectasia has occurred in hyperopic eyes, thick corneas, and eyes that otherwise appeared "normal," but these eyes could have been excluded for surgery by close topographic pattern analysis alone.

Putting It All Together: Corneal Biomechanical Analysis

Figure 3-13 provides an overview strategy for corneal biomechanical evaluation, taking into account the variety of screening strategies discussed in this chapter, along with other previously mentioned patient variables.

Summary and Take Home Points

A variety of testing modalities are currently available to assess corneal biomechanics and a patient's suitability for refractive surgery. Among these, Placido-based curvature remains the best understood and validated technique; however, tomographic measurements obtained through Scheimpflug imaging or high-resolution OCT are becoming increasingly utilized. Future testing modalities may prove additive to current screening strategies.

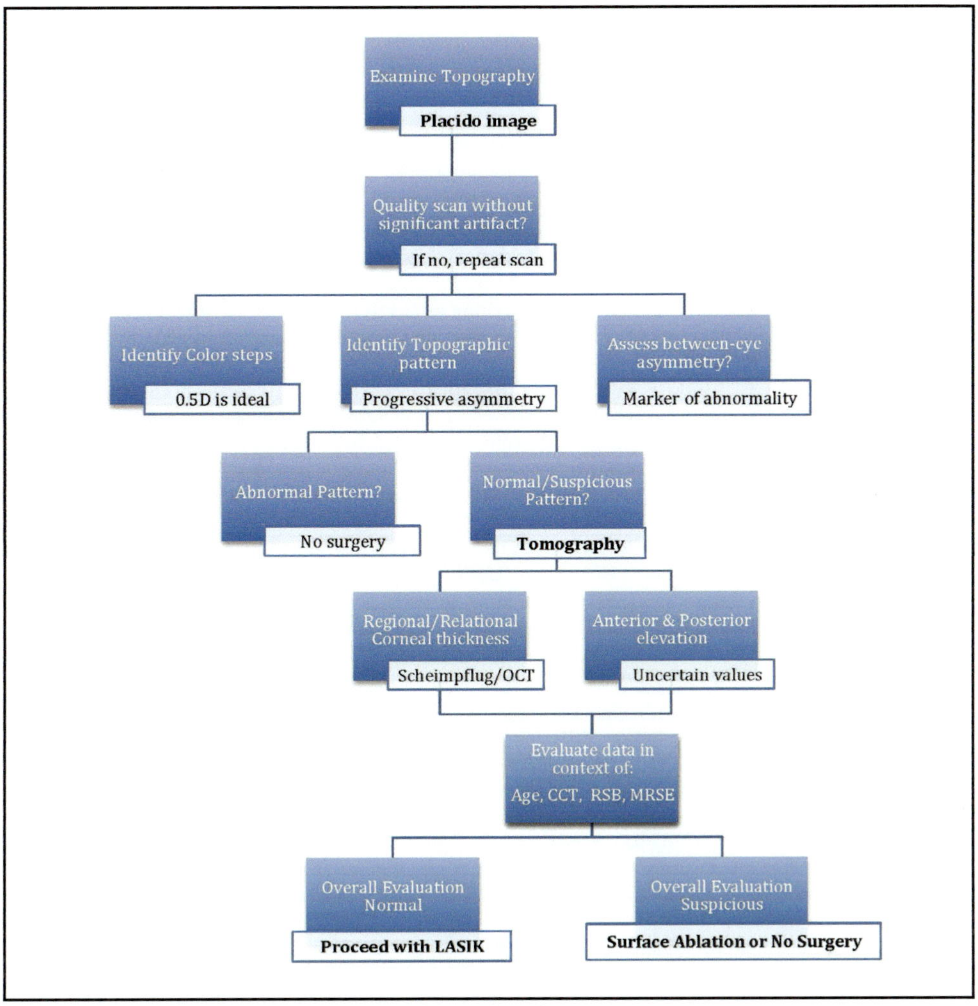

Figure 3-13. Flow sheet of corneal biomechanical evaluation.

Bibliography

Ambrósio R Jr, Alonso RS, Luz A, Coca Velarde LG. Corneal-thickness spatial profile and corneal-volume distribution: tomographic indices to detect keratoconus. *J Cataract Refract Surg.* 2006;32(11):1851-1859.

Ambrósio R Jr, Caiado AL, Guerra FP, et al. Novel pachymetric parameters based on corneal tomography for diagnosing keratoconus. *J Refract Surg.* 2011;27(10):753-758.

Ambrósio R Jr, Klyce SD, Wilson SE. Corneal topographic and pachymetric screening of keratorefractive patients. *J Refract Surg.* 2003;19(1):24-29.

Ambrósio R Jr, Nogueira LP, Caldas DL, et al. Evaluation of corneal shape and biomechanics before LASIK. *Int Ophthalmol Clin.* 2011;51(2):11-38.

Belin MW, Khachikian SS. An introduction to understanding elevation-based topography: how elevation data are displayed a review. *Clin Experiment Ophthalmol.* 2009;37(1):14-29.

De Paiva CS, Harris LD, Pflugfelder SC. Keratoconus-like topographic changes in keratoconjunctivitis sicca. *Cornea.* 2003;22(1):22-24.

Fontes BM, Ambrósio R Jr, Jardim D, Velarde GC, Nosé W. Corneal biomechanical metrics and anterior segment parameters in mild keratoconus. *Ophthalmology.* 2010;117(4):673-679.

Guilbert E, Saad A, Grise-Dulac A, Gatinel D. Corneal thickness, curvature, and elevation readings in normal corneas: combined Placido-Scheimpflug system versus combined Placido-scanning-slit system. *J Cataract Refract Surg.* 2012;38(7):1198-1206.

Klyce SD. Computer-assisted corneal topography. High-resolution graphic presentation and analysis of keratoscopy. *Invest Ophthalmol Vis Sci.* 1984;25(12):1426-1435.

Klyce SD, Wilson SE. Methods of analysis of corneal topography. Refract Corneal Surg. 1989;5(6):368-371.

Li Y, Meisler DM, Tang M, et al. Keratoconus diagnosis with optical coherence tomography pachymetry mapping. *Ophthalmology.* 2008;115(12):2159-2166.

Liu Z, Huang AJ, Pflugfelder SC. Evaluation of corneal thickness and topography in normal eyes using the Orbscan corneal topography system. *Br J Ophthalmol.* 1999;83(7):774-778.

Maeda N, Klyce SD, Smolek MK. Comparison of methods for detecting keratoconus using videokeratography. *Arch Ophthalmol.* 1995;113(7):870-874.

Rabinowitz YS, McDonnell PJ. Computer-assisted corneal topography in keratoconus. *Refract Corneal Surg.* 1989;5(6):400-408.

Rabinowitz YS. Videokeratographic indices to aid in screening for keratoconus. *J Refract Surg.* 1995;11(5):371-379.

Rabinowitz YS, Yang H, Brickman Y, et al. Videokeratography database of normal human corneas. *Br J Ophthalmol.* 1996;80(7):610-616.

Randleman JB, Dawson DG, Grossniklaus HE, McCarey BE, Edelhauser HF. Depth-dependent cohesive tensile strength in human donor corneas: implications for refractive surgery. *J Refract Surg.* 2008;24(1):S85-S89.

Randleman JB, Russell B, Ward MA, Thompson KP, Stulting RD. Risk factors and prognosis for corneal ectasia after LASIK. *Ophthalmology.* 2003;110(2):267-275.

Randleman JB, Woodward M, Lynn MJ, Stulting RD. Risk assessment for ectasia after corneal refractive surgery. *Ophthalmology.* 2008;115(1):37-50.

Randleman JB, Trattler WB, Stulting RD. Validation of the ectasia risk assessment score system for preoperative laser in situ keratomileusis screening. *Am J Ophthalmol.* 2008;145(5):813-818.

Randleman JB. Pre-refractive surgery topographic evaluation. In Wang M, ed. *Corneal Topography: A Guide for Clinical Application in the Wavefront Era. 2nd ed.* Thorofare, NJ: SLACK Incorporated; 2011:231-242.

Randleman JB, Woodward MA. Evaluation and diagnosis of postoperative corneal ectasia. Hafezi F, Randleman JB (eds). *Corneal Collagen Cross Linking.* Thorofare, NJ: SLACK Incorporated; 2013:31-38.

Reinstein DZ, Gobbe M, Archer TJ, Silerman RH, Coleman DJ. Epithelial, stromal, and total corneal thickness in keratoconus: three-dimensional display with artemis very-high frequency digital ultrasound. *J Refract Surg.* 2010;26(4):259-271.

Reinstein DZ, Archer TJ, Gobbe M. Corneal epithelial thickness profile in the diagnosis of keratoconus. *J Refract Surg.* 2009;25(7):604-610.

Rocha KM, Perez-Straziota CE, Stulting RD, Randleman JB. SD-OCT analysis of regional epithelial thickness profiles in keratoconus, postoperative corneal ectasia, and normal eyes. *J Refract Surg.* 2013;29(3):173-179.

Saad A, Gatinel D. Topographic and tomographic properties of forme fruste keratoconus corneas. *Invest Ophthalmol Vis Sci.* 2010;51(11):5546-5555.

Saad A, Gatinel D. Evaluation of total and corneal wavefront high order aberrations for the detection of forme fruste keratoconus. *Invest Ophthalmol Vis Sci.* 2012;17;53(6):2978-2992.

Saad A, Lteif Y, Azan E, Gatinel D. Biomechanical properties of keratoconus suspect eyes. *Invest Ophthalmol Vis Sci.* 2010;51(6):2912-2916.

Smolek MK, Klyce SD, Hovis JK. The Universal Standard Scale: proposed improvements to the American National Standards Institute (ANSI) scale for corneal topography. *Ophthalmology.* 2002;109(2):361-369.

Sonmez B, Doan MP, Hamilton DR. Identification of scanning slit-beam topographic parameters important in distinguishing normal from keratoconic corneal morphologic features. *Am J Ophthalmol.* 2007;143(3):401-408.

Varssano D, Kaiserman I, Hazarbassanov R. Topographic patterns in refractive surgery candidates. *Cornea.* 2004;23(6):602-607.

Please visit www.routledge.com/ 9781617110368
to access additional material.

4

Basic Techniques for Refractive Surgical Procedures

Chapter Highlights

- Excimer laser surgery surgical steps
  - ◊ Surface ablation specific steps
  - ◊ LASIK specific steps
- Phakic intraocular lens surgical steps
- Refractive lens exchange surgical steps

This chapter is intended to orient the reader to the basic steps for the most common refractive surgical procedures, including surface ablation, LASIK, phakic intraocular lens (PIOL) implantation, and refractive lens exchange. Some surgical details are specific to different femtosecond and excimer laser platforms, whereas other steps may be unique for each surgical location. Therefore, the reader is cautioned to become completely familiar with all aspects of each surgery in the environment where they will be operating.

Basic Surgical Technique: Excimer Laser Ablation

Most of the steps required for both surface ablation and LASIK excimer laser procedures are identical; however, the primary difference between procedures is the creation of a partial-thickness lamellar flap for LASIK or epithelial removal and preparation of Bowman's layer for surface ablation. Table 4-1 provides a step-by-step guide for surface ablation and LASIK procedures. Essential steps for all excimer laser procedures include laser calibration and confirmation that

Randleman JB.
Refractive Surgery: An Interactive Case-Based Approach (pp. 39-43).

Table 4-1. Step-by-Step Surface Ablation and LASIK Procedures

PROCEDURE TYPE	SURFACE ABLATION	LASIK
Step 1	Excimer laser calibration	Excimer laser calibration
Step 2	Obtain WFG measurements[a]	Obtain WFG measurements[a]
Step 3	Program laser with surgical plan	Program laser with surgical plan
Step 4	Prep the patient	Prep the patient
Step 5	Review the programmed surgical plan	Review the programmed surgical plan
Step 6	Epithelial removal	Flap creation
Step 7	Prepare stromal bed for laser	Prepare stromal bed for laser
Step 8	Excimer laser ablation	Excimer laser ablation
Step 9	Irrigate surface	Irrigate flap interface
Step 10	Mitomycin C application[b]	Smooth flap
Step 11	Irrigate	
Step 12	TBCL placement	

Abbreviation: TBCL, therapeutic bandage contact lens; WFG, wavefront-guided.

[a] This step is necessary only for WFG treatments.
[b] Mitomycin C application is applied at this time if used for the surgery.

all surgical data are entered correctly into the excimer laser. Although technicians frequently perform these 2 steps, both are ultimately the surgeon's responsibility to confirm and both require establishing a reproducible system, similar to a pilot's preflight checklist, to confirm each step is performed accurately for every surgery.

Every laser device has its own calibration schedule, and this calibration is usually performed at the beginning of each surgical day and between a specified number of eyes or patients, to assure the appropriate beam profile is being generated. Many surgeons utilize an individualized nomogram to determine laser ablation profiles for the patient's refraction. If wavefront-guided treatment is performed, the data must be accurately transferred from the aberrometers to the laser. The surgical plan will also include setting an optical zone for treatment.

Most surgeons use 5% to 10% povidone-iodine solution or alcohol wipes to prepare the patient's eyelids. Laser vision correction is considered a "clean" rather than a sterile procedure; therefore, specific patient preparation steps may vary slightly from surgeon to surgeon.

Epithelial Removal for Surface Ablation Procedures

For surface ablation, including photorefractive keratectomy (PRK), laser-assisted subepithelial keratomileusis (LASEK), and epipolis laser in situ keratomileusis (epi-LASIK), Bowman's layer is prepared for treatment by epithelial removal or displacement. Ethanol (20%), mechanical removal, automated brush systems, mechanical microkeratome with an epithelial separator, or transepithelial ablation with some excimer lasers can all be used to displace the epithelium, and the majority of literature reports demonstrate equivalence in final outcomes among these techniques.

Flap Creation for LASIK

Anterior stromal, hinged corneal flaps can be created with either a mechanical microkeratome, using a high-oscillating blade, or the femtosecond laser. With both devices, suction is applied to fixate the globe, and intraocular pressure (IOP) increases significantly for the brief period of flap creation. Confirmation of appropriate suction, through confirming fixation of eye movement, checking for increased IOP (above 60 mm Hg), and/or confirming that vision has become dark for the patient is necessary before proceeding with flap creation to assure a high quality flap. Many modern microkeratomes and all femtosecond lasers create thin, reproducible flaps with nearly planar architecture. Some femtosecond lasers create a side "cut" separate from the lamellar tissue cleavage, whereas others create both through the same mechanism. The presence or absence of a side cut upon initiation of the flap creation determines the probability of generating an opaque bubble layer (see Chapter 5 for more information). After flap creation with either device, the flap is separated from the posterior stroma and reflected out of the ablation zone.

Excimer Laser Ablation

Patient positioning during ablation is critical. Cyclotorsion can occur and can be clinically relevant if large amounts of astigmatism correction or wavefront-guided ablations are being performed. Some surgeons mark the patient when he or she is sitting in an upright position to be able to identify the 0- and 180-degree meridians when the patient is supine. Modern excimer lasers employ tracking devices to account for microsaccades during ablation; however, the patient must still cooperate with fixation, and the surgeon must confirm this fixation throughout the ablation.

If peripheral ablations are planned, including hyperopic, astigmatic, or highly myopic ablations with a large treatment zone, care should be taken to cover the LASIK flap hinge to prevent double ablation on the adjacent underside of the flap and posterior stroma.

Immediate Postablation Measures

After surface ablation, most surgeons use chilled balanced salt solution (BSS) to irrigate and cool the corneal surface. After LASIK, the posterior stromal bed and interface are irrigated to remove any particles from the tear film that lodged under the flap.

Most surgeons advocate use of mitomycin C (MMC) 0.05% for prophylaxis to prevent visually significant haze after surface ablation. Some surgeons advocate use only in patients with higher ablations, whereas others recommend prophylactic use in all patients. Mitomycin C was initially used for up to 2 minutes; however, recent studies have found no difference in efficacy between longer and shorter application times (12 seconds) when used prophylactically. If MMC is used and copious irrigation is applied to thoroughly rinse the corneal surface, most surgeons will then apply a therapeutic bandage contact lens (TBCL) to facilitate comfort and epithelial healing over the first few postoperative days.

For LASIK, after ablation the flap is smoothed and confirmed to be on good position. After these steps, topical antibiotics, topical steroids, and frequently topical nonsteroidal anti-inflammatory (NSAIDs) drops are administered. It is important not to apply topical NSAIDs before TBCL placement after surface ablation, as some NSAIDs have been associated with delayed epithelial healing and haze formation if applied to the bare stroma (see Figure 5-5).

Surgical Technique: Phakic Intraocular Lens Implantation

Phakic intraocular lenses are available for the treatment of higher degrees of myopia (see Table 1-3) and currently are available in two varieties in the United States: iris-fixated IOLs (Artisan; Ophtec BV and Verisyse; Abbott Medical Optics Inc) made of rigid poly methyl methacrylate (PMMA) and sulcus-fixated (Visian ICL; STAAR Surgical Co) made of a flexible collamer material. Additional varieties of these PIOLs are available outside of the United States, including a foldable variety of the iris-fixated PIOL (Artiflex, Ophtec BV or Veriflex, Abbott Medical Optics Inc), and toric implantable contact lenses (ICLs). Anterior chamber-fixated PIOLs are also in various stages of clinical trials and may be approved in the near future. Outside of the United States, PIOLs are also available to treat hyperopia.

Phakic IOLs are implanted through either a 6-mm incision for the iris-fixated PIOL or through a 3-mm or smaller wound for the ICL. Throughout the procedures, it is critical to maintain significant anterior chamber depth with viscoelastic to protect both the corneal endothelium and the crystalline lens. After implantation and appropriate PIOL positioning, all viscoelastic is removed. The iris-fixated PIOL usually require sutures for incision closure, whereas the ICL usually does not.

Surgical Technique: Refractive Lens Exchange

From a technical standpoint, refractive lens exchange is identical to standard cataract surgery. A variety of IOL styles are utilized depending on the patient's goals, desires, and ocular conditions. Currently in the United States, these IOL styles include standard monofocal (spheric or aspheric), toric, multifocal, and pseudoaccommodating. Outside of the United States, there are a multitude of IOLs that address presbyopia through a variety of different mechanisms, and some accommodating IOLs may soon be approved for use in the United States.

Bibliography

Buratto L, Slade SG. *PRK: The Past, Present, and Future of Surface Ablation.* Thorofare, NJ: SLACK Incorporated; 2012

Buratto L, Slade SG, Hauranieh N. *Phakic IOLs: State of the Art.* Thorofare, NJ: SLACK Incorporated; 2012

Buratto L, Slade SG, Tavolato M. *LASIK: The Evolution of Refractive Surgery.* Thorofare, NJ: SLACK Incorporated; 2012.

Davison JA, Johnson SC. Intraoperative complications of LASIK flaps using the intralase femtosecond laser in 3009 cases. *J Refract Surg.* 2010;26(11):851-857.

Durrie DS, Kezirian GM. Femtosecond laser versus mechanical keratome flaps in wavefront-guided laser in situ keratomileusis: prospective contralateral eye study. *J Cataract Refract Surg.* 2005;31(1):120-126.

Güell JL, Morral M, Kook D, Kohnen T. Phakic intraocular lenses part 1: historical overview, current models, selection criteria, and surgical techniques. *J Cataract Refract Surg.* 2010;36(11):1976-1993.

Lim T, Yang S, Kim M, Tchah H. Comparison of the IntraLase femtosecond laser and mechanical microkeratome for laser in situ keratomileusis. *Am J Ophthalmol.* 2006;141(5):833-839.

Majmudar PA, Forstot SL, Dennis RF, et al. Topical mitomycin-C for subepithelial fibrosis after refractive corneal surgery. *Ophthalmology.* 2000;107(1):89-94.

Patel SV, Maguire LJ, McLaren JW, Hodge DO, Bourne WM. Femtosecond laser versus mechanical microkeratome for LASIK: a randomized controlled study. *Ophthalmology.* 2007;114(8):1482-1490.

Rocha KM, Randleman JB, Stulting RD. Analysis of microkeratome thin flap architecture using Fourier-domain optical coherence tomography. *J Refract Surg.* 2011;27(10):759-763.

Tran DB, Sarayba MA, Bor Z, et al. Randomized prospective clinical study comparing induced aberrations with IntraLase and Hansatome flap creation in fellow eyes: potential impact on wavefront-guided laser in situ keratomileusis. *J Cataract Refract Surg.* 2005;31(1):97-105.

Virasch VV, Majmudar PA, Epstein RJ, Vaidya NS, Dennis RF. Reduced application time for prophylactic mitomycin C in photorefractive keratectomy. *Ophthalmology.* 2010;117(5):885-889.

Please visit www.routledge.com/ 9781617110368 to access additional material.

5

Overview of Refractive Surgical Complications

Chapter Highlights

- Complications of excimer laser corneal refractive procedures
- Complications of phakic intraocular lens implantation
- Complications of refractive lens exchange

Refractive surgery is uniquely successful among both ocular surgeries and elective surgeries. Fortunately, severe complications are rare and have become less common over time, now occurring in approximately less than 0.5% of cases. However, the rarity of significant complications makes the diagnosis of specific complications challenging, as one is unlikely to see many cases of any particular disorder. Further, some complications are unique to refractive surgery, such as irregular ablations and LASIK interface disorders.

Complications can be categorized based on functional outcome (visual acuity loss, foreign body sensation), etiology (scar, infection, biomechanical weakening), anatomical location (ocular surface, LASIK interface), or relative severity (mild, including residual ametropia amenable to retreatment and mild dry eye; or serious, including infection and ectasia). Table 5-1 provides a comparative overview of the relative frequency of a variety of potential complications between LASIK and advanced surface ablation (ASA); overall complication rates are equivalent between techniques, but the etiologies differ significantly.

Randleman JB.
Refractive Surgery: An Interactive Case-Based Approach (pp. 45-68).

Table 5-1. Comparative Frequency of Corneal Refractive Surgical Complications

COMPLICATION	LASIK	SURFACE ABLATION
Vision loss	*	*
Aberrations	*	*
Retreatment	*	*
Dry eye	**	*
Corneal haze	*	***
Infection	*	***
Flap complications	***	N/A
Inflammatory complications	**	*
Irregular astigmatism	*	*
Ectasia	***	*

The asterisks indicate a relative risk (considering both severity and comparative possibility of occurring) for each complication per procedure as compared to the alternative surgical option. * = low; ** = moderate; *** = high

Complications of Excimer Laser Corneal Refractive Procedures

Complications can arise from a variety of mechanisms, as highlighted in the breakout box.

Complications of Corneal Refractive Procedures

- Residual ametropia and visual aberrations
- Ocular surface issues
- Diplopia
- Infectious keratitis
- LASIK flap complications
- LASIK interface complications
- Irregular astigmatism (limited)
- Ectasia (progressive)

Residual Ametropia

Retreatment (or enhancement) rates after excimer laser procedures vary by indication and patient expectations but generally are less than 5% for all procedures. Patients with hyperopia or high astigmatism have a higher likelihood of requiring retreatment than patients with myopia. Reported enhancement rates among publications and refractive centers differ based on their criteria for retreatment. Also, there is discrepancy in the literature regarding enhancement rates for patients selecting monovision, but these individuals may be more sensitive to smaller degrees of ametropia in their distance eye and thus have a higher retreatment rate than patients corrected bilaterally for distance vision.

Visual Aberrations

Visual aberrations take many forms and descriptions, including glare, halos, starbursts, and (a more generic term) *night vision disturbances* or *complaints* (NVC). Visual aberrations are most frequently associated with residual ametropia. Other causes include dry eye syndrome, preoperative higher-order aberrations in significantly aberrated eyes, induction of higher-order aberrations after surgery, and irregular astigmatism. Pupil size has not been correlated with increased risk of visual aberrations; however, reducing pupil size may have beneficial effects

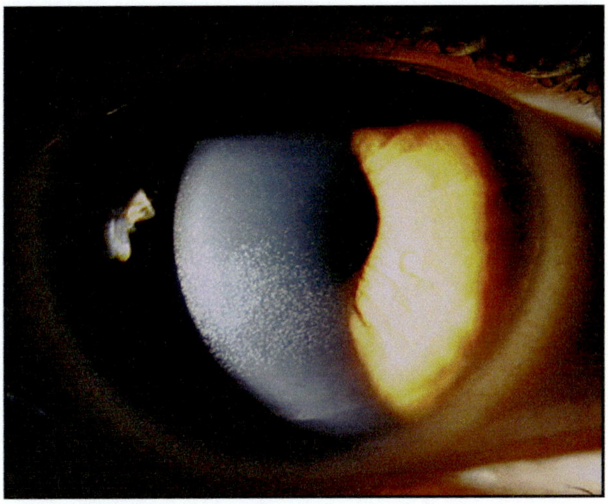

Figure 5-1. Slit-lamp image demonstrating punctate epitheliopathy in a patient with dry eye after LASIK.

if symptoms do occur. Treatments vary by etiology but include retreatment with wavefront-optimized or wavefront-guided ablation patterns for routine ametropia, or topography-guided ablation patterns for some irregular errors, including decentered or small optical zones and mild irregular astigmatism. Topical brimonidine (Bausch & Lomb) may be effective for night vision disturbances by minimizing pupil dilation at night.

Dry Eye Syndrome

Most patients experience transient dry eye symptoms in the early postoperative period after PRK and LASIK, which usually resolves; however, some patients develop significant dry eye postoperatively (Figure 5-1). Estimates vary, but up to 30% of patients experience at least moderate, transient dry eye symptoms; the percentage drops considerably for more significant symptoms and longer follow-up. Patients with dry eye signs and symptoms preoperatively are at higher risk for chronic dry eye after surgery, and these individuals should be carefully screened and appropriately counseled before undergoing surgery, and in some instances declined surgery. Effective treatment strategies include aggressive lubrication with artificial tear supplements and ointments, topical cyclosporine drops, punctual occlusion, and, rarely, more aggressive treatments such as serum tears and moisture chamber glasses.

Diplopia After Laser Ablation

Diplopia is a rare complication that may arise after corneal refractive surgery, most commonly manifesting as monocular diplopia from irregular astigmatism. This can occur from a variety of mechanisms, including surface healing issues, flap complications or interface complications leading to scarring in LASIK, or irregular excimer laser ablations. Specific entities will be discussed under their respective subheadings within this chapter.

Binocular diplopia can arise from the dissociation of long-standing phorias, most commonly in association with monovision refractive outcomes. Any patient with a history of strabismus or significant amblyopia who is not successfully wearing longstanding monovision correction should be excluded from monovision surgical correction. To screen for at-risk individuals beyond this, a careful evaluation of muscle balance and movements are necessary, as well as inspection of current spectacles, because some individuals may be wearing prism spectacles and not mention or not know it. Although not definitive, spectacles may control phorias better than contact lenses, and extra care should be given to individuals with phorias who use only spectacle correction. Cycloplegic refraction is critical in identifying at-risk individuals in the following instances:

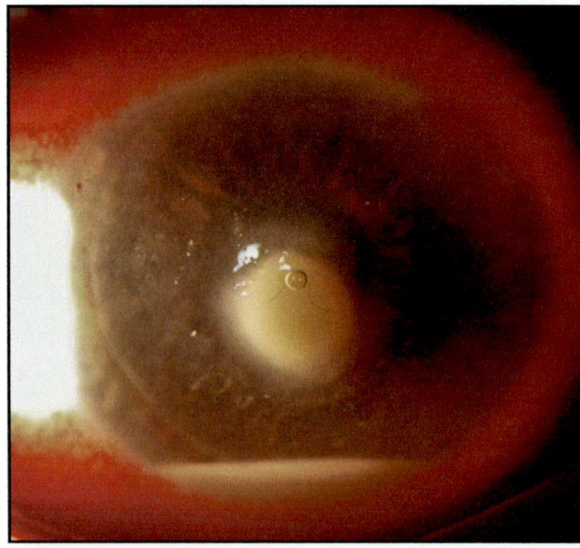

Figure 5-2. Infectious keratitis after LASIK with central infiltrate and hypopyon.

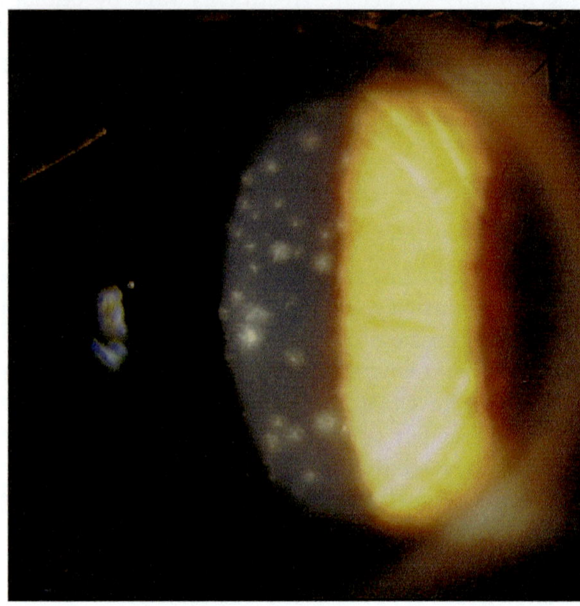

Figure 5-3. Subepithelial infiltrates from adenovirus reactivation after LASIK.

myopes with exophorias and hyperopes with esophorias who achieve orthophoria, in addition to emmetropia, with their spectacles if the myopic individual has a spectacle prescription more myopic than his or her cycloplegic refraction, or if a hyperopic individual is earning the maximal hyperopic refraction with maximal relaxation of accommodation. If significant doubt exists, an extended contact lens trial with the planned refractive goal may be warranted.

Infectious Keratitis

Infectious keratitis is a rare but potentially devastating complication, occurring in approximately 0.02% to 0.2% of surface ablation cases and 0.03% to 0.1% of LASIK cases (Figure 5-2). A variety of organisms can cause postoperative keratitis, including viruses (Adenovirus and herpes simplex virus) (Figure 5-3), bacteria (*Staphylococcus* species and *Pseudomonas*), atypical

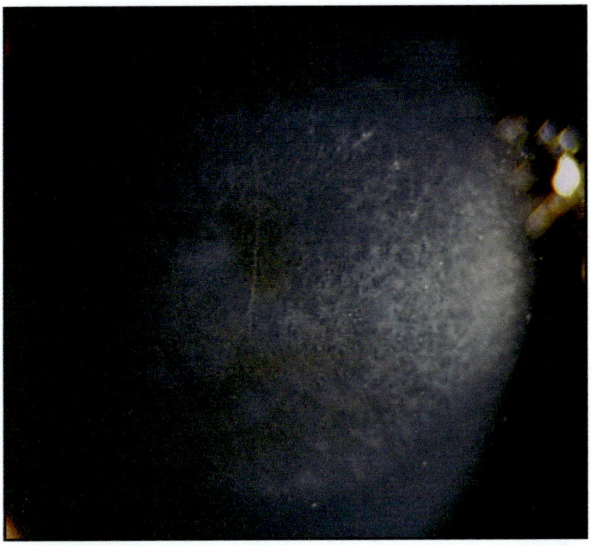

Figure 5-4. High-magnification image demonstrating anterior corneal haze following surface ablation.

mycobacteria, fungi, and *Acanthamoeba*. Adenovirus usually has a relatively benign course with ultimately good acuity, whereas herpes simplex virus can lead to loss of best acuity after PRK or LASIK.

The most common nonviral cause of infectious keratitis is *Staphylococcus aureus*, followed by *Mycobacterium, Pseudomonas*, fungal infections, and *Acanthamoeba. Staphylococcus* infections and *Pseudomonas* usually present within the first 2 to 7 days postoperatively, whereas the other organisms generally present between 2 and 3 weeks postoperatively. *Methicillin-resistant Staphylococcus aureus* (MRSA) is becoming a more common infectious organism in corneal refractive surgical procedures.

In the initial phase of treatment, LASIK flaps should be lifted, cultures taken, the flap bed irrigated with fortified antibiotics, and broad-spectrum topical antibiotics started. For infections with a delayed onset, the use of empiric amikacin may be beneficial in treating atypical mycobacteria. Surface ablation infections can be managed similarly to routine corneal ulcers; however, in nonresponsive LASIK infections, flap amputation may be necessary to facilitate antibiotic penetration. Most infections resolve with mild to moderate loss of best acuity, but, rarely, therapeutic penetrating keratoplasty is necessary. More details will be provided in the LASIK Interface section of this chapter.

Corneal Haze and Scarring

Although postoperative corneal haze is a potential complication of any corneal refractive procedure, in practice, PRK has the greatest potential to induce haze due to the increased healing response and growth factors exposed to the bare stroma after epithelial removal and ablation of Bowman's layer (Figure 5-4). Haze can occur many months postoperatively, and it is more commonly associated with greater tissue ablations.

In the past decade, the incidence of haze after PRK has decreased dramatically due to changes in excimer laser ablation profiles and the prophylactic use of mitomycin C (MMC). Although there remains some controversy about the safety of MMC, specifically in terms of endothelial cell loss, most studies have found no or minimal effects on the endothelium with short-term use.

Delayed corneal healing resulting in haze also has been reported with the use of some nonsteroidal anti-inflammatory drugs when applied to the bare stroma prior to bandage contact lens

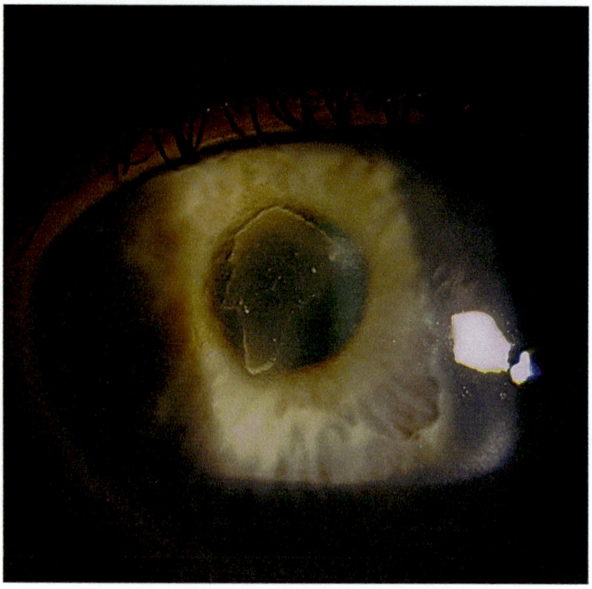

Figure 5-5. Slit-lamp photo showing delayed corneal healing and central haze following nepafenac (topical nonsteroidal) use after surface ablation.

Table 5-2. Comparative Frequency of Flap Complications With Mechanical Microkeratomes and Femtosecond Lasers

COMPLICATION	MICROKERATOME	FEMTOSECOND
Suction loss	*	*
Free cap	***	*
Partial flap	**	*
Buttonhole flap	***	
Vertical gas breakthrough		***
Opaque bubble layer		*
Epithelial defects	***	*

The asterisks indicate a relative risk (considering both severity and comparative possibility of occurring) for each complication per procedure as compared to the alternative surgical option. * = low; ** = moderate; *** = high

placement after surface ablation (Figure 5-5). To avoid this, bandage contact lens placement should always occur prior to drop administration in surface ablation cases.

LASIK Flap Complications

- Epithelial defects
- Opaque bubble layer
- Vertical gas breakthrough
- Buttonhole flap
- Free cap
- Flap dislocation
- Flap striae

Flap Complications

LASIK flaps may be created with a mechanical microkeratome or a femtosecond (FS) laser. As a result of modern technology, flap-related complications occur much less frequently and, if they do occur, most are relatively minor. However, the potential exists for serious complications of flaps that are created with either type of device (Table 5-2 and Figure 5-6).

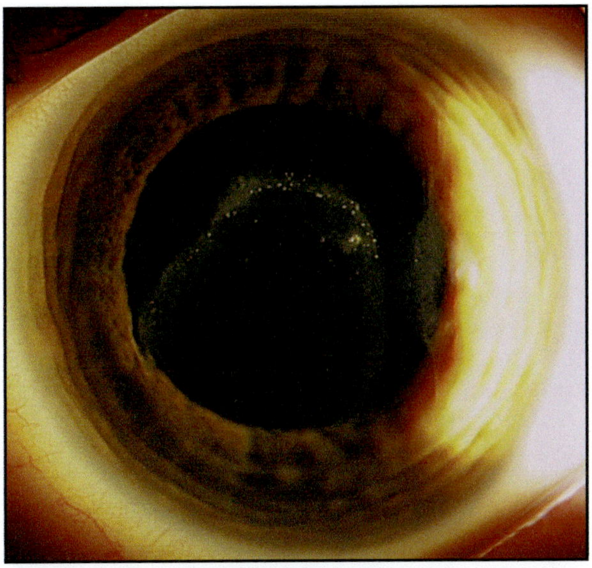

Figure 5-6. Slit-lamp image with corneal scarring from a severe buttonhole LASIK flap, where 2 partial flaps were created during the microkeratome pass.

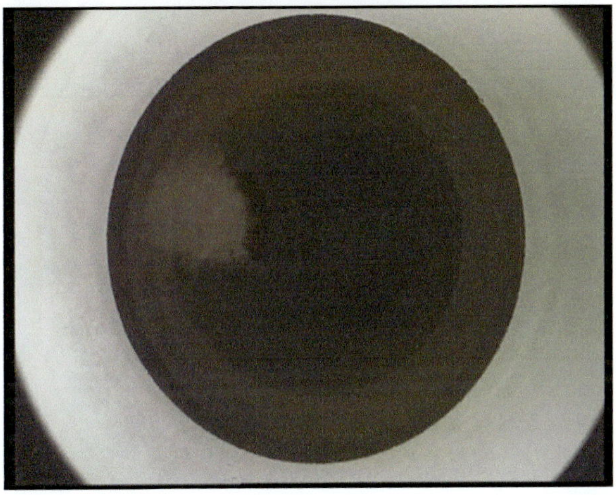

Figure 5-7. Opaque bubble layer from LASIK flap creation with a femtosecond laser. (Reprinted with permission of Sonia Yoo, MD.)

Complications include epithelial defects, which occur more frequently using a mechanical microkeratome than using FS laser devices, and an opaque bubble layer, which is unique to some FS lasers that create the stromal bed dissection prior to side cuts (Figure 5-7). Although epithelial defect formation is usually not visually significant in itself, it does predispose the patient to postoperative interface inflammation, generally called *diffuse lamellar keratitis* (DLK), and creates the potential for recurrent erosions with recurrent bouts of interface inflammation. Epithelial defect formation is more common in individuals with epithelial basement membrane dystrophy (EBMD), and all patients should be carefully screened for this epithelial abnormality. If there is a history of previous epithelial trauma or any report of recurrent erosion symptoms, evaluation of the epithelium and search for grossly loose areas using a Q-tip may be warranted.

The most significant flap complications include a free cap, whereby the hinge is nonexistent, and the flap is therefore completely separated from the underlying stroma; a partial flap; a decentered flap; and a buttonhole flap (Figure 5-8), which is caused by the mechanical microkeratome "skipping" over a portion of the cornea, leaving a small amount of uncut tissue. Free caps can occur with either a microkeratome or FS laser; however, they are more common with a microkeratome. Partial and decentered flaps may be created using either device. In these

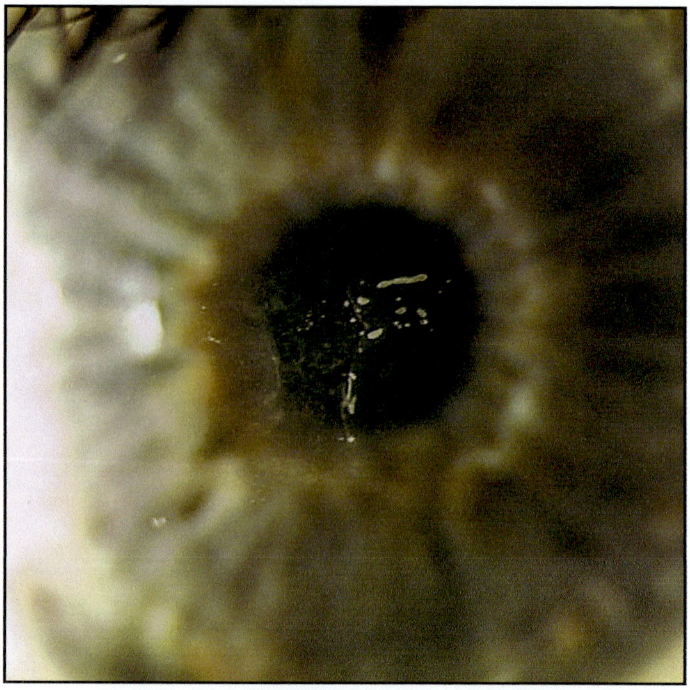

Figure 5-8. LASIK buttonhole flap created with a microkeratome.

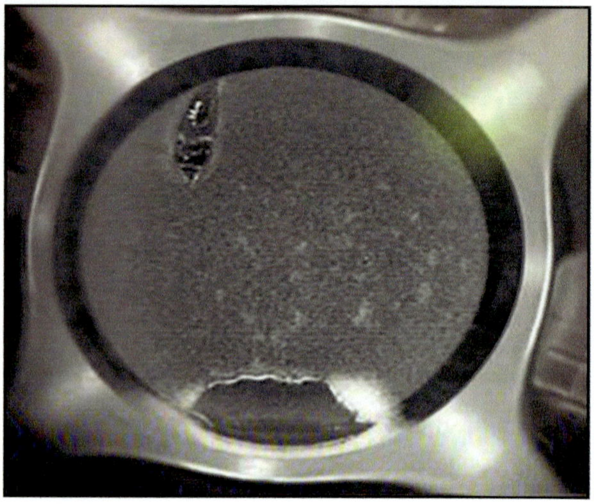

Figure 5-9. Vertical gas breakthrough (upper left portion of the image) from LASIK flap creation with a femtosecond laser. (Reprinted with permission of Sonia Yoo, MD.)

cases, ablation may proceed if there is adequate stromal bed exposure for full, centered ablation to occur; if insufficient exposure is attained the flap should be replaced without performing ablation. True buttonhole flaps are unique to microkeratomes. An analogous complication can occur with the FS laser vertical gas breakthrough and may mimic a buttonhole flap if it occurs in a large enough area (Figure 5-9). Cases with buttonhole flaps or vertical gas breakthrough should not have ablation performed.

Early postoperative complications include dislocated flaps, which require repositioning, and flap striae, which may be insignificant microstria (usually a result of epithelial sloughing) or macrostria in the visual axis that require flap repositioning (Figure 5-10). Epithelial defects may also present in the early postoperative period, increasing the risk of infection, as well as predisposing the eye to interface inflammation.

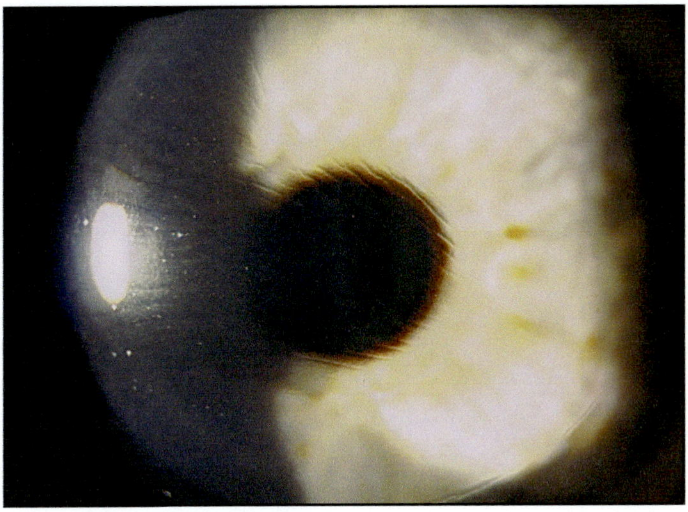

Figure 5-10. LASIK flap striae.

Transient light sensitivity and rainbow glare are phenomena that are unique to FS laser flap creation and are technically flap-related complications, although they appear in the early postoperative period. Transient light sensitivity is in some ways analogous to, but less significant than, DLK and may require more frequent steroid dosing in the early postoperative period. Rainbow glare is a poorly understood phenomena that occurs with some cases with FS laser flap creation but without excimer laser ablation due to the case being aborted for some reason, such as a persistent opaque bubble layer or anterior chamber gas bubbles that prevent excimer laser tracking. Rainbow glare likely results from the FS laser bed ablation not being "smoothed" by excimer laser ablation. Although rare, this phenomenon may be challenging to treat.

Interface Complications

LASIK Interface Complications

- Diffuse lamellar keratitis (DLK)
- Pressure-induced stromal keratopathy (PISK)
- Central toxic keratopathy (CTK)
- Infectious keratitis
- Epithelial ingrowth

A variety of complications, with overlapping clinical features, can present in the LASIK interface, but they each have unique mechanisms, time courses, and management strategies. These complications are rare, but due to their overlapping clinical appearance and uniqueness to LASIK, they are essential to understand for all practitioners managing postoperative refractive patients; thus, they are covered in relatively greater detail in this chapter.

Interface disorders can have a focal or diffuse appearance, can have conjunctival erythema or not, foreign body sensation or not, and can present from 1 day to 3 to 4 weeks postoperatively or beyond, such as in the case of epithelial ingrowth. Each interface disorder behaves quite differently when treated with topical or oral steroids, and this response can confirm the diagnosis or redirect therapy if the response is not as anticipated. Close attention to these specific features should rapidly lead the clinician to the appropriate diagnosis and ultimate management. However, all of these entities are relatively rare, occurring in approximately 1 of 1000 eyes, which makes the initial diagnosis increasingly challenging for less experienced surgeons and clinicians.

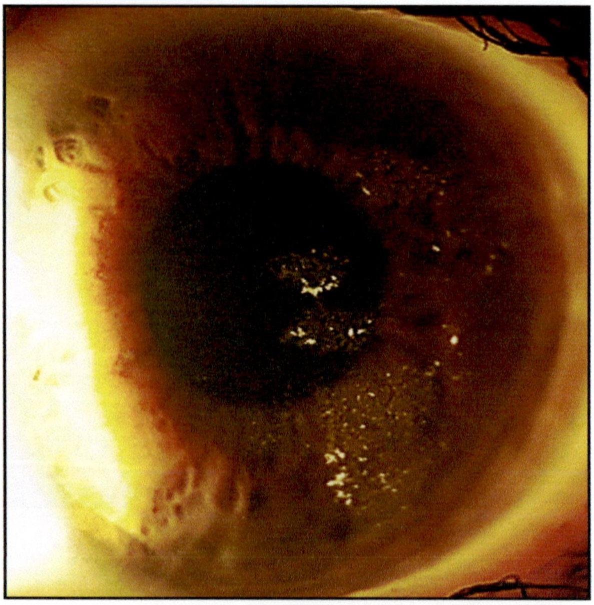

Figure 5-11. Composite image of LASIK interface disorders. (A) Benign interface debris in the LASIK interface. *(continued)*

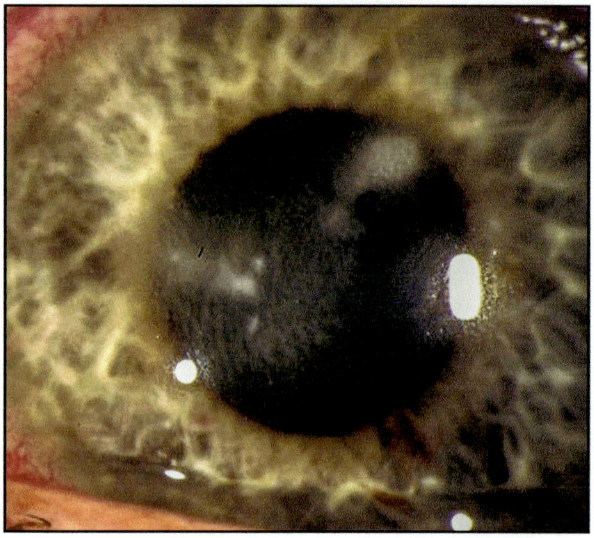

Figure 5-11 (continued). (B) Infectious keratitis.

Among these rare entities, DLK is the most common (Figure 5-11) and can occur in clusters or outbreaks; thus, most interface presentations are initially diagnosed and managed as DLK. Further, because the clinical appearance of DLK evolves from a mild, diffuse appearance to a dense, focal scar (Figure 5-12), DLK can mimic other entities at its various stages of development. Complicating the clinical scenario, a higher proportion of patients have benign, inconsequential interface debris, and this finding, combined with unrelated but routine complaints of mild foreign body sensation that naturally accompany LASIK in the early postoperative period, may lead the clinician to a diagnosis of DLK and the initiation of inappropriate treatment.

Differentiating between these interface disorders is critical to rapid, appropriate diagnosis, treatment, and ultimate visual outcome. Although initial similarities exist, taking a careful history of symptoms and onset, combined with a focused clinical examination, allows for accurate diagnosis and treatment on presentation. Table 5-3 presents a comparative overview of these disorders.

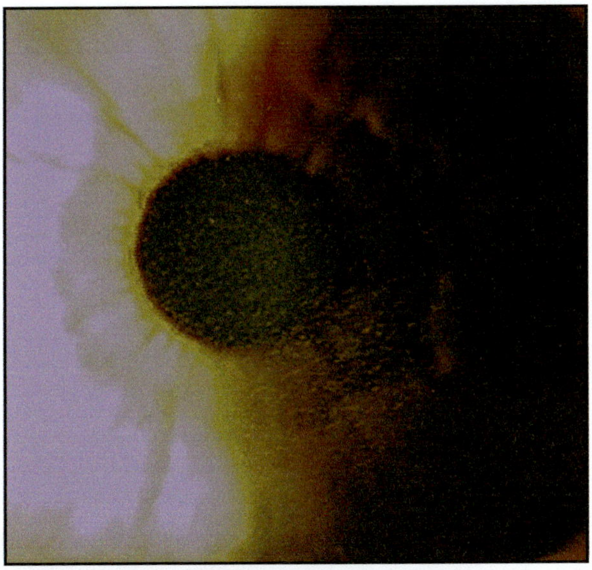

Figure 5-11 (continued). (C) DLK, stage 3. Note the diffuse, granular haze throughout the central cornea.

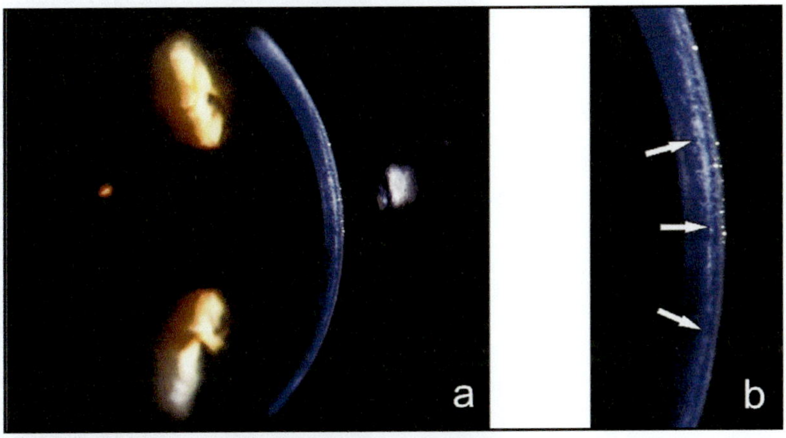

Figure 5-11 (continued). (D) PISK. The interface fluid visible in figure A is highlighted in higher magnification as a line of opacification in figure B (white arrows).

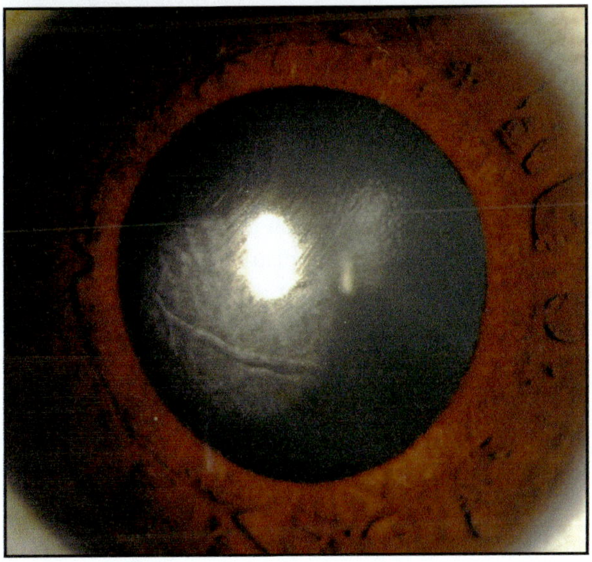

Figure 5-11 (continued). (E) Central toxic keratopathy.

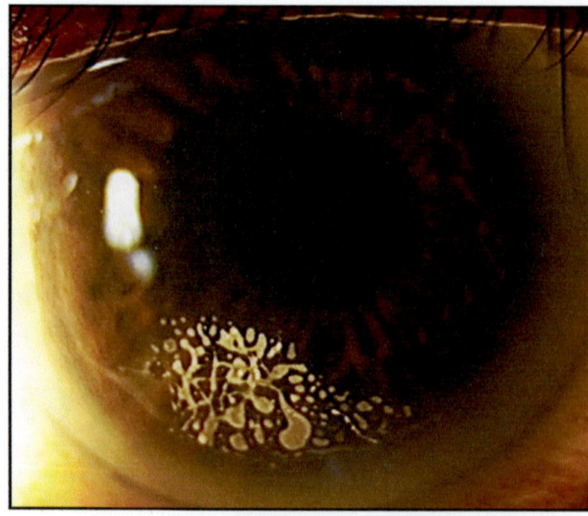

Figure 5-11 (continued). (F) Epithelial ingrowth. (All figures in 5-11 reprinted with permission from Randleman JB, Shah RD. LASIK interface complications: etiology, management, and outcomes. *J Refract Surg.* 2012;28(8):575-588.)

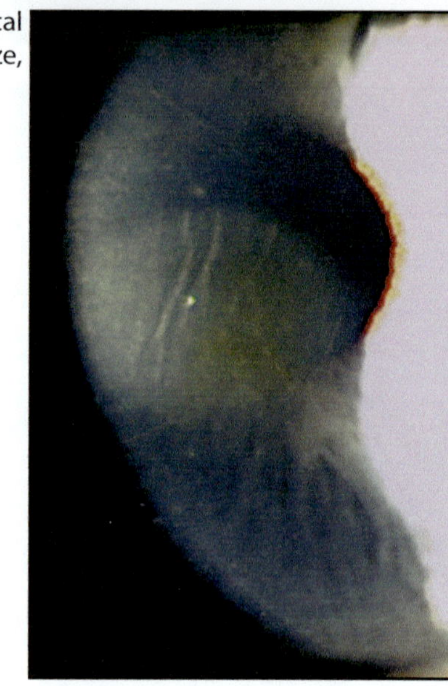

Figure 5-12. DLK, stage 4. (A) Slit-lamp image demonstrating focal corneal haze with a striate appearance within the center of the haze, similar to the appearance of central toxic keratopathy. *(continued)*

Interface Disorders: Etiology

DLK is an inflammatory response in the LASIK interface to a variety of stimuli, with a typical white blood cell buildup in the interface that coalesces as the condition advances. Central toxic keratopathy (CTK) is a noninflammatory focal opacification that appears at its most advanced stage almost immediately on presentation and gradually fades over time (see Figure 5-11). Pressure-induced stromal keratopathy (PISK) is a steroid response, resulting in high intraocular pressure (IOP), with ensuing fluid accumulation in the interface (Figure 5-13). The amount of fluid present may be relatively small, resulting in a diffuse haziness in the interface, or it may be large, resulting in a visible fluid cleft separating the anterior flap from the posterior residual bed. Infectious keratitis can occur from a variety of different organisms, including bacteria, fungi, and *Mycobacterium*, and the organism will influence the onset of signs and symptoms, which may occur from the first 3 to 5 postoperative days to more than 2 weeks after LASIK. Epithelial ingrowth occurs when a fistula develops under the flap, allowing epithelial cell growth into the interface (see Figure 5-11). This disorder usually occurs much later, generally weeks to months

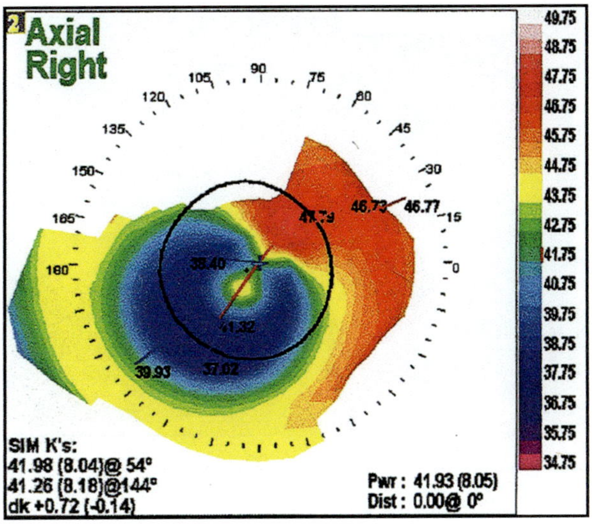

Figure 5-12 (continued). (B) Corresponding topography with notable focal flattening corresponding to the focal haze.

Table 5-3. Signs and Symptoms of Interface Disorders Over Time

DAY	DIFFUSE LAMELLAR KERATITIS	CENTRAL TOXIC KERATOPATHY	PRESSURE-INDUCED STROMAL KERATOPATHY	INFECTIOUS KERATITIS
1	FBS ± WBC's peripherally (stage 1)	None	None	None
2 to 3	Increased WBC's (stage 2)	Dense central opacification	None	None
4 to 7	More dense, coalescing (stage 2 to 3)	Stable opacification	None	FBS, redness, infiltrate (bacterial)
8 to 14	Coalescence to focal opacity ± scarring (stage 3 to 4)	Stable	None	Worsening of symptoms (bacterial), onset of symptoms (fungal)
15 to 21	Final coalescence to stage 4 or resolution	Stable	Onset of haze	Worsening of symptoms (bacterial, fungal), onset of symptoms (mycobacterial)
22 to 35	Final outcome	Slow resolution	Worsening haze ± fluid cleft	Variable, depending on organism and treatment

FBS: foreign body sensation; WBC: white blood cell

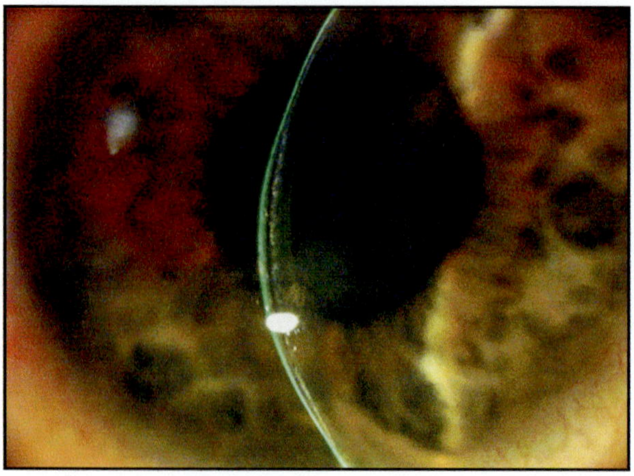

Figure 5-13. PISK with an obvious fluid cleft. (Reprinted with permission from Randleman JB, Shah RD. LASIK interface complications: etiology,management, and outcomes. *J Refract Surg*. 2012;28(8):575-588.)

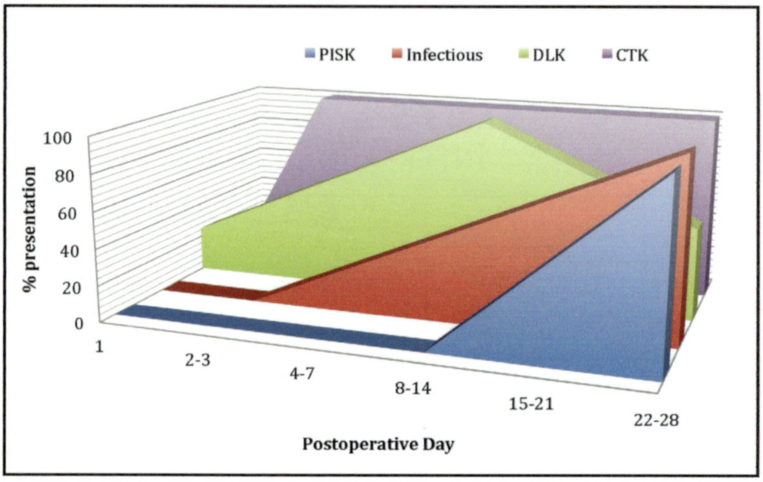

Figure 5-14. Relative presentation time points for LASIK interface complications. The Y-axis represents that time point by which that relative percentage of cases will present, and a decline in percentage on the Y-axis for DLK indicates the likelihood that DLK should begin to evolve and resolve with appropriate management over that time course.

after LASIK, and the distinct appearance is usually not confused with other interface disorders, but it has been related in the literature to atypical DLK and PISK.

Time of Onset and Symptoms at Presentation

Time of onset of interface disorders is a key differentiator, although it may be more challenging to exactly determine if the symptoms begin in between regularly scheduled visits because only patient-reported timing is available. Figure 5-14 graphically represents relative time of onset for each interface disorder.

DLK generally presents in the first few days after LASIK, typically in the first 1 to 5 days, usually first with increased foreign body sensation and subtle, diffuse, granular interface opacity but with minimal visual changes. If left untreated, DLK frequently increases in severity and can progress to a dense, coalesced, focal scar with significant visual loss.

Central toxic keratopathy also typically presents within the first week; however, there is usually no accompanying foreign body sensation, but early significant visual loss is common, and there is no diffuse haze on clinical examination. Central toxic keratopathy rarely progresses beyond its initial clinical appearance unless a flap lift is performed, which can exacerbate flap necrosis and ultimate scarring.

Infectious keratitis can also occur within the first week, but it usually takes at least a few days to develop. Infectious etiologies are accompanied by increased foreign body sensation; some degree of visual reduction; and increased conjunctival erythema, which is unique among interface disorders and has a more coalesced infiltrate.

PISK does not appear within the first 1 to 2 weeks postoperatively, as it takes some time for the IOP response to steroids to develop, which precedes interface fluid accumulation and the diffusely hazy appearance

Clinical Appearance: Diffuse or Focal Haze

DLK and PISK both present initially with diffuse interface haze. However, over their course, DLK either improves or progresses to a more focal scar, but it does not remain diffuse indefinitely, whereas PISK maintains its diffuse appearance and never coalesces. In contrast, CTK presents from its onset as a focal scar and is not diffuse at any time point. Infectious keratitis may have some accompanying diffuse haze due to white blood cell accumulation, but it is almost always accompanied by a more focal infiltrate at some location from onset. Early DLK and PISK may overlap clinically, whereas late DLK may mimic CTK.

Clinical Appearance: Evolution

DLK has the most potential for evolution in appearance, and at various stages it may mimic benign interface debris (stage 1), PISK (stage 2 to 3), and CTK (stage 4). However, DLK does evolve in clinical appearance relatively rapidly (over the course of days to weeks), as opposed to the other conditions, which exhibit minimal changes over time. Interface debris will be constant, unchanging, and asymptomatic. Central toxic keratopathy will present abruptly as deep, central, focal haze mimicking stage 4 DLK. PISK will present with diffuse granular interface haze with or without demonstrable interface fluid, and this appearance will change little until appropriate treatment is initiated. Infectious keratitis will evolve in appearance over time, but rapidly looks less and less like these other conditions due to its focal nature, increasing ocular redness, and coalescence into more localized, denser infiltrates.

Response to Topical or Oral Steroids

DLK is highly sensitive to steroids, and it responds to topical steroids for mild cases and to a combination of topical and oral steroids in moderate cases. In contrast, CTK exhibits no response to topical or oral steroids, and PISK progressively worsens with continued topical steroid use. The response of infectious keratitis to steroids is variable, but the infection will certainly not resolve with steroids alone.

Management

Management of DLK includes topical and/or oral steroids for early stages and flap lift with irrigation plus continued steroid use for more advanced cases. Central toxic keratopathy requires only observation, as no interventions have been found to be useful. PISK requires lowering IOP with glaucoma medications and cessation of steroid use. Infectious keratitis requires antibiotics administration specific to the infecting organism; thus, gram stains and cultures should be obtained, even if this requires flap lift. Some advocate irrigation with antibiotics under the flap.

Irregular Astigmatism From Laser Ablation

Irregular astigmatism due to laser ablation can arise from decentered ablation, including flap hinge ablation, and central islands. Decentered ablations can occur as a result of LASIK flap decentration (Figure 5-15), improper treatment alignment due to improper initial laser alignment

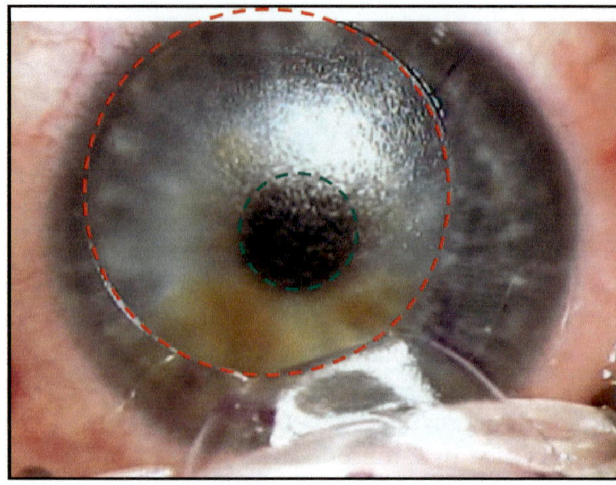

Figure 5-15. Intraoperative image demonstrating a decentered flap. The flap edge is highlighted in red broken lines, and the pupil is highlighted in green broken lines. (Reprinted with permission of Sonia Yoo, MD.)

or tracking registration, significant patient movement during surgery, or ineffective laser tracking, resulting in significant topographic irregularity over the central pupil (Figure 5-16). Decentered ablations may be more functionally significant after hyperopic ablations (see Figure 5-16). However, modern laser trackers and iris registration software have significantly reduced the incidence of this complication.

Central island patterns occur secondary to the broad-beam laser treating in a nonhomogeneous manner, a central blockage of the laser treatment by laser plume, the central accumulation of fluid on the cornea, or, occasionally, as a result of agents on the laser head itself that block the appropriate laser beam profile. The utilization of flying spot lasers and improved plume evacuation has significantly reduced the incidence of central island formation. Central islands can result in significant irregular astigmatism that is not readily amenable to further ablation. Ablation of both the stromal bed and flap hinge results in effectively double ablation in that focal region. This irregularity generally dissipates over time with corneal remodeling.

Postoperative Corneal Ectasia

Corneal ectasia after excimer laser surgery, usually LASIK, is a progressive steepening and thinning of the cornea, with resultant irregular astigmatism that reduces uncorrected and often best spectacle-corrected visual acuity (Figure 5-17). This steepening usually occurs inferiorly and usually in eyes with preoperative topographic abnormalities corresponding to the area of postoperative steepening.

Postoperative corneal ectasia remains a rare but feared complication of usually uneventful corneal refractive surgery. Since the first reports in 1998, numerous cases have been described in small series. Rather than representing a specific disease entity, postoperative ectasia, which is similar to naturally occurring ectatic diseases such as keratoconus or pellucid marginal corneal degeneration, is an end-stage manifestation of biomechanical weakening, resulting in corneal warpage. Corneal warpage arises from a variety of specific causes, including surgery in patients who are destined to develop keratoconus in their lifetime, preoperatively weak corneas that may not have developed keratoconus but decompensated after surgical intervention, and potentially otherwise normal corneas that have been excessively weakened postoperatively from the creation of a residual stromal bed too thin to maintain structural integrity.

Estimates of the incidence of ectasia can vary widely, from 0.04% to 0.2% in modern reports; however, the actual incidence remains undetermined and could be higher or lower than these

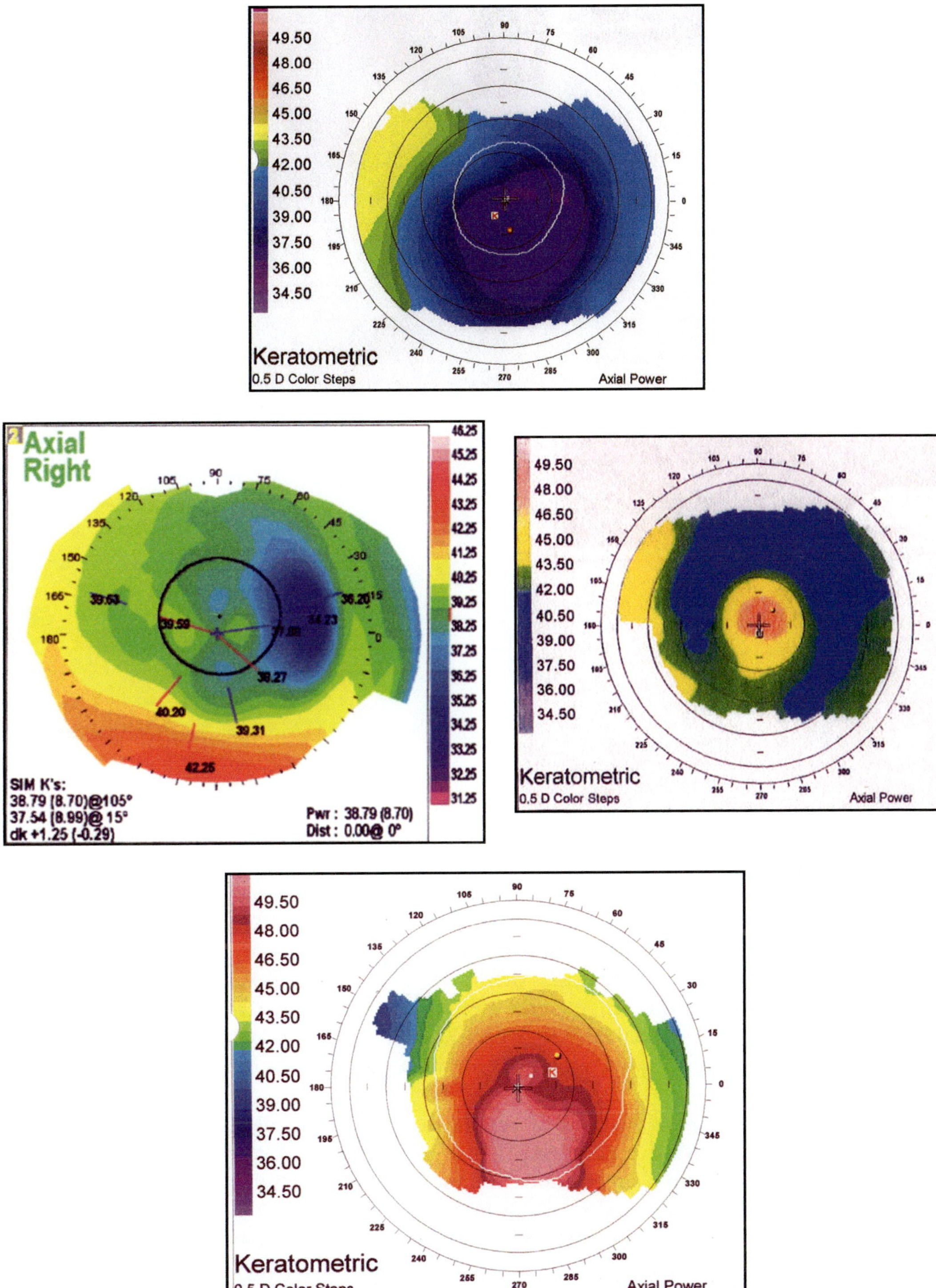

Figure 5-16. Irregular astigmatism from irregular laser ablations. (A) Decentered ablation, myopic LASIK. (B) Flap hinge ablation. (C) Central island. (D) Decentered ablation, hyperopic LASIK.

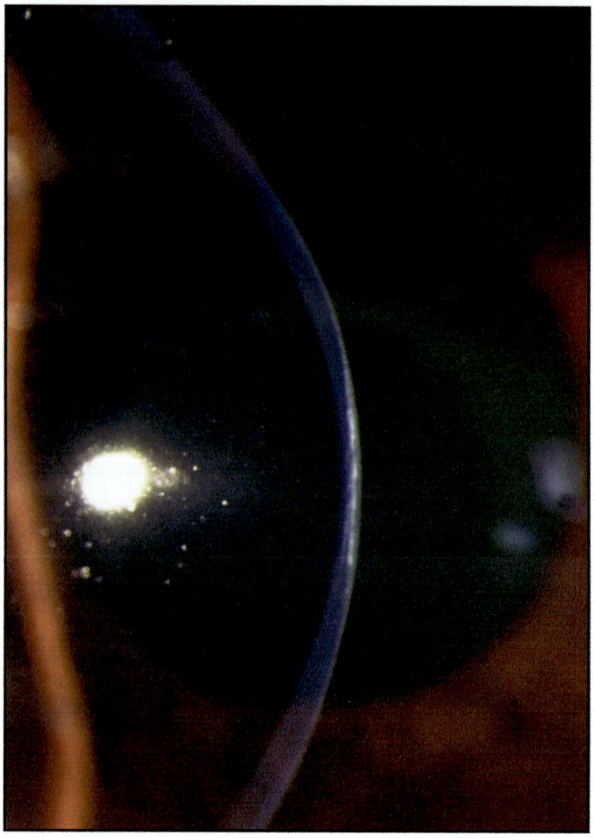

Figure 5-17. Postoperative corneal ectasia. (A) Slit-lamp image with notable central focal corneal thinning. *(continued)*

reported figures. The incidence of ectasia does appear to be significantly decreasing based on more recent publications, as diligent screening strategies (discussed in Chapter 3) are being utilized.

Wide variability exists in the preoperative presentation of patients who develop ectasia (Table 5-4). Such individuals tend to be younger, more myopic, have thinner corneas preoperatively, have lesser postoperative residual stromal bed thickness (RSB), and more frequently have abnormal preoperative topographies, compared with patients who do not develop ectasia. However, there is no single criterion that definitively predicts the development of ectasia, and cases have presented from wide ranges of the aforementioned parameters. One critical screening issue is the estimation of residual RSB after LASIK. Although no absolute cutoff exists, 250 μm has been set as a generally accepted minimum threshold, and RSB less than 300 μm may carry an increased risk.

The earliest clinical manifestations of ectasia can be subtle and require a high index of suspicion for diagnosis. Most patients experience increasing myopia and astigmatism, which can be misinterpreted as simple regression. In these early stages, topographic changes may also be quite subtle. Posterior float and elevation maps are inherently unreliable postoperatively to determine absolute differences compared with preoperative maps; however, significant increases in elevations noted on serial topography after surgery may indicate early ectatic changes. Advanced cases are clinically indistinguishable from keratoconus or pellucid marginal corneal degeneration.

The onset of presentation is also highly variable. Approximately 25% of cases present by 3 months, 50% by 12 months, and 80% by 2 years postoperatively; however, cases have presented as early as 1 week and as late as 5 or more years after LASIK and more than 10 years after PRK.

Progressive ectatic changes induce significant irregular astigmatism with a corresponding reduction in corrected distance visual acuity. Less than 10% of eyes can be visually rehabilitated

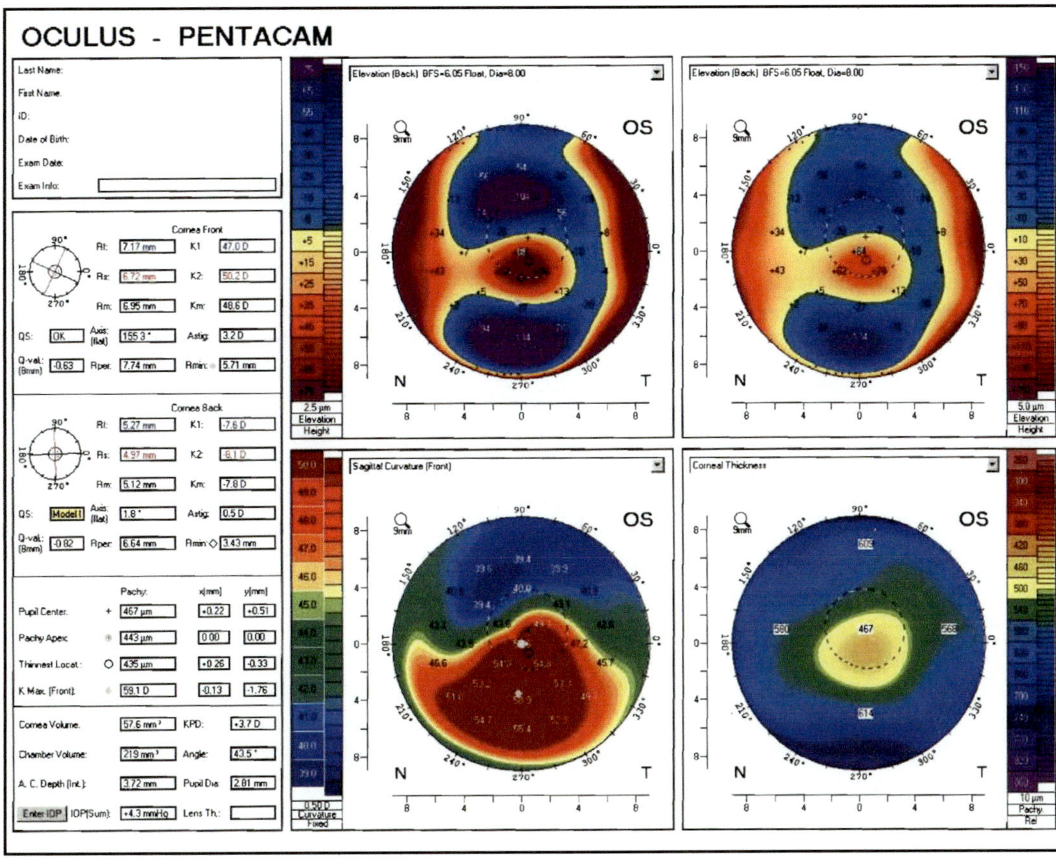

Figure 5-17 (continued). (B) Corresponding topographic appearance.

Table 5-4. Summary of Ectasia Patient Demographics		
DEMOGRAPHIC	AVERAGE	RANGE
Age (y)	35	18 to 62
Sex (% male)	60	
Manifest refraction (diopters)	-8.00	+5.00 to -24.00
Corneal thickness (µm)	520	406 to 597
Residual stromal bed (µm)	260	170 to 419
Abnormal preoperative topography (%)	45	

to an acceptable level with spectacles alone, and most patients require rigid gas permeable contact lenses for best acuity. In the past, approximately 8% of ectatic eyes required corneal transplantation; however, with the advent of corneal collagen cross-linking, this number appears to be dramatically decreasing, as this treatment halts and may partially reverse the ectatic process in the majority of eyes.

Complications From Intraocular Refractive Surgical Procedures

Complications of Phakic Intraocular Lens Implantation

Surgical Complications for Phakic Intraocular Procedures

- Endothelial cell loss
- Cataract formation
- Pupillary block

Primary concerns for phakic intraocular lens (PIOL) implantation include persistent anterior chamber inflammation (Figure 5-18), corneal endothelial cell loss (Figure 5-19), IOP spikes, PIOL detachment (Figure 5-20), and cataract formation (Figure 5-21). Other complications of intraocular surgery, including wound healing issues (more common for nonfoldable poly methyl methacrylate PIOLs), endophthalmitis, and retinal detachment are possible but rare. Small hyphemas from iris manipulation are possible with certain PIOLs. Phakic IOLs may become dislodged spontaneously or from trauma (see Figure 5-20) and require refixation, but this is rare. Persistent inflammation, IOP issues, or endothelial cell loss may require explantation.

Residual ametropia, especially astigmatism, is not uncommon for PIOLs, as toric PIOLs are not currently available in the United States. In many cases, planned bioptics, combining PIOL implantation with corneal refractive surgery, may provide the best unaided acuity. Thus, all PIOL candidates should be screened for corneal surgery before PIOL implantation if bioptics are considered.

Complications of Refractive Lens Exchange

Surgical Complications for Pseudophakic Intraocular Procedures

- Residual ametropia, especially astigmatism
- Visual aberrations
- Regular risks of cataract surgery

General complications for refractive lens exchange (RLE) include all possible complications for cataract surgery, including postoperative inflammation, wound leak, cystoid macular edema (CME), retinal detachment, and choroidal hemorrhage, among others. In addition, RLE is associated with enhanced attention to refractive outcomes; therefore, residual ametropia, especially astigmatism, and any IOL calculation errors are magnified with these procedures. Other specific complications for RLE depend on the IOL style implanted.

For monofocal IOLs, residual astigmatism is possible and may require excimer laser surgery for correction. In all cases where PRK or LASIK is contemplated after cataract extraction, a full topographic and corneal thickness evaluation is necessary before surgery to ensure that the patient is a good candidate for corneal surgery if it is required. If monovision is the surgical goal, patients should understand the rare potential for diplopia to occur postoperatively due to the dissociation of undiagnosed phorias.

For toric IOLs, major concerns are IOL malpositioning at the time of surgery due to the incorrect identification of the appropriate steep meridian, errors during patient marking, or lens rotation. Toric IOLs require in-the-bag placement due to currently available IOL designs for rotational stability; thus, in cases with capsule compromise, toric IOL implantation will not be

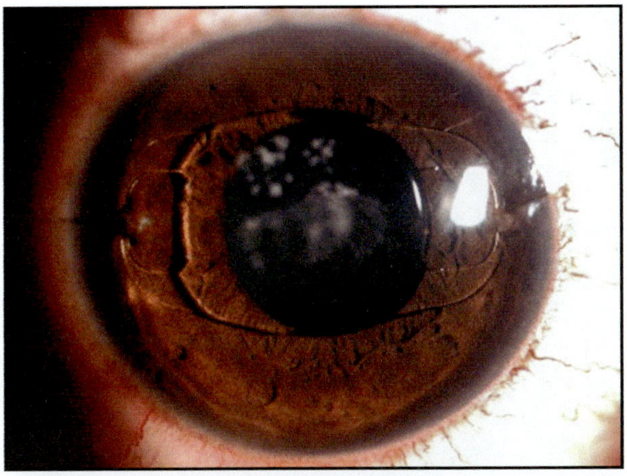

Figure 5-18. Slit-lamp image demonstrating significant inflammatory debris deposited on the surface of the phakic IOL.

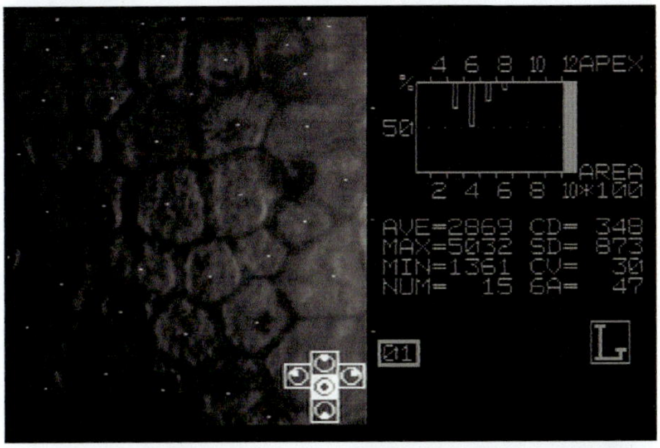

Figure 5-19. Specular microscopic image demonstrating low endothelial cell density (348) with significant cell polymegathism.

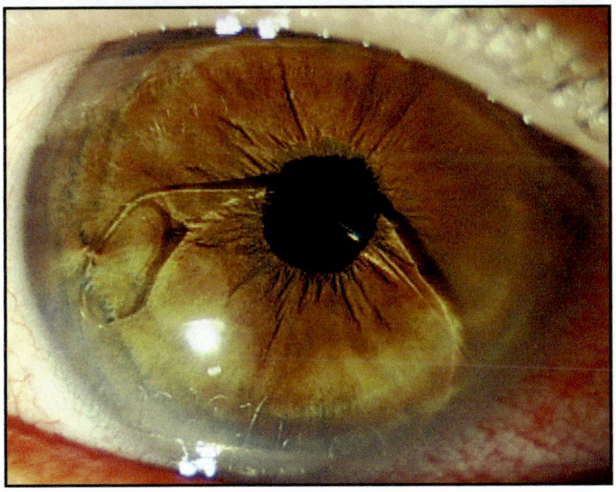

Figure 5-20. Detached iris-claw PIOL. One portion of the PIOL is still fixated to the iris, whereas the other has become dislodged after trauma.

possible. Postoperatively, IOL rotation is uncommon but does occur, and for higher power toric IOLs, this may lead to symptomatic residual astigmatism.

For multifocal IOLs, residual astigmatism of more than 0.50 diopters is unlikely to be well tolerated and may necessitate corneal refractive surgery, with the same caveats mentioned previously. Specifically, patients who undergo multifocal IOL implantation should be screened for laser vision correction options prior to lens implant so that all refractive options are known

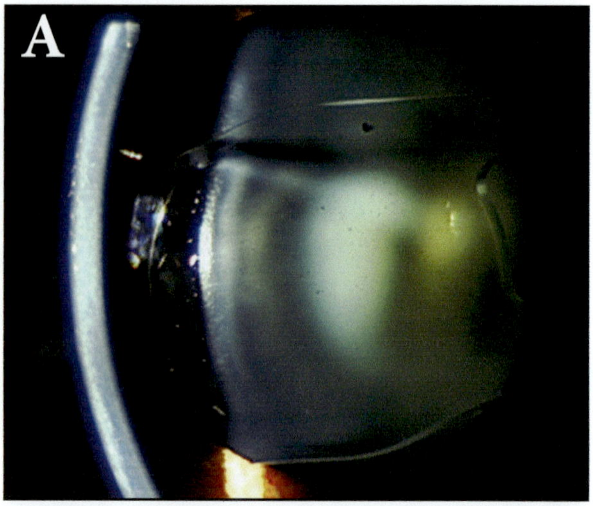

Figure 5-21. (A) Cataract formation following PIOL implantation with iris-fixated PIOL

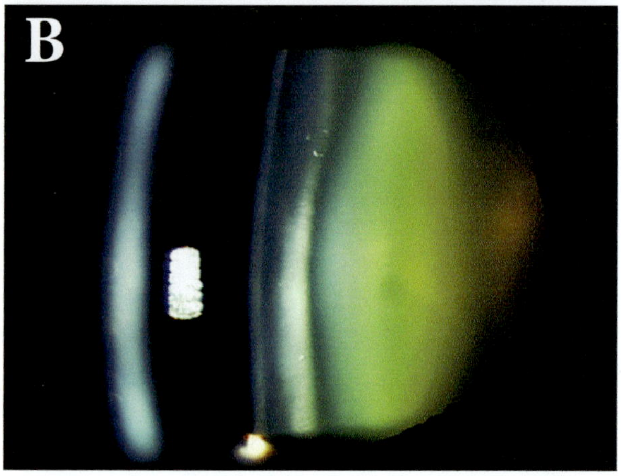

Figure 5-21. (B) Cataract formation following PIOL implantation with sulcus PIOL.

preoperatively. Multifocal IOLs are sensitive to IOL centration and may require intervention, either IOL repositioning or iris manipulation, to improve centration in certain cases. Most multifocal IOLs perform poorly in patients with very small pupils, and this should be determined prior to implantation. These lenses are highly sensitive to any other mild issues that may compromise visual function, including corneal guttae or any maculopathy, and posterior capsule opacification. Many patients report glare, halos, and other related visual aberrations, especially at night. Most of these aberrations are tolerable, but a small proportion of patients does not adapt and feel that their night vision is severely compromised. For all of these reasons, some patients simply do not adapt to multifocal IOLs and require explantation. This is thought to occur in approximately 1% of patients, although the actual number is unknown. Therefore, although posterior capsule opacification is easy to treat, an intact capsule should be maintained until it is certain that the IOL will remain in the eye.

Pseudoaccommodative IOLs vary widely in reported functional outcomes. These lenses have few of the multifocal-specific complications, but they also have less ability to improve unaided near acuity. Current pseudoaccommodative IOLs are dependent on z-axis positioning and may get into improper z-axis orientation, which requires intervention. These IOLs are designed and expected to be implanted in an intact capsule, although reports of sulcus implantation with no apparent short-term complications exist.

Summary and Take Home Points

Refractive surgery enjoys a low complication rate; however, familiarity with the possible mechanisms for complications is critical to appropriately diagnose and manage complications if they occur. The most common postoperative problems after laser vision correction include residual ametropia, dry eye, and visual aberrations, whereas the most serious complications include infectious keratitis, scarring, and LASIK interface disorders from a variety of etiologies. Phakic IOLs have a unique subset of complications, including accelerated endothelial cell loss, PIOL detachment, and cataract formation. Complications after RLE are identical to those after cataract surgery.

Bibliography

Bamba S, Rocha KM, Ramos-Esteban JC, Krueger RR. Incidence of rainbow glare after laser in situ keratomileusis flap creation with a 60-kHz femtosecond laser. *J Cataract Refract Surg.* 2009;35(6):1082-1086.

Bühren J, Martin T, Kühne A, Kohnen T. Correlation of aberrometry, contrast sensitivity, and subjective symptoms with quality of vision after LASIK. *J Refract Surg.* 2009;25(7):559-568.

Chalita MR, Chavala S, Xu M, Krueger RR. Wavefront analysis in post-LASIK eyes and its correlation with visual symptoms, refraction, and topography. *Ophthalmology.* 2004;111(3):447-453.

Chan A, Manche EE. Effect of preoperative pupil size on quality of vision after wavefront-guided LASIK. *Ophthalmology.* 2011;118(4):736-741.

Chayet A, Bains HS. Prospective, randomized, double-blind, contralateral eye comparison of myopic LASIK with optimized aspheric or prolate ablations. *J Refract Surg.* 2012;28(2):112-119.

Chen S, Feng Y, Stojanovic A, Jankov MR II, Wang Q. IntraLase femtosecond laser vs mechanical microkeratomes in LASIK for myopia: a systematic review and meta-analysis. *J Refract Surg.* 2012;28(1):15-24.

Donnenfeld ED, Kim T, Holland EJ, et al; American Society of Cataract and Refractive Surgery Cornea Clinical Committee. ASCRS white paper: management of infectious keratitis following laser in situ keratomileusis. *J Cataract Refract Surg.* 2005;31(10):2008-2011.

Edwards JD, Burka JM, Bower KS, Stutzman RD, Sediq DA, Rabin JC. Effect of brimonidine tartrate 0.15% on night-vision difficulty and contrast testing after refractive surgery. *J Cataract Refract Surg.* 2008;34(9):1538-1541.

Golas L, Manche EE. Dry eye after laser in situ keratomileusis with femtosecond laser and mechanical keratome. *J Cataract Refract Surg.* 2011;37(8):1476-1480.

Goldsberry DH, Epstein RJ, Majmudar PA, et al. Effect of mitomycin C on the corneal endothelium when used for corneal subepithelial haze prophylaxis following photorefractive keratectomy. *J Refract Surg.* 2007;23(7):724-727.

Hessert D, Tanzer D, Brunstetter T, Kaupp S, Murdoch D, Mirzaoff M. Topical cyclosporine A for postoperative photorefractive keratectomy and laser in situ keratomileusis. *J Cataract Refract Surg.* 2013;39(4):539-547.

Jabbur NS, Sakatani K, O'Brien TP. Survey of complications and recommendations for management in dissatisfied patients seeking a consultation after refractive surgery. *J Cataract Refract Surg.* 2004;30(9):1867-1874.

Jalali S, Yuen LH, Boxer Wachler BS. Effect of nepafenac sodium 0.1% on delayed corneal epithelial healing and haze after photorefractive keratectomy: retrospective comparative study. *J Cataract Refract Surg.* 2008;34(9):1542-1545.

Lee JH, You YS, Choe CM, Lee ES. Efficacy of brimonidine tartrate 0.2% ophthalmic solution in reducing halos after laser in situ keratomileusis. *J Cataract Refract Surg.* 2008;34(6):963-967.

Levinson BA, Rapuano CJ, Cohen EJ, Hammersmith KM, Ayres BD, Laibson PR. Referrals to the Wills Eye Institute Cornea Service after laser in situ keratomileusis: reasons for patient dissatisfaction. *J Cataract Refract Surg.* 2008;34(1):32-39.

Mian SI, Li AY, Dutta S, Musch DC, Shtein RM. Dry eyes and corneal sensation after laser in situ keratomileusis with femtosecond laser flap creation Effect of hinge position, hinge angle, and flap thickness. *J Cataract Refract Surg.* 2009;35(12):2092-2098.

Mian SI, Shtein RM, Nelson A, Musch DC. Effect of hinge position on corneal sensation and dry eye after laser in situ keratomileusis using a femtosecond laser. *J Cataract Refract Surg.* 2007;33(7):1190-1194.

Moshirfar M, Welling JD, Feiz V, Holz H, Clinch TE. Infectious and noninfectious keratitis after laser in situ keratomileusis: occurrence, management, and visual outcomes. *J Cataract Refract Surg.* 2007;33(3):474-483.

Netto MV, Mohan RR, Medeiros FW, et al. Femtosecond laser and microkeratome corneal flaps: comparison of stromal wound healing and inflammation. *J Refract Surg.* 2007;23(7):667-676.

Nettune GR, Pflugfelder SC. Post-LASIK tear dysfunction and dysesthesia. Ocul Surf. 2010;8(3):135-145.

Parkhurst GD, Psolka M, Kezirian GM. Phakic intraocular lens implantation in United States military warfighters: a retrospective analysis of early clinical outcomes of the Visian ICL. *J Refract Surg.* 2011;27(7):473-481.

Perez-Straziota CE, Randleman JB, Stulting RD. Visual Outcomes with wavefront-guided and wavefront-optimized LASIK. *J Cataract and Refract Surg.* 2010; 36(3):437-441.

Randleman JB. Etiology and clinical presentations of irregular astigmatism after keratorefractive surgery. In: Wang M, ed. *Irregular Astigmatism: Diagnosis and Treatment.* Thorofare, NJ: SLACK Incorporated; 2007:79-90.

Randleman JB. Corneal ectasia: prevention and detection. In Krachmer JH, Mannis MJ, Holland ED, eds. *Cornea. 3rd ed.* London, United Kingdom; Elsevier Ltd; 2010:1883-1888.

Randleman JB, Lynn MJ, Banning CS, Stulting RD. Risk factors for epithelial defect formation during laser in situ keratomileusis. *J Cataract Refract Surg.* 2007;33(10):1738-1743.

Randleman JB, Shah RD. LASIK interface complications: etiology, management, and outcomes. *J Refract Surg.* 2012;28(8):575-588.

Randleman JB, White AJ Jr, Lynn MJ, Hu MH, Stulting RD Incidence, outcomes, and risk factors for enhancement after wavefront-optimized advanced surface ablation and laser in situ keratomileusis. *J Refract Surg.* 2009;25(3):273-276.

Salomão MQ, Ambrósio R Jr, Wilson SE. Dry eye associated with laser in situ keratomileusis: Mechanical microkeratome versus femtosecond laser. *J Cataract Refract Surg.* 2009;35(10):1756-1760.

Schallhorn SC, Amesbury EC, Tanzer DJ. Avoidance, recognition, and management of LASIK complications. *Am J Ophthalmol.* 2006;141(4):733-739.

Schallhorn SC, Kaupp SE, Tanzer DJ, Tidwell J, Laurent J, Bourque LB. Pupil size and quality of vision after LASIK. *Ophthalmology.* 2003;110(8):1606-1614.

Schallhorn SC, Tanzer DJ, Kaupp SE, Brown M, Malady SE. Comparison of night driving performance after wavefront-guided and conventional LASIK for moderate myopia. *Ophthalmology.* 2009;116(4):702-709.

Srinivasan S, Rootman DS. Anterior chamber gas bubble formation during femtosecond laser flap creation for LASIK. *J Refract Surg.* 2007;23(8):828-830.

Sugar A, Rapuano CJ, Culbertson WW, et al. Laser in situ keratomileusis for myopia and astigmatism: safety and efficacy: a report by the American Academy of Ophthalmology. *Ophthalmology.* 2002;109(1):175-187.

Tan J, Simon D, Mrochen M, Por YM. Clinical results of topography-based customized ablations for myopia and myopic astigmatism. *J Refract Surg.* 2012;28(11 Suppl):S829-S836.

Varley GA, Huang D, Rapuano CJ, Schallhorn S, Boxer Wachler BS, Sugar A; Ophthalmic Technology Assessment Committee Refractive Surgery Panel, American Academy of Ophthalmology. LASIK for hyperopia, hyperopic astigmatism, and mixed astigmatism: a report by the American Academy of Ophthalmology. *Ophthalmology.* 2004;111(8):1604-1617.

Watanabe K, Negishi K, Kawai M, Torii H, Kaido M, Tsubota K. Effect of experimentally induced astigmatism on functional, conventional, and low-contrast visual acuity. *J Refract Surg.* 2013;29(1):19-24.

Watson SL, Bunce C, Allan BD. Improved safety in contemporary LASIK. *Ophthalmology.* 2005;112(8):1375-1380.

Woodward MA, Randleman JB, Stulting RD. Reasons for patient dissatisfaction in eyes after phacoemulsification with multifocal intraocular lens implantation. *J Cataract Refract Surg.* 2009;35(6):992-997.

Zhang ZH, Jin HY, Suo Y, et al. Femtosecond laser versus mechanical microkeratome laser in situ keratomileusis for myopia: Metaanalysis of randomized controlled trials. *J Cataract Refract Surg.* 2011;37(12):2151-2159.

6

Refractive Surgery
The Decision-Making Process

Chapter Highlights

- Surgical decisions based on preoperative refractive error
- Surgical decisions based on minimizing complications for specific indications
- Relative comparison of refractive surgical procedures
- Refractive surgery decision tree analysis

Surgical decision making is too complex and multifactorial in nature to put into a simple table or flow diagram. Beyond the numerous issues discussed in the chapters on procedure overview, biomechanical considerations, and surgical complications, one must always keep the patient's choice and his or her desires at the forefront of every surgical decision.

For many patients, more than one surgical option exists, and the same visual outcomes may be achieved through different procedures for many of them. For other patients, no surgery is recommended, even when considering the diversity of surgical options available. For some patients, one particular procedure will have the most advantageous risk/benefit profile and will most likely generate the best outcome.

Some general guidelines can be followed to help navigate the surgical decision process. This process has been categorized based first on refractive error, followed by procedure choice based on minimizing risk of complications. These are guidelines only, not dictums to follow absolutely, and these guidelines are subject to interpretation. They inevitably represent my subjective experience and interpretation of the available data; thus, other surgeons may structure this list differently.

Surgical Decisions Based on Preoperative Refractive Error

Indications and "best" treatment ranges for different procedures vary significantly. Treatment ranges are based on spherical error only (myopia and hyperopia), as there does not appear to be significant differences in outcomes for regular astigmatic correction among currently available

Randleman JB.
Refractive Surgery: An Interactive Case-Based Approach (pp. 69-75).

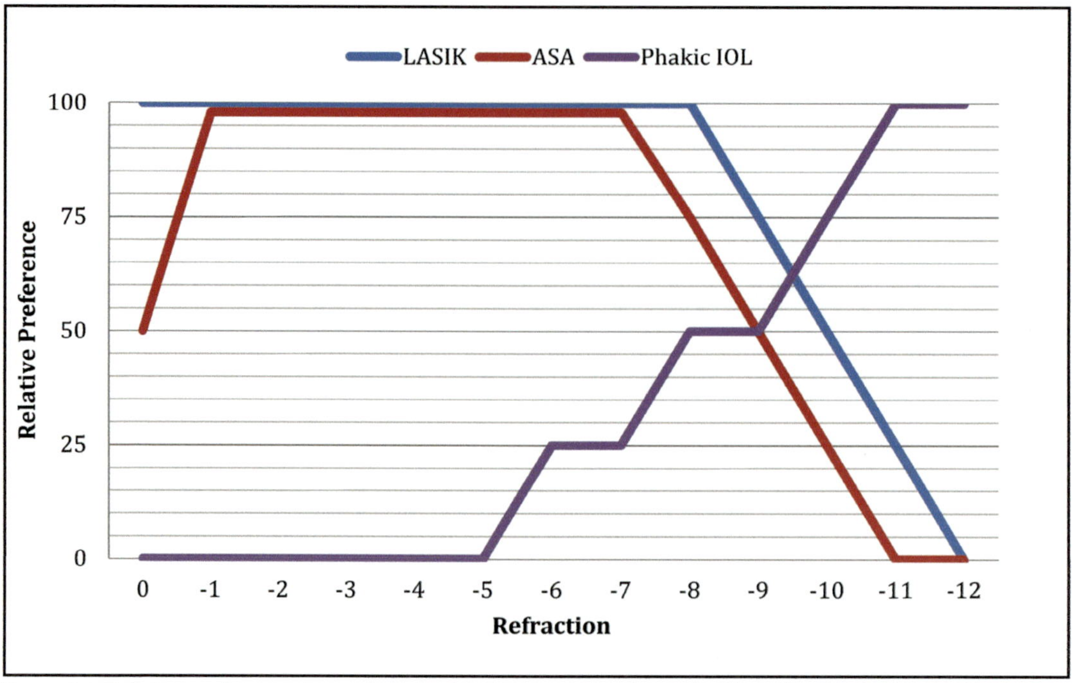

Figure 6-1. Relative preference for each procedure by amount of myopia. Note that for the interval between -1D and -7D ASA and LASIK overlap. At higher errors, advanced surface ablation (ASA) falls off in preference more rapidly due to decreased predictability and increased chance for corneal haze. All preferences assume otherwise normal exams, including biomechanical analysis and residual stromal bed thickness.

excimer laser procedures, and toric phakic intraocular lenses (PIOLs) are not currently available within the United States.

Figure 6-1 represents my relative preferences for the treatment of myopia based solely on the level of myopia. Note the direct overlap between LASIK and surface ablation from approximately -1.00 to -7.00 diopters (D), as both procedures appear equally efficacious within this treatment range. Significant fluctuations in choice of procedure occurs for myopia between -8.00 and -12.00 D, and this is one of the more controversial areas of refractive surgery, with multiple procedures available but no procedure clearly superior for the average patient. Most excimer laser platforms are approved for much higher treatments than demonstrated in Figure 6-1. For many surgeons, the range of "appropriate" treatment has narrowed over the years; however, treating up to the approved treatment ranges is still acceptable practice for certain patients. The FDA approval of new technology, especially additional PIOL models and toric PIOLs, could significantly influence surgical planning in the United States, especially for moderate myopia.

Figure 6-2 represents my relative preferences for the treatment of hyperopia based solely on the level of hyperopia. Again, note the direct overlap between LASIK and surface ablation from approximately +1.00 to +4.00 D, as both procedures appear equally efficacious within this treatment range. Controversy exists regarding the most appropriate treatment for hyperopic patients, especially those above +4.00 D, and age frequently plays a significant role in the decision process. Phakic IOLs are not currently approved for the correction of hyperopia in the United States; however, refractive lens technology continues to advance, so this remains a dynamic area of surgical decision making that is likely to change rapidly as technological advances become available.

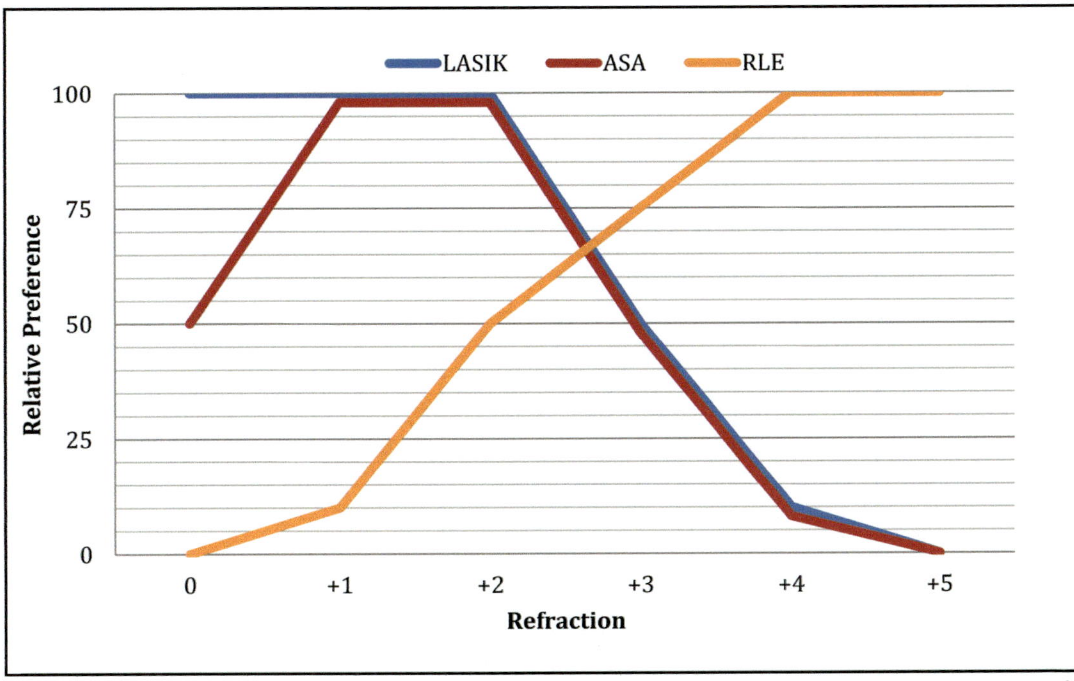

Figure 6-2. Relative preference for each procedure by amount of hyperopia. All preferences assume otherwise normal exams, including biomechanical analysis and residual stromal bed thickness, and a clear crystalline lens

Surgical Decisions Based on Minimizing Complications

When the available treatments have been determined based on refractive error, specific patient-related issues should be considered. The most critical areas were highlighted in the preceding chapters; thus Tables 6-1 and 6-2 outline procedures based on these issues.

Ectasia-susceptible patients are not good LASIK candidates; however, their eligibility for surface ablation remains hotly debated. Although most patients have similar infection risk profiles, those in the health care field or other related fields may be more susceptible to infection; thus, surface ablation for these individuals may not be desirable or, at minimum, caution should be taken in the early postoperative period if surface ablation is performed. Extremely large pupil size is a topic that must be discussed with potential PIOL patients because these individuals may have a dilated pupil size that exceeds the IOL optic. However, the patient may still opt for treatment of their myopia, but he or she should understand the increased incidence of glare and halos he or she may encounter.

Older age, specifically patients with early nuclear sclerotic lens changes, is an issue influencing the surgical decision making process for most patients aged >60 years and some patients aged >50 years; however, some older patients are candidates for corneal procedures.

Table 6-1. Screening Algorithm for Refractive Surgery				
PROCEDURE	LASIK	PHOTOREFRACTIVE KERATECTOMY	PHAKIC INTRAOCULAR LENS IMPLANTATION	REFRACTIVE LENS EXCHANGE
Does patient have a treatable refraction?	+3.00 to -12.00 D, ≤+6.00 D astigmatism	+3.00 to -8.00 D, ≤+6.00 D astigmatism	-5.00 to -20.00 D, ≤2.00 D astigmatism	Any spherical error, up to +4.00 D corneal astigmatism[a]
Does patient correct to 20/20?	Usually	Usually	Variable**	Variable
If acuity is not 20/20, is there an identifiable reason?	Yes	Yes	Yes	Yes
Is corneal thickness adequate for laser vision correction?	>480 µm, residual stromal bed thickness >250 µm	>450 µm, residual stromal bed thickness >250 µm	Any	Any
Any abnormal physical examination findings?	No	No	No	Cataract only
Topographic evaluation	Normal	Normal to mild suspect	Normal-suspicious, stable topography	Normal-suspicious, stable topography

[a] Depending on IOL style being used.

**Some high myopes do not correct to 20/20 unrelated to pathology that would contraindicate surgery.

Putting it All Together: Surgical Decision-Tree Analysis

Figures 6-3 and 6-4 combine refractive error and patient-specific details into decision-tree analyses for myopia and hyperopia, respectively. Although patient desire will ultimately drive this decision, these figures provide a framework for the decision analysis.

Table 6-2. Most Common Refractive Surgical Procedures and Their Relative Strengths and Weaknesses

PROCEDURE	BETTER FOR	WORSE FOR
LASIK	Primary myopia and low hyperopia treatment Infection risk Surface healing issues	Ectasia susceptible Thinner corneas Flap trauma Epithelial abnormalities (epithelial basement membrane dystrophy)
Surface ablation	Primary myopia and low hyperopia treatment Epithelial basement membrane dystrophy Thinner corneas Flap trauma risk Ectasia susceptible	Haze and scarring risk Infection risk
Phakic intraocular lens	High myopia Ectasia susceptible Severe dry eye/surface issues	Endothelial dysfunction Large pupils Early lens changes
Refractive lens exchange	Higher hyperopia Early lens changes Presbyopia correction	Retinal detachment risk Precise visual outcomes

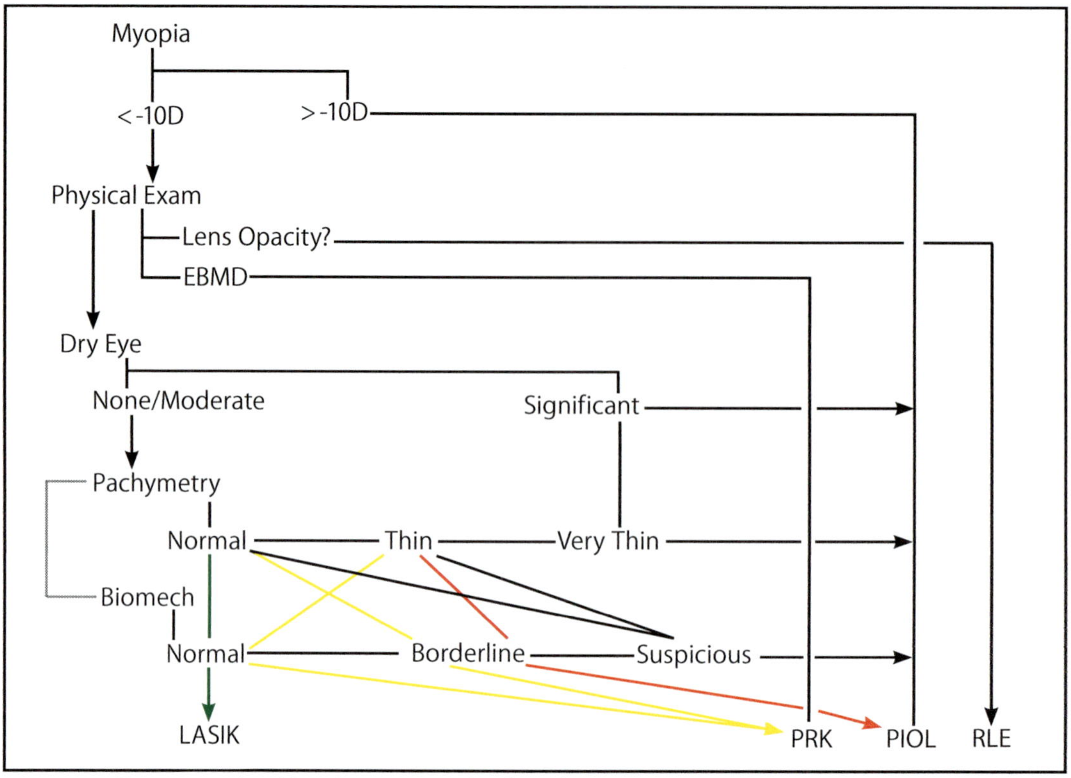

Figure 6-3. Treatment algorithm for myopia. The flow diagram incorporates the elements that influence surgical technique choice, including refractive error, physical exam findings, corneal thickness, and corneal biomechanics. For pachymetry, "Normal" = approximately 500 microns or more, "Thin" = approximately 480 microns, "Very Thin = approximately 450 microns or less. In general, the color-coded lines signify "Green = Go", "Yellow = Caution", and "Red = Danger" in the decision-making process. Black lines indicate firm recommendations.

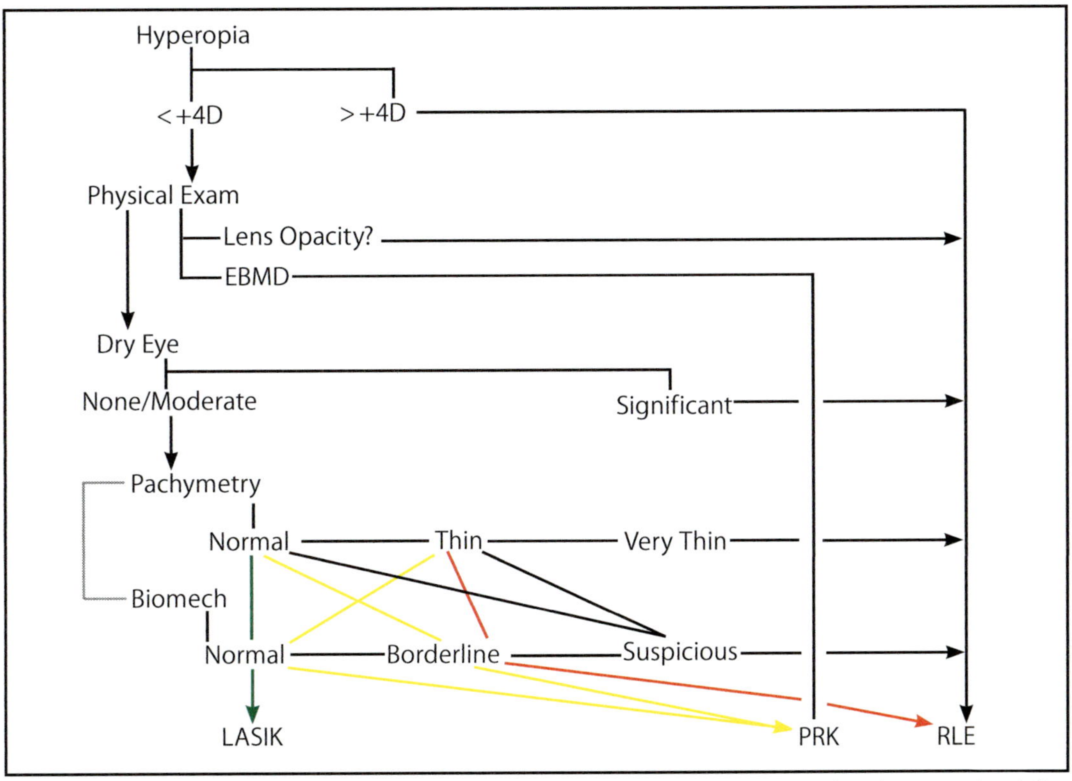

Figure 6-4. Treatment algorithm for hyperopia. The flow diagram incorporates the elements that influence surgical technique choice, including refractive error, physical exam findings, corneal thickness, and corneal biomechanics. For pachymetry, "Normal" = approximately 500 microns or more, "Thin" = approximately 480 microns, "Very Thin = approximately 450 microns or less. In general, the color-coded lines signify "Green = Go", "Yellow = Caution", and "Red = Danger" in the decision-making process. Black lines indicate firm recommendations.

Bibliography

Farjo AA, Sugar A, Schallhorn SC, et al. Femtosecond lasers for LASIK flap creation: a report by the American Academy of Ophthalmology. *Ophthalmology.* 2013;120(3):e5-e20.

Huang D, Schallhorn SC, Sugar A, et al. Phakic intraocular lens implantation for the correction of myopia: a report by the American Academy of Ophthalmology. *Ophthalmology.* 2009;116(11):2244-2258.

Nanavaty MA, Daya SM. Refractive lens exchange versus phakic intraocular lenses. *Curr Opin Ophthalmol.* 2012;23(1):54-61.

Schallhorn SC, Farjo AA, Huang D, et al; American Academy of Ophthalmology. Wavefront-guided LASIK for the correction of primary myopia and astigmatism a report by the American Academy of Ophthalmology. *Ophthalmology.* 2008;115(7):1249-1261.

Sugar A, Rapuano CJ, Culbertson WW, et al. Laser in situ keratomileusis for myopia and astigmatism: safety and efficacy: a report by the American Academy of Ophthalmology. *Ophthalmology.* 2002;109(1):175-187.

Varley GA, Huang D, Rapuano CJ, et al; Ophthalmic Technology Assessment Committee Refractive Surgery Panel, American Academy of Ophthalmology. LASIK for hyperopia, hyperopic astigmatism, and mixed astigmatism: a report by the American Academy of Ophthalmology. *Ophthalmology.* 2004;111(8):1604-1617.

Please visit www.routledge.com/ 9781617110368 to access additional material.

Section II
Case Studies in Refractive Surgery

Introduction (or Things You Need to Know Before Tackling These Cases!)

Now, armed with core information from the previous chapters that form the basis of patient evaluation and surgical decision making, the following cases are designed to challenge your diagnostic skills and fundamental understanding of refractive surgical procedures. Each case provides all, or most, of the information needed to counsel patients appropriately and to make sound surgical decisions. Each case is accompanied by a list of questions that are designed to shape your thinking about the specific case, which will be presented in a real-world way to facilitate your thought process but will not lead you directly to the answers. As in real life, patient evaluations do not come with a how-to guide; therefore, you must identify the most important information for each case and make your decisions for treatment accordingly.

Each case has an accompanying explanation of the concepts presented therein, along with a bibliography to guide you toward additional relevant materials. Although the cases that follow can be approached in a variety of ways, it is hoped that you will fully digest the material presented and fully answer each question before moving onto the case discussion, as this process will likely yield the best learning experience.

Notes About the Examination

For each case, assume that any information not included in the presentation is normal or noncontributory, unless the questions specifically ask what additional information you would need to evaluate the case at hand. Slit-lamp and fundus examinations should be considered unremarkable unless specific details or images are provided. Consider cycloplegic and manifest refractions to be equivalent for normal, non-diagnostic situations. All patients have had a sufficient time interval from contact lens wear for their refraction to be stable unless otherwise noted. Estimated flap thickness = 110 μm for all LASIK cases. All cases will be provided with estimated ablation depths related to the refractive error from which estimated residual stromal bed thickness can be calculated by using the thin flap thickness estimations described previously.

Topographic and Biomechanical Analysis

Most cases will include accompanying topographies, and some will have additional testing available. In clinical practice, all patients will have topography that is available at the time of evaluation, and interpretation of these diagnostic images, specifically when they are and are not particularly relevant to the patient at hand, is one of the most challenging aspects of modern refractive surgical evaluations. It will be up to you to decide if the important case information lies in the topographic images and when they are essentially normal and/or noncontributory to your evaluation.

The scans presented have not been digitally altered; however, some cases represent composite imaging for teaching purposes, rather than actual scans from individual patients. Therefore, slight discrepancies in data, such as keratometry values or corneal thickness measures may be present between the case values and imaging devices. These differences are not meant to trick or confuse you; values should be interpreted as equivalent unless otherwise specified.

Questions

Many of the questions are worded in a similar manner, and this is for two reasons. First, the goal of the questions is to make you think about the case without unduly biasing you in a specific direction or leading you to the answer. Patients do not present with the answers and neither will these cases! Second, there are a finite number of questions that are relevant before and after refractive surgery to assist you in best evaluating and treating patients; therefore, the same questions are logically posed for a variety of unique presentations.

A Word About the Bibliographies

The structure of this book is quite different from most other books, and that difference continues into the bibliography sections at the end of each case. Instead of being a list of citations, the bibliographies are intended to help guide individual searches for more information. All bibliographies list books and articles alphabetically by the first author's surname. These lists are not exhaustive; rather, they are intended to support the concepts presented and serve as a starting point for further individual review. Effort has been made to minimize duplications; however, some citations are essential reading for a variety of different topics and are thus duplicated.

Online Companion Video Cases

In addition to the cases contained herein, there are nine video-based cases contained online at the accompanying website: www.routledge.com/9781617110368

These cases include surgical videos to guide you through the cases analysis process. Detailed explanation is available at the website.

Disclaimer About the Cases

Innumerable clinical presentations before and after refractive surgery exist; thus, the cases that follow are, by definition, an incomplete coverage of the field. Straightforward cases have been omitted. This omission includes both the 30-year-old low myope with a normal examination and the patient who develops moderate dry eye symptoms after LASIK because, although significant, their management is not complicated or controversial. Although not every case that follows is complicated or controversial, many are. Finally, the opinions expressed are also those of only this author.

PART 1
Preoperative Evaluations

—CASE 1—

A 36-year-old male desires refractive surgical correction. He has no significant family, past medical, or ocular history.

CASE HISTORY		
	Right Eye	**Left Eye**
Present correction method	CTL	CTL
Manifest refraction	-7.00 +1.25 x 095	-6.75 +1.25 x 100
CDVA (current)	20/20	20/20
UNVA (current)	20/20	20/20
Dominant eye	Right	
Ocular alignment	Orthophoric	Orthophoric
Keratometry		
Flat K	43.75 @ 180	43.75 @ 180
Steep K	44.25 @ 90	44.50 @ 90
Pupil size (bright)	4.7 mm	4.0 mm
Pupil size (dim)	6.6 mm	6.7 mm
Central corneal thickness	535 µm	530 µm
Physical examination	Normal	Normal
Estimated ablation depth	105 µm	100 µm

QUESTIONS

1. Is this patient a candidate for refractive surgery? If so, what treatment options are available?
2. Considering all factors, what procedure would you recommend and why?
3. What are the most likely patient complaints in the early postoperative period for each potential treatment option?
4. What are the most significant potential complications for each procedure for this patient?
5. What special considerations are there for this patient regarding potential retreatment for postoperative ametropia?

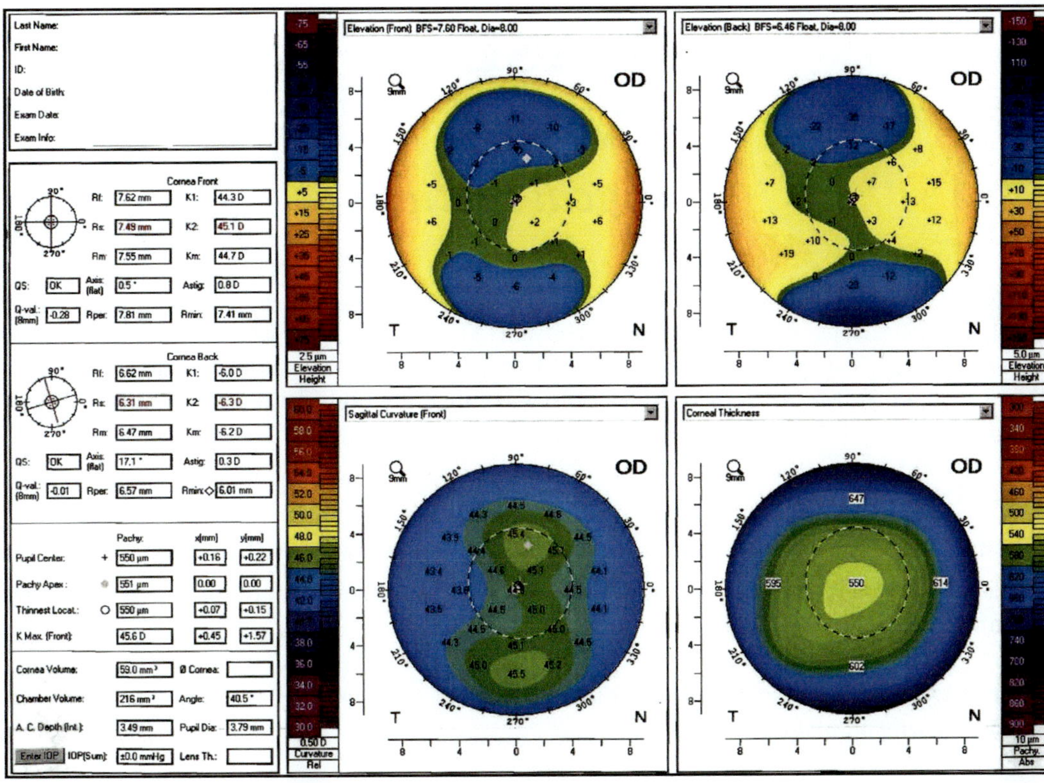
Last Name:
First Name:
ID:
Date of Birth:
Exam Date:
Exam Info:
Cornea Front
Rf: 7.62 mm K1: 44.3 D
Rs: 7.49 mm K2: 45.1 D
Rm: 7.55 mm Km: 44.7 D
QS: OK Axis (flat) 0.5° Astig: 0.8 D
Q-val. (8mm) -0.28 Rper: 7.81 mm Rmin: 7.41 mm
Cornea Back
Rf: 6.62 mm K1: -6.0 D
Rs: 6.31 mm K2: -6.3 D
Rm: 6.47 mm Km: -6.2 D
QS: OK Axis (flat) 17.1° Astig: 0.3 D
Q-val. (8mm) -0.01 Rper: 6.57 mm Rmin: 6.01 mm
Pachy: x[mm] y[mm]
Pupil Center: + 550 µm +0.16 +0.22
Pachy Apex: 551 µm 0.00 0.00
Thinnest Locat.: O 550 µm +0.07 +0.15
K Max. (Front): 45.6 D +0.45 +1.57
Cornea Volume: 59.0 mm³ Ø Cornea:
Chamber Volume: 216 mm³ Angle: 40.5°
A. C. Depth (Int.): 3.49 mm Pupil Dia: 3.79 mm
Enter IOP IOP(Sum): ±0.0 mmHg Lens Th.:
Elevation (Front) BFS=7.60 Float, Dia=8.00
OD
2.5 µm Elevation Height
Elevation (Back) BFS=6.46 Float, Dia=8.00
OD
5.0 µm Elevation Height
Sagittal Curvature (Front)
OD
0.50 D Curvature Rel
Corneal Thickness
OD
647
595
550
614
602
10 µm Pachy. Abs
T
N

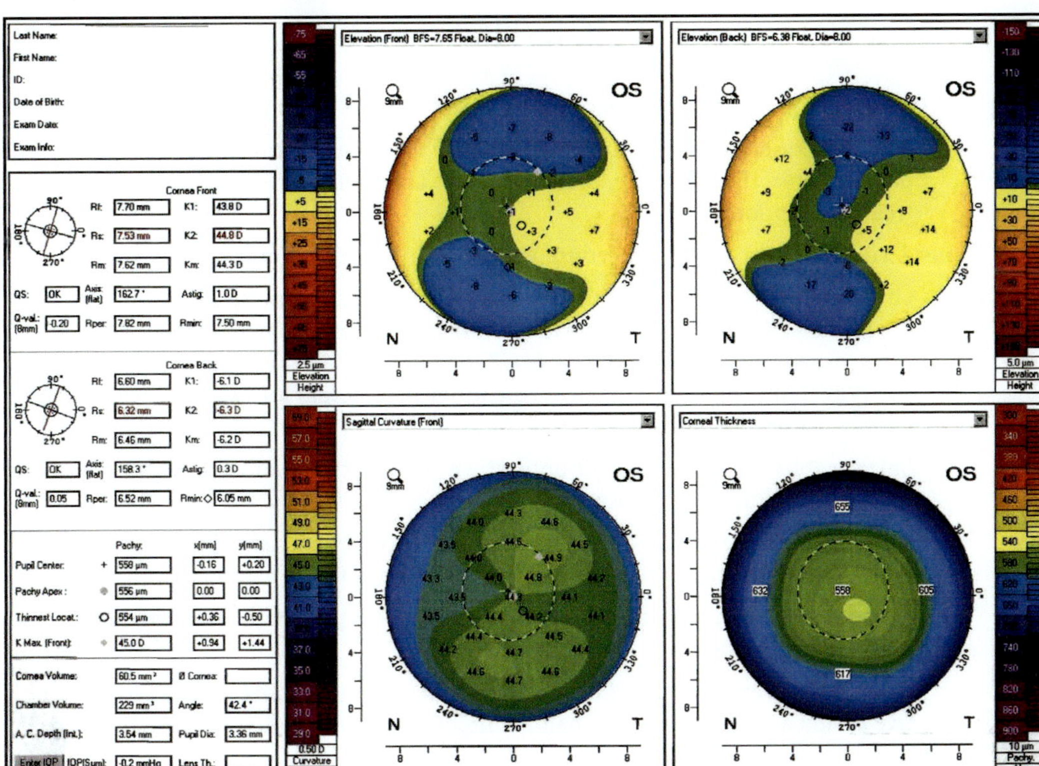
Last Name:
First Name:
ID:
Date of Birth:
Exam Date:
Exam Info:
Cornea Front
Rf: 7.70 mm K1: 43.8 D
Rs: 7.53 mm K2: 44.8 D
Rm: 7.62 mm Km: 44.3 D
QS: OK Axis (flat) 162.7° Astig: 1.0 D
Q-val. (8mm) -0.20 Rper: 7.82 mm Rmin: 7.50 mm
Cornea Back
Rf: 6.60 mm K1: -6.1 D
Rs: 6.32 mm K2: -6.3 D
Rm: 6.46 mm Km: -6.2 D
QS: OK Axis (flat) 158.3° Astig: 0.3 D
Q-val. (8mm) 0.05 Rper: 6.52 mm Rmin: 6.05 mm
Pachy: x[mm] y[mm]
Pupil Center: + 558 µm -0.16 +0.20
Pachy Apex: 556 µm 0.00 0.00
Thinnest Locat.: O 554 µm +0.36 -0.50
K Max. (Front): 45.0 D +0.94 +1.44
Cornea Volume: 60.5 mm³ Ø Cornea:
Chamber Volume: 229 mm³ Angle: 42.4°
A. C. Depth (Int.): 3.54 mm Pupil Dia: 3.36 mm
Enter IOP IOP(Sum): -0.2 mmHg Lens Th.:
Elevation (Front) BFS=7.65 Float, Dia=8.00
OS
2.5 µm Elevation Height
Elevation (Back) BFS=6.38 Float, Dia=8.00
OS
5.0 µm Elevation Height
Sagittal Curvature (Front)
OS
0.50 D Curvature Rel
Corneal Thickness
OS
655
632
558
605
617
10 µm Pachy. Abs
N
T

—Case 1—
Myopia
Surgical Options

Myopia is the most common indication for refractive surgery. Primary treatment options include LASIK, surface ablation, and phakic intraocular lens (PIOL) implantation for higher myopia. The best surgical option depends on the patient's screening evaluation and degree of myopia. Higher myopia requires increased diligence in screening and consideration of multiple surgical options.

Case Analysis

- Estimated residual stromal bed (RSB) thickness is approximately 310 to 320 μm in both eyes.
- Case Figures show normal topographies with symmetric bowtie patterns and good corneal thickness.

Pearl: *Myopia is the most common refractive error presenting for surgery. Become familiar and comfortable with all treatment options!*

Questions

1. Is this patient a candidate for refractive surgery? If so, what treatment options are available?

   Yes, this patient appears to be a reasonable candidate for refractive surgery. In the patient's prescription range, LASIK, surface ablation, and PIOL implantation are all treatment options.

2. Considering all factors, what procedure would you recommend and why?

   Given a normal topography and an otherwise normal examination, thin-flap LASIK is a reasonable option. For this patient, estimated RSB is approximately 310 to 330 μm [RSB = central corneal thickness (CCT; 535 μm) – flap thickness (100 to 120 μm) – ablation (100 to 105 μm)]. None of the other risk factors for ectasia, including topographic pattern, age, or CCT are of concern.

   Surface ablation is a treatment option: An increased risk of haze with high myopia treatment should be considered.

   Phakic IOL is a reasonable treatment option: Intraocular risks should be considered, and PIOL implantation will not fully address the patient's astigmatism.

3. What are the most likely patient complaints in the early postoperative period for each potential treatment option?

   Most patients experience mild to moderate dry eye symptoms in the early postoperative period as well as glare and halos at night. These phenomena are usually transient.

4. What are the most significant potential complications for each procedure for this patient?

   Although serious complications are unlikely, the greatest concerns are postoperative ectasia after LASIK, corneal haze after surface ablation, and endothelial cell loss and early cataract formation after PIOL implantation.

5. What special considerations are there for this patient regarding potential retreatment for postoperative ametropia?

   Due to the amount of tissue being removed, if this patient undergoes LASIK and subsequently needs retreatment, surface ablation may be a better retreatment option. If the patient initially has surface ablation, then repeat surface ablation would be the best retreatment option. If the patient has PIOL implantation, then either LASIK or surface ablation may be a reasonable retreatment option.

Refractive Surgery for Myopia

LASIK and surface ablation are both FDA approved for up to -14.00 diopters (D) of myopic treatment for most laser platforms, although most surgeons have a lower practical cutoff for both procedures. Phakic IOLs are approved for use from -3.00 D to more than -20.00 D depending on IOL style. For more information on approval ranges, see Chapter 1. The currently available PIOL options in the United States include the Visian Implantable Collamer Lens (STAAR Surgical Co), which is implanted in the ciliary sulcus, and the Artisan IOL (Ophtec BV) or the Verisyse PIOL (Abbott Medical Optics Inc), both of which are fixated to the iris and called iris-claw IOLs.

Figure 6-1 demonstrates the author's procedure preference for treating myopia when all other factors are equivalent. Note that all 3 procedures are viable options in this patient's treatment range. The relative risks and benefits for each procedure are discussed in the remaining sections of this case.

LASIK

LASIK has excellent predictability and rapid healing in this prescription range. With high myopia, postoperative biomechanical issues are the most concerning potential problem; therefore, confirmation of adequate RSB thickness through intraoperative pachymetric measurement is critical. Many modern microkeratomes and femtosecond lasers have the ability to create thin, reproducible flaps between 100 to 110 μm ±10 μm. At higher degrees of treatment, postoperative glare and halos are more common than in lower myopic treatments.

Surface Ablation

Surface ablation is also an excellent option for myopia up to -10.00 D; however, there may be a reduction in accuracy for myopia above -8.00 D, and there is an increased risk for visually significant haze. The use of mitomycin C for prophylaxis mitigates this risk. Routine concerns, including delayed healing, postoperative discomfort, and infection are similar, regardless of the level of myopia being treated. At higher degrees of myopia treatment, postoperative glare and halos are more common than for lower myopic treatments.

Phakic Intraocular Lens

Phakic IOLs provide excellent visual acuity in high myopia patients. In many studies, patients preferred the visual acuity achieved from a PIOL than that achieved with LASIK for high myopia. However, PIOLs carry increased risk of more significant complications, including endothelial cell loss; early cataract formation, which is more problematic for patients with high myopia; and intraocular infection, although infection is exceptionally rare. Patients considering PIOL implantation must have an endothelial cell count performed with either specular or confocal microscopy, as there are specific minimum values listed for each PIOL, stratified by patient age.

Retreatment Options and Bioptics

Patients with high myopia may have an increased likelihood of residual ametropia necessitating retreatment, although recent studies have found minimal differences between low and moderate to high myopes.

If retreatment is desired after surface ablation, repeat surface ablation is most reasonable. If primary LASIK is performed, either LASIK or surface ablation may be an option; however, if there is question about adequate RSB thickness, then surface ablation performed on the flap is the best option. Although this appears slightly less accurate than primary surface ablation, there is theoretically no biomechanical effect, as the flap is already functionally decoupled from the underlying stroma.

In retreatment or planned initial surgery, combining PIOL implantation with either LASIK or surface ablation, termed *bioptics*, may provide the best accuracy and visual acuity, although the patient is undertaking risks from both procedures when choosing this option.

Bibliography

Chen SH, Feng YF, Stojanovic A, Wang QM. Meta-analysis of clinical outcomes comparing surface ablation for correction of myopia with and without 0.02% mitomycin C. *J Refract Surg.* 2011;27(7):530-541.

Huang D, Schallhorn SC, Sugar A, et al. Phakic intraocular lens implantation for the correction of myopia: a report by the American Academy of Ophthalmology. *Ophthalmology.* 2009;116(11):2244-2258.

Malecaze FJ, Hulin H, Bierer P, et al. A randomized paired eye comparison of two techniques for treating moderately high myopia: LASIK and Artisan phakic lens. *Ophthalmology.* 2002;109(9):1622-1630.

Parkhurst GD, Psolka M, Kezirian GM. Phakic intraocular lens implantation in United States military warfighters: a retrospective analysis of early clinical outcomes of the Visian ICL. *J Refract Surg.* 2011;27(7):473-481.

Randleman JB, Loft ES, Banning CS, Lynn MJ, Stulting RD. Outcomes of wavefront-optimized surface ablation. *Ophthalmology.* 2007;114(5):983-988.

Randleman JB, White AJ, Hu MH, Stulting RD. Incidence, outcomes, and risk factors for enhancement after wavefront-optimized advanced surface ablation and laser in situ keratomileusis. *J Refract Surg.* 2009;25(3):273-276.

Randleman JB, Woodward M, Lynn MJ, Stulting RD. Risk assessment for ectasia after corneal refractive surgery. *Ophthalmology.* 2008;115(1):37-50.

Reinstein DZ, Archer TJ, Gobbe M, Johnson N. Accuracy and reproducibility of Artemis central flap thickness and visual outcomes of LASIK with the Carl Zeiss Meditec VisuMax femtosecond laser and MEL 80 excimer laser platforms. *J Refract Surg.* 2010;26(2):107-119.

Rocha KM, Randleman JB, Stulting RD. Analysis of microkeratome thin flap architecture using Fourier-domain optical coherence tomography. *J Refract Surg.* 2011;27(10):759-763.

Rosman M, Alió JL, Ortiz D, Pérez-Santonja JJ. Refractive stability of LASIK with the Visx 20/20 excimer laser vs ZB5m phakic iol implantation in patients with high myopia (>-10.00 D): a 10-year retrospective study. *J Refract Surg.* 2011;27(4):279-286.

Sánchez-Galeana CA, Smith RJ, Rodriguez X, Montes M, Chayet AS. Laser in situ keratomileusis and photorefractive keratectomy for residual refractive error after phakic intraocular lens implantation. *J Refract Surg.* 2001;17(3):299-304.

Schallhorn S, Tanzer D, Sanders DR, Sanders ML. Randomized prospective comparison of Visian toric implantable collamer lens and conventional photorefractive keratectomy for moderate to high myopic astigmatism. *J Refract Surg.* 2007;23(9):853-867.

Schallhorn SC, Farjo AA, Huang D, et al; American Academy of Ophthalmology. Wavefront-guided LASIK for the correction of primary myopia and astigmatism a report by the American Academy of Ophthalmology. *Ophthalmology.* 2008;115(7):1249-1261.

Slade SG, Durrie DS, Binder PS. A prospective, contralateral eye study comparing thin-flap LASIK (sub-Bowman keratomileusis) with photorefractive keratectomy. *Ophthalmology.* 2009;116(6):1075-1082.

Sugar A, Rapuano CJ, Culbertson WW, et al. Laser in situ keratomileusis for myopia and astigmatism: safety and efficacy: a report by the American Academy of Ophthalmology. *Ophthalmology.* 2002;109(1):175-187.

Vilaseca M, Padilla A, Pujol J, Ondategui JC, Artal P, Güell JL. Optical quality one month after verisyse and Veriflex phakic IOL implantation and Zeiss MEL 80 LASIK for myopia from 5.00 to 16.50 diopters. *J Refract Surg.* 2009;25(8):689-698.

—Case 2—

A 51-year-old male desires refractive surgical correction, ideally for uncorrected distance visual acuity (UDVA) and uncorrected near visual acuity (UNVA), although he feels distance is most important. The patient is an avid golfer and frequently drives at night. He has no significant family, past medical, or ocular history.

CASE HISTORY		
	Right Eye	**Left Eye**
Present correction method	Spectacles and CTL	Spectacles and CTL
Manifest refraction	+2.75 +1.50 x 095	+3.25 +2.50 x 079
CDVA (current)	20/20	20/25
CNVA (current)	20/20	20/20
Near add	+2.25 D	+2.25 D
Dominant eye	Right	
Keratometry		
Flat K	42.0 @ 002	41.75 @ 168
Steep K	44.25 @ 092	45.25 @ 075
Pupil size (bright)	4.1 mm	3.8 mm
Pupil size (dim)	5.7 mm	5.5 mm
Central corneal thickness	605 µm	615 µm
Physical examination	Normal	Normal
Estimated ablation depth	40 µm	45 µm

Questions

1. Is this patient a candidate for refractive surgery? If so, what treatment options are available?
2. Considering all factors, what procedure(s) would you recommend and why?
3. What are the most significant potential complications for each procedure available for this patient based on his examination?
4. How stable is this patient's refraction likely to be for the various treatment options?
5. What special considerations are there for this patient regarding potential retreatment for postoperative ametropia?

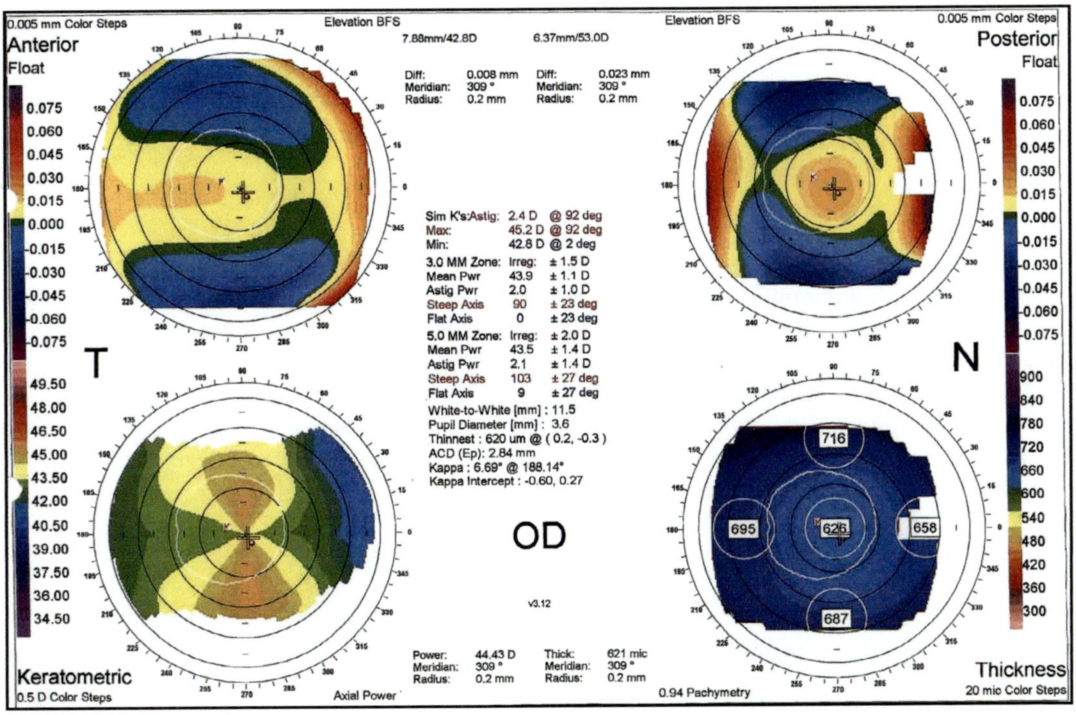
0.005 mm Color Steps
Anterior
Float
Elevation BFS
7.88mm/42.8D
6.37mm/53.0D
Elevation BFS
0.005 mm Color Steps
Posterior
Float
Diff: 0.008 mm Meridian: 309 ° Radius: 0.2 mm
Diff: 0.023 mm Meridian: 309 ° Radius: 0.2 mm
0.075 0.060 0.045 0.030 0.015 0.000 -0.015 -0.030 -0.045 -0.060 -0.075
Sim K's:Astig: 2.4 D @ 92 deg
Max: 45.2 D @ 92 deg
Min: 42.8 D @ 2 deg
3.0 MM Zone: Irreg: ± 1.5 D
Mean Pwr 43.9 ± 1.1 D
Astig Pwr 2.0 ± 1.0 D
Steep Axis 90 ± 23 deg
Flat Axis 0 ± 23 deg
5.0 MM Zone: Irreg: ± 2.0 D
Mean Pwr 43.5 ± 1.4 D
Astig Pwr 2.1 ± 1.4 D
Steep Axis 103 ± 27 deg
Flat Axis 9 ± 27 deg
White-to-White [mm] : 11.5
Pupil Diameter [mm] : 3.6
Thinnest : 620 um @ (0.2, -0.3)
ACD (Ep): 2.84 mm
Kappa : 6.69° @ 188.14°
Kappa Intercept : -0.60, 0.27
T
N
OD
v3.12
49.50 48.00 46.50 45.00 43.50 42.00 40.50 39.00 37.50 36.00 34.50
900 840 780 720 660 600 540 480 420 360 300
716
695
626
658
687
Power: 44.43 D Meridian: 309 ° Radius: 0.2 mm
Thick: 621 mic Meridian: 309 ° Radius: 0.2 mm
Keratometric
0.5 D Color Steps
Axial Power
0.94 Pachymetry
Thickness
20 mic Color Steps

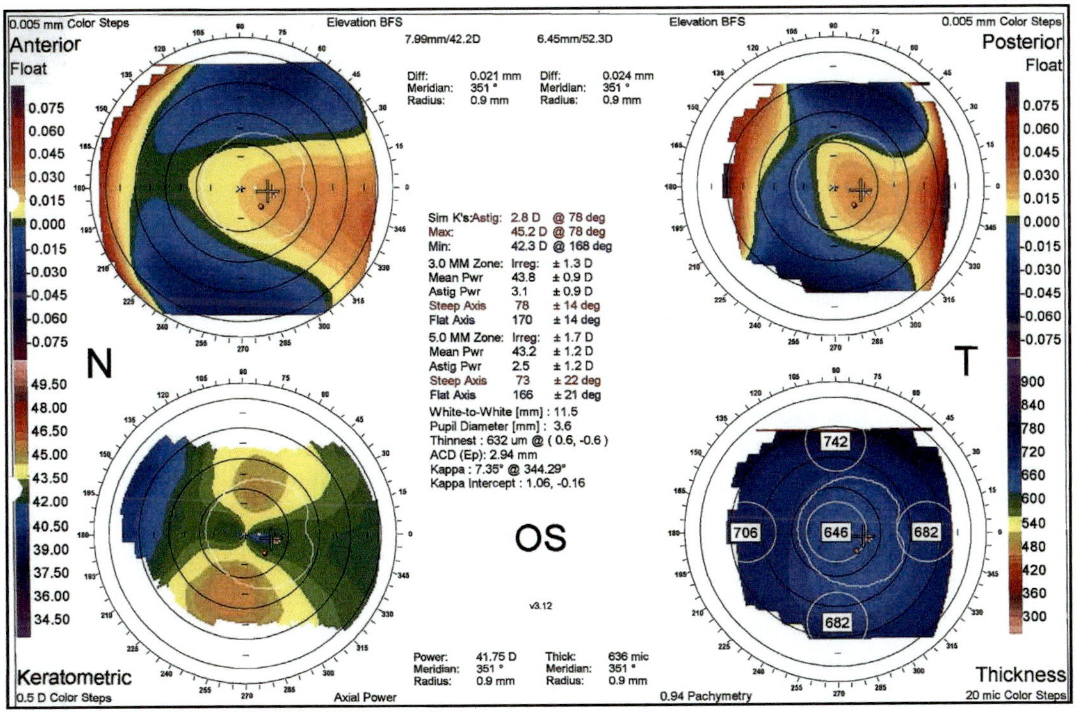
0.005 mm Color Steps
Anterior
Float
Elevation BFS
7.99mm/42.2D
6.45mm/52.3D
Elevation BFS
0.005 mm Color Steps
Posterior
Float
Diff: 0.021 mm Meridian: 351 ° Radius: 0.9 mm
Diff: 0.024 mm Meridian: 351 ° Radius: 0.9 mm
0.075 0.060 0.045 0.030 0.015 0.000 -0.015 -0.030 -0.045 -0.060 -0.075
Sim K's:Astig: 2.8 D @ 78 deg
Max: 45.2 D @ 78 deg
Min: 42.3 D @ 168 deg
3.0 MM Zone: Irreg: ± 1.3 D
Mean Pwr 43.8 ± 0.9 D
Astig Pwr 3.1 ± 0.9 D
Steep Axis 78 ± 14 deg
Flat Axis 170 ± 14 deg
5.0 MM Zone: Irreg: ± 1.7 D
Mean Pwr 43.2 ± 1.2 D
Astig Pwr 2.5 ± 1.2 D
Steep Axis 73 ± 22 deg
Flat Axis 166 ± 21 deg
White-to-White [mm] : 11.5
Pupil Diameter [mm] : 3.6
Thinnest : 632 um @ (0.6, -0.6)
ACD (Ep): 2.94 mm
Kappa : 7.35° @ 344.29°
Kappa Intercept : 1.06, -0.16
N
T
OS
v3.12
49.50 48.00 46.50 45.00 43.50 42.00 40.50 39.00 37.50 36.00 34.50
900 840 780 720 660 600 540 480 420 360 300
742
706
646
682
682
Power: 41.75 D Meridian: 351 ° Radius: 0.9 mm
Thick: 636 mic Meridian: 351 ° Radius: 0.9 mm
Keratometric
0.5 D Color Steps
Axial Power
0.94 Pachymetry
Thickness
20 mic Color Steps

—Case 2—
Hyperopia
Surgical Options

Hyperopia is less common than myopia but generally more visually disabling, especially with age. Primary hyperopia treatment options include LASIK, surface ablation (together termed *laser vision correction* [LVC]), and refractive lens exchange (RLE). Although a variety of collagen-shrinking technologies are available (laser thermal keratoplasty and conductive keratoplasty), these have generally fallen out of use due to their significant regression of refractive effect. The best surgical option for hyperopia depends on the patient's screening evaluation, degree of hyperopia, and the patient's goals and desires.

Case Analysis

- Estimated residual stromal bed (RSB) thickness is > 300 μm for both eyes.
- Case Figures show normal topographies with symmetric bowtie patterns and normal corneal thickness

Pearl: *Hyperopia is significantly more challenging to treat; look to avoid high hyperopic laser ablations and consider lens-based surgery much earlier!*

Questions

1. Is this patient a candidate for refractive surgery? If so, what treatment options are available?

   Yes, this patient appears to be a reasonable candidate for refractive surgery. In his prescription range, LASIK, surface ablation, and RLE are all potential options.

2. Considering all factors, what procedure would you recommend and why?

   Given this patient's age, preoperative keratometry values, and visual goals, refractive lens exchange with a toric IOL to minimize astigmatism for distance acuity, or planned bioptics (RLE ± LVC) has the greatest likelihood of achieving his visual goals. Primary LVC is possible but unlikely to remain stable over time, and the patient is likely to develop cataractous changes in the relatively near future.

3. What are the most significant potential complications for each procedure available for this patient based on his examination?

   The greatest concerns for LVC are decentered ablations or irregular astigmatism from flap ablation in hyperopes, and standard cataract surgical complications with RLE. Further, given the patient's central keratometry reading approximately 44.00 diopters (D) in both eyes, he may have a less optimal results from primary LVC.

4. How stable is this patient's refraction likely to be for the various treatment options?

   If the patient elects RLE, then refractive error is unlikely to change significantly over time. However, LVC has an increased risk of regression for hyperopic treatments, increasing relative to the refractive error treated.

5. What special considerations are there for this patient regarding potential retreatment for postoperative ametropia?

   Given the patient's astigmatism, he is likely to need subsequent LVC following RLE. If he opts for primary LVC, then he is likely to require retreatment in the future for regressed hyperopia.

Refractive Surgery for Hyperopia

LASIK and surface ablation are both FDA approved for up to +6.00 D of hyperopic treatment for most laser platforms, although most surgeons have a lower practical cutoff for both procedures, usually between +3.00 and +4.00 D. RLE can correct any amount of spherical error, although its accuracy is currently less than with excimer laser procedures. Phakic intraocular lenses (IOLs) are not approved in the United States for hyperopia, and their use is limited by reduced anterior chamber depth common in hyperopic eyes.

Figure 6-2 demonstrates this author's procedure preference for hyperopia when all other factors are equivalent. Note that all 3 procedures are viable options in this patient's treatment range. For hyperopia, the relative risks and benefits are discussed in the remaining sections of this case.

LASIK and Surface Ablation

LASIK has excellent initial predictability and rapid healing in the patient's prescription range. However, regression is common with higher refractions. Because laser ablation occurs peripherally, care must be taken to protect the LASIK flap hinge to avoid undersurface ablation, with resulting irregular astigmatism (see Figure 5-10). Surface ablation is also an excellent option but carries the same general risks of regression for higher prescriptions. Anecdotally, there appears to be greater haze formation with peripheral surface ablation; however, this is unlikely to be visually significant, as it usually occurs outside the visual axis.

Recent studies have demonstrated that steeper corneas preoperatively have poorer visual outcomes after LASIK and surface ablation, and hyperopic ablation may be less effective in patients with keratometry greater than 44.00 D. Hyperopic ablations are also more sensitive to centration issues, and even moderately decentered ablations may have a significant effect on acuity, inducing irregular astigmatism in the visual axis.

Refractive Lens Exchange

RLE provides an excellent alternative to laser vision correction for many hyperopic patients, especially anyone with any degree of cataract development. Refractive accuracy is lower than that with excimer laser treatment, but long-term stability is significantly better. RLE carries more significant potential risks than LVC. Further, multifocal IOLs may cause significant glare and halos, usually at night, which may be intolerable for rare patients. Intraocular lens exchange for multifocal IOLs occurs in approximately 1% of patients, and all patients should be counseled about this preoperatively.

Currently, toric multifocal IOLs are not available in the United States, but this may soon change. Pseudoaccommodating IOLs are available in the United States (recently approved in a toric version), and multiple functionally accommodating IOLs are in various stages of development and approval in the United States.

Monofocal IOLs targeted for distance focus with planed LVC for residual astigmatism is also a reasonable option for this patient. The patient may opt for this choice, given his desire for best visual acuity when golfing and driving at night.

Retreatment Options and Bioptics

Retreatment (enhancement) rates after primary LVC are significantly higher for patients with hyperopia than those with myopia. Patients with hyperopia and astigmatism frequently require bioptics for maximal refractive error correction, especially for astigmatism management. Patients with multifocal IOL implantation are especially intolerant of even low amounts of astigmatism. For most patients, LASIK or surface ablation is a reasonable option; however, this necessitates appropriate screening prior to RLE to assure that LVC will be an option postoperatively.

Bibliography

Alfonso JF, Fernández-Vega L, Baamonde MB, Montés-Micó R. Prospective visual evaluation of apodized diffractive intraocular lenses. *J Cataract Refract Surg.* 2007;33(7):1235-1243.

Bababeygy SR, Zoumalan CI, Chien FY, Manche EE. Wavefront-guided laser in situ keratomileusis retreatment for consecutive hyperopia and compound hyperopic astigmatism. *J Cataract Refract Surg.* 2008;34(8):1260-1266.

de Vries NE, Webers CA, Montés-Micó R, Ferrer-Blasco T, Nuijts RM. Visual outcomes after cataract surgery with implantation of a +3.00 D or +4.00 D aspheric diffractive multifocal intraocular lens: Comparative study. *J Cataract Refract Surg.* 2010;36(8):1316-1322.

Durrie DS, Smith RT, Waring GO IV, Stahl JE, Schwendeman FJ. Comparing conventional and wavefront-optimized LASIK for the treatment of hyperopia. *J Refract Surg.* 2010;26(5):356-363.

Fine IH, Hoffman RS, Packer M. Refractive lens exchange: the quadruple win and current perspectives. *J Refract Surg.* 2007;23(8):819-824.

Gil-Cazorla R, Teus MA, de Benito-Llopis L, Mikropoulos DG. Femtosecond laser vs mechanical microkeratome for hyperopic laser in situ keratomileusis. *Am J Ophthalmol.* 2011;152(1):16-21.e2.

Kashani S, Rajan M, Gartry D. Wavefront-guided retreatment after primary wavefront-guided laser in situ keratomileusis in myopes and hyperopes: long-term follow-up. *Am J Ophthalmol.* 2009;147(3):417-423.e2.

Keir NJ, Simpson T, Hutchings N, Jones L, Fonn D. Outcomes of wavefront-guided laser in situ keratomileusis for hyperopia. *J Cataract Refract Surg.* 2011;37(5):886-893.

Kezirian GM, Moore CR, Stonecipher KG. Four-year postoperative results of the US ALLEGRETTO WAVE clinical trial for the treatment of hyperopia. *J Refract Surg.* 2008;24(4):S431-S438.

Llovet F, Galal A, Benitez-del-Castillo JM, Ortega J, Martin C, Baviera J. One-year results of excimer laser in situ keratomileusis for hyperopia. *J Cataract Refract Surg.* 2009;35(7):1156-1165.

Packer M, Hoffman RS, Fine IH, Dick HB. Refractive lens exchange. *Int Ophthalmol Clin.* 2006 Summer;46(3):63-82.

Randleman JB, White AJ Jr, Lynn MJ, Hu MH, Stulting RD. Incidence, outcomes, and risk factors for retreatment after wavefront-optimized ablations with PRK and LASIK. *J Refract Surg.* 2009;25(3):273-276.

Williams LB, Dave SB, Moshirfar M. Correlation of visual outcome and patient satisfaction with preoperative keratometry after hyperopic laser in situ keratomileusis. *J Cataract Refract Surg.* 2008;34(7):1083-1088.

Young JJ, Schallhorn SC, Brown MC, Hettinger KA. Effect of keratometry on visual outcomes 1 month after hyperopic LASIK. *J Refract Surg.* 2009;25(7 Suppl):S672-S676.

—CASE 3—

A 32-year-old male desires refractive surgical correction. He has no significant family, past medical, or ocular history.

CASE HISTORY		
	Right Eye	**Left Eye**
Present correction method	Toric soft CTL	Toric soft CTL
Manifest refraction	-7.25 +4.50 x 095	-7.50 +4.75 x 081
CDVA (current)	20/25	20/25
UNVA (current)	20/20	20/20
Dominant eye	Right	
Cycloplegic refraction	-7.25 +4.50 x 091	-7.25 +4.75 x 080
Keratometry		
Flat K	39.7 @ 005	39.9 @ 179
Steep K	43.4 @ 095	43.7 @ 089
Pupil size (bright)	4.4 mm	4.1 mm
Pupil size (dim)	6.1 mm	6.3 mm
Central corneal thickness	561 µm	554 µm
Physical exam	Normal	Normal
Estimated ablation depth	120 µm	120 µm

QUESTIONS

1. Is this patient a candidate for refractive surgery? If so, what treatment options are available?
2. Considering all factors, what procedure would you recommend and why?
3. What are the most significant potential complications for each procedure available for this patient based on his examination?
4. What special considerations are there when considering lase vision correction (LVC) in this patient?
5. What special considerations are there for this patient regarding potential retreatment for postoperative ametropia?

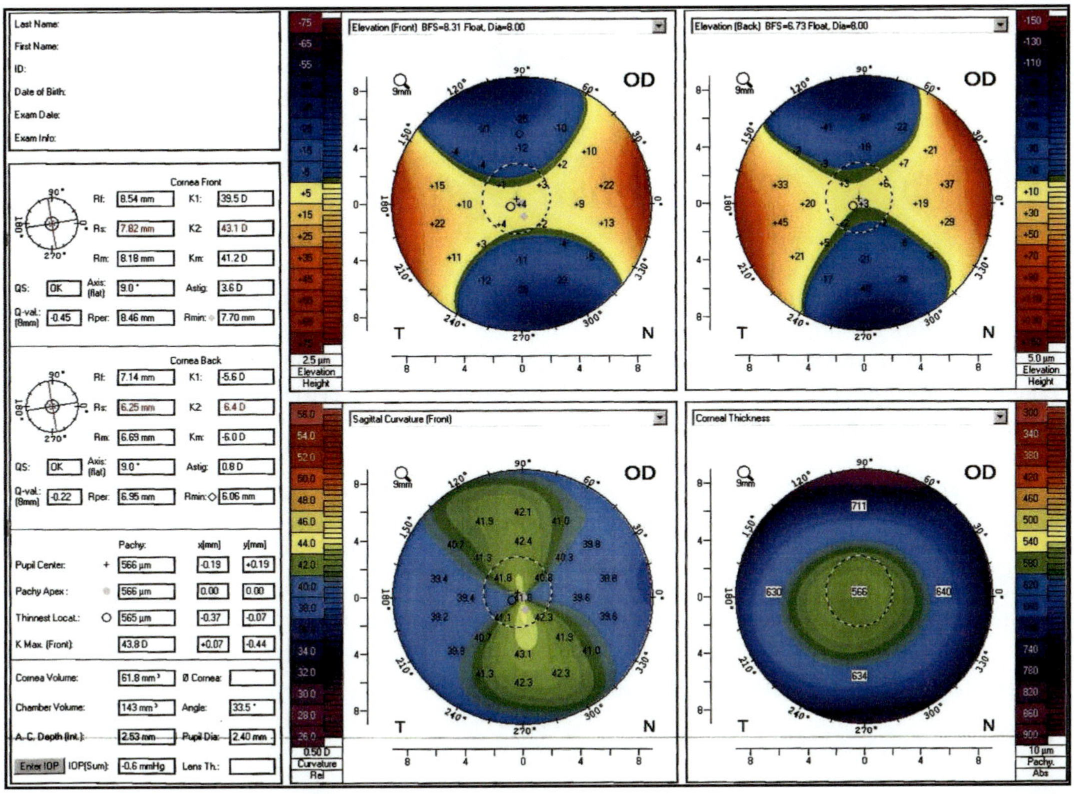
Last Name:
First Name:
ID:
Date of Birth:
Exam Date:
Exam Info:
Cornea Front
Rf: 8.54 mm K1: 39.5 D
Rs: 7.82 mm K2: 43.1 D
Rm: 8.18 mm Km: 41.2 D
QS: OK Axis (flat): 9.0° Astig: 3.6 D
Q-val. (8mm): -0.45 Rper: 8.46 mm Rmin: 7.70 mm
Cornea Back
Rf: 7.14 mm K1: -5.6 D
Rs: 6.25 mm K2: -6.4 D
Rm: 6.69 mm Km: -6.0 D
QS: OK Axis (flat): 9.0° Astig: 0.8 D
Q-val. (8mm): -0.22 Rper: 6.95 mm Rmin: 6.06 mm
Pachy: x[mm] y[mm]
Pupil Center: + 566 µm -0.19 +0.19
Pachy Apex: 566 µm 0.00 0.00
Thinnest Locat.: O 565 µm -0.37 -0.07
K Max. (Front): 43.8 D +0.07 -0.44
Cornea Volume: 61.8 mm³ Ø Cornea:
Chamber Volume: 143 mm³ Angle: 33.5°
A. C. Depth (Int.): 2.53 mm Pupil Dia: 2.40 mm
Enter IOP IOP(Sum): -0.6 mmHg Lens Th.:
Elevation (Front) BFS=8.31 Float, Dia=8.00
Elevation (Back) BFS=6.73 Float, Dia=8.00
Sagittal Curvature (Front)
Corneal Thickness
OD
T N
2.5 µm Elevation Height
5.0 µm Elevation Height
0.50 D Curvature Rel
10 µm Pachy. Abs

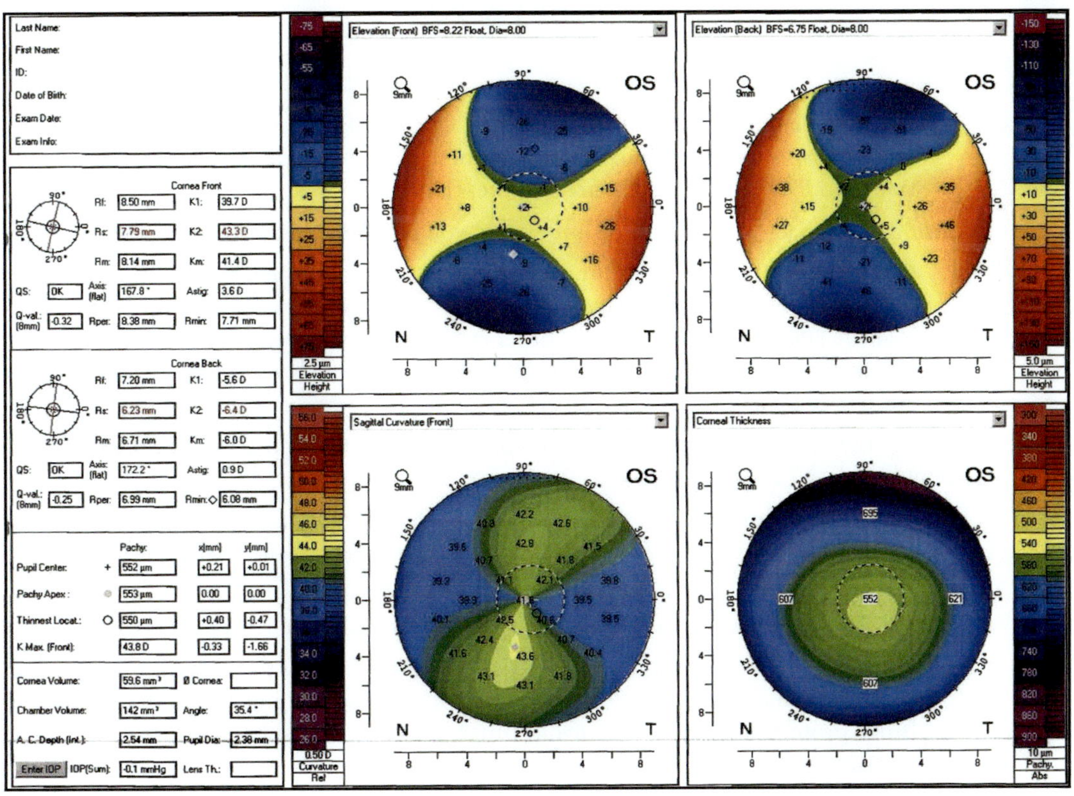
Last Name:
First Name:
ID:
Date of Birth:
Exam Date:
Exam Info:
Cornea Front
Rf: 8.50 mm K1: 39.7 D
Rs: 7.79 mm K2: 43.3 D
Rm: 8.14 mm Km: 41.4 D
QS: OK Axis (flat): 167.8° Astig: 3.6 D
Q-val. (8mm): -0.32 Rper: 8.38 mm Rmin: 7.71 mm
Cornea Back
Rf: 7.20 mm K1: -5.6 D
Rs: 6.23 mm K2: -6.4 D
Rm: 6.71 mm Km: -6.0 D
QS: OK Axis (flat): 172.2° Astig: 0.9 D
Q-val. (8mm): -0.25 Rper: 6.99 mm Rmin: 6.08 mm
Pachy: x[mm] y[mm]
Pupil Center: + 552 µm +0.21 +0.01
Pachy Apex: 553 µm 0.00 0.00
Thinnest Locat.: O 550 µm +0.40 -0.47
K Max. (Front): 43.8 D -0.33 -1.66
Cornea Volume: 59.6 mm³ Ø Cornea:
Chamber Volume: 142 mm³ Angle: 35.4°
A. C. Depth (Int.): 2.54 mm Pupil Dia: 2.38 mm
Enter IOP IOP(Sum): -0.1 mmHg Lens Th.:
Elevation (Front) BFS=8.22 Float, Dia=8.00
Elevation (Back) BFS=6.75 Float, Dia=8.00
Sagittal Curvature (Front)
Corneal Thickness
OS
N T
2.5 µm Elevation Height
5.0 µm Elevation Height
0.50 D Curvature Rel
10 µm Pachy. Abs

—Case 3—
Astigmatism
Surgical Options

Astigmatism is less common than myopia but generally more visually disabling at all distances. Primary treatment options for astigmatism include LASIK, surface ablation (together termed *laser vision correction*), and toric phakic intraocular lens (PIOL) implantation outside the United States. When considering treatment options for high astigmatism, it is critical to differentiate regular astigmatism from irregular astigmatism.

Case Analysis

- Estimated residual stromal bed thickness (RSB) is 315 to 335 µm for both eyes.
- Case Figures show normal topographies with symmetric bowtie pattern in the right eye and mildly asymmetric pattern in the left eye, with good corneal thickness in both eyes.

Pearl: *High astigmatism can be effectively treated, but beware of treating (or inducing) irregular astigmatism!*

Questions

1. Is this patient a candidate for refractive surgery? If so, what treatment options are available?

   Yes, this patient appears to be a reasonable candidate for refractive surgery, as his topography is not suspicious. In the patient's prescription range, LASIK, surface ablation, and PIOL implantation are all potential options.

2. Considering all factors, what procedure would you recommend and why?

   Given the patient's topography and an otherwise normal examination, I would opt for thin-flap LASIK or surface ablation. For this patient, the estimated RSB thickness is above 300 µm, and there are no other risk factors for ectasia. Surface ablation is also a reasonable option. Currently available PIOLs are also an option, but they cannot address the patient's astigmatism.

3. What are the most significant potential complications for each procedure available for this patient based on his examination?

   The greatest concerns are irregular astigmatism for any LVC, postoperative ectasia with LASIK (unlikely), corneal haze with surface ablation (unlikely), and endothelial cell loss and early cataract formation with PIOLs.

4. What special considerations are there when considering LVC in this patient?

   For high astigmatic ablations, patient alignment is critical to maximize astigmatism correction and minimize the occurrence of induced astigmatism. For LASIK, flap hinge protection is critical to avoid hinge ablation with subsequent irregular astigmatism.

5. What special considerations are there for this patient regarding potential retreatment for postoperative ametropia?

    Due to the amount of tissue being removed, if this patient undergoes LASIK and subsequently needs retreatment, it may be best to offer surface ablation. If the patient initially has surface ablation, then repeat surface ablation would be the best retreatment option. If the patient has PIOL implantation, then either LASIK or surface ablation is a reasonable retreatment option. Given the patient's astigmatism, he would definitely need subsequent LVC following PIOL implantation.

Refractive Surgery for Astigmatism

LASIK and surface ablation are both FDA approved for up to 6.00 diopters (D) of astigmatism correction for most laser platforms. In contrast to hyperopic ablation, astigmatic ablation appears more accurate and stable over time, even for higher refractive errors. Phakic IOLs are approved for use between -3.00 and -20.00 D, depending on IOL style, but are not yet available in toric versions in the United States. For more information about approval ranges see Chapter 1. Critical issues when considering treatment for high astigmatism include ensuring accurate ocular alignment, avoiding cyclotorsion, and differentiating between regular and irregular astigmatism.

LASIK and Surface Ablation

LASIK has excellent predictability and rapid healing for moderate to high astigmatism. However, residual refractive error and retreatment rates are higher with higher cylinder corrections than myopic ablations. Because laser ablation occurs peripherally in a certain meridian, care must be taken to protect the LASIK flap hinge to avoid undersurface ablation, with resulting irregular astigmatism if treatment occurs in the meridian of the hinge (see Figure 5-10). Surface ablation is also an excellent option, but it has the same increased rate of residual error and retreatment as myopic ablation, and it has the same risk of visually insignificant peripheral haze as it does with hyperopic ablation.

Phakic Intraocular Lens

Phakic IOLs provide excellent visual acuity in highly myopic patients, but it should be undertaken only as a planned bioptics procedure, if needed, in individuals with significant astigmatism. Outside of the United States, toric phakic intraocular lenses are available, and these may be available at some point within the United States. Given the ability to correct this patient's error with LVC and the definitive need for LVC following PIOL, there is a limited role for spherical PIOLs for high astigmatism, unless there is some need to reduce the refractive error but still have reliance on visual aids, such as a career that requires some moderate level of uncorrected acuity.

Retreatment Options and Bioptics

Retreatment (enhancement) rates after primary LVC are higher for astigmatism >2.00 D than for lower amounts of astigmatism or myopia. If retreatment is desired after surface ablation, repeat surface ablation is most reasonable. If primary LASIK is performed, either LASIK or surface ablation may be options; however, if there is question about adequate RSB thickness, then surface ablation performed on the flap may be the best option. Although this appears slightly less accurate than primary surface ablation, there is theoretically no biomechanical effect because the flap is already functionally decoupled from the underlying stroma. Combining PIOLs with either LASIK or surface ablation, termed *bioptics*, may provide the best accuracy and visual acuity, although the patient is undertaking risks from both procedures when choosing this route.

Ocular Alignment for Astigmatism Correction

Accurate ocular alignment is key to correcting higher amounts of astigmatism. Initial patient alignment is the most critical step and can minimize most treatment problems. Having the patient positioned under the laser with both eyes open is effective to assure appropriate alignment.

Ocular cyclotorsion up to 20 degrees can occur when patients assume the supine position under the laser, and this must be taken into account to avoid treatment on the incorrect meridian. Some lasers have advanced detection systems, including iris registration; however, the benefit of this is debatable. Many surgeons utilize some form of limbal marking when the patient is in the upright position, usually at the slit lamp, to accurately identify the 0- and 180-degree meridians so that they can be aligned when the patient is supine. Many lasers have "crosshairs" to facilitate alignment with these predetermined marks or other anatomic landmarks.

Differentiating Regular and Irregular Astigmatism

Regular astigmatism has a symmetric pattern on topography, with reproducible refractions and visual acuity usually correctable to 20/20, although some patients have meridional amblyopia that may limit their best-corrected visual acuity without any corneal abnormality or irregular astigmatism. Irregular astigmatism has an asymmetric topographic pattern, and in more significant cases acuity is not correctable to 20/20 with refraction or spectacles. In these cases, rigid gas permeable contact lens over refraction may yield improved acuity. Mild degrees of irregular astigmatism in an otherwise biomechanically normal cornea may still achieve good outcomes after LVC. Significant irregular astigmatism should be excluded from standard LVC due to the unpredictable visual outcomes; topography-guided laser ablation may be able to achieve better outcomes for these individuals in the future. Irregular astigmatism may also be a marker of biomechanical instability; thus, all patients with any irregular astigmatism should be thoroughly screened prior to considering LVC.

Bibliography

Bhikoo R, Rayner S, Gray T. Toric implantable collamer lens for patients with moderate to severe myopic astigmatism: 12-month follow-up. *Clin Experiment Ophthalmol.* 2010;38(5):467-674.

Choi SH, Lee MO, Chung ES, Chung TY. Comparison of the toric implantable collamer lens and bioptics for myopic astigmatism. *J Refract Surg.* 2011;27(2):91-97.

Febbraro JL, Koch DD, Khan HN, Saad A, Gatinel D. Detection of static cyclotorsion and compensation for dynamic cyclotorsion in laser in situ keratomileusis. *J Cataract Refract Surg.* 2010 Oct;36(10):1718-23.

Hasegawa A, Kojima T, Isogai N, Tamaoki A, Nakamura T, Ichikawa K. Astigmatism correction: Laser in situ keratomileusis versus posterior chamber collagen copolymer toric phakic intraocular lens implantation. *J Cataract Refract Surg.* 2012;38:574-81

Moshirfar M, Chen MC, Espandar L, Meyer JJ, Christensen D, Christiansen SM, Dave SB, Bedke B, Kurz C. Effect of iris registration on outcomes of LASIK for myopia with the VISX CustomVue platform. *J Refract Surg.* 2009 Jun;25(6):493-502.

Neuhann IM, Lege BA, Bauer M, Hassel JM, Hilger A, Neuhann TF. Static and dynamic rotational eye tracking during LASIK treatment of myopic astigmatism with the Zyoptix laser platform and Advanced Control Eye Tracker. *J Refract Surg.* 2010 Jan;26(1):17-27.

Prakash G, Agarwal A, Ashok Kumar D, Jacob S, Agarwal A. Comparison of laser in situ keratomileusis for myopic astigmatism without iris registration, with iris registration, and with iris registration-assisted dynamic rotational eye tracking. *J Cataract Refract Surg.* 2011;37(3):574-581.

Randleman JB, White AJ, Hu MH, Stulting RD. Incidence, outcomes, and risk factors for enhancement after wavefront-optimized advanced surface ablation and laser in situ keratomileusis. *J Refract Surg.* 2009;25(3):273-276.

Sanders DR, Sanders ML. Comparison of the toric implantable collamer lens and custom ablation LASIK for myopic astigmatism. *J Refract Surg.* 2008;24(8):773-778.

Schallhorn S, Tanzer D, Sanders DR, Sanders ML. Randomized prospective comparison of Visian toric implantable collamer lens and conventional photorefractive keratectomy for moderate to high myopic astigmatism. *J Refract Surg.* 2007;23(9):853-867.

Schallhorn SC, Farjo AA, Huang D, et al; American Academy of Ophthalmology. Wavefront-guided LASIK for the correction of primary myopia and astigmatism a report by the American Academy of Ophthalmology. *Ophthalmology.* 2008;115(7):1249-1261.

Shen EP, Chen WL, Hu FR. Manual limbal markings versus iris-registration software for correction of myopic astigmatism by laser in situ keratomileusis. J *Cataract Refract Surg.* 2010;36(3):431-436.

Stonecipher KG, Kezirian GM, Stonecipher K. LASIK for mixed astigmatism using the ALLEGRETTO WAVE: 3- and 6-month results with the 200- and 400-Hz platforms. *J Refract Surg.* 2010;26(10):S819-S823.

Sugar A, Rapuano CJ, Culbertson WW, et al. Laser in situ keratomileusis for myopia and astigmatism: safety and efficacy: a report by the American Academy of Ophthalmology. *Ophthalmology.* 2002;109(1):175-187.

Wang TJ, Lin YH, Chang DC, Chou HC, Wang IJ. Comparison of the effects of cylindrical correction with and without iris recognition technology in wavefront laser-assisted in situ keratomileusis. *Clin Experiment Ophthalmol.* 2012;40(3):239-246.

—Case 4—

A 46-year-old male desires refractive surgical correction, ideally to see clearly at all distances. His hobbies include golf, and he is a certified helicopter pilot. He has no significant family, past medical, or ocular history.

CASE HISTORY		
	Right Eye	**Left Eye**
Present correction method	CTL	CTL
Manifest refraction	-3.50 sphere	-3.75 sphere
CDVA (current)	20/20	20/20
CNVA (current)	20/20	20/20
Add	+1.50	+1.50
Dominant eye	Right	
Ocular alignment	Orthophoric	Orthophoric
Keratometry		
Flat K	47.2 @ 176	47.3 @ 170
Steep K	48.0 @ 086	48.3 @ 080
Pupil size (bright)	3.2 mm	3.6 mm
Pupil size (dim)	5.1 mm	5.1 mm
Central corneal thickness	561 µm	562 µm
Physical examination	Normal	Normal
Estimated ablation depth	55 µm	60 µm

Questions

1. What special considerations are there for this patient regarding visual acuity outcomes?
2. What are the most important factors to use in assisting the patient to make the appropriate decision regarding surgical goals?
3. What are the most likely patient complaints in the early postoperative period for this individual?
4. What special considerations are there for this patient regarding potential retreatment for postoperative ametropia?
5. What is the major long-term concern for this patient if he opts for the treatment that provides the broadest available range of visual acuity?

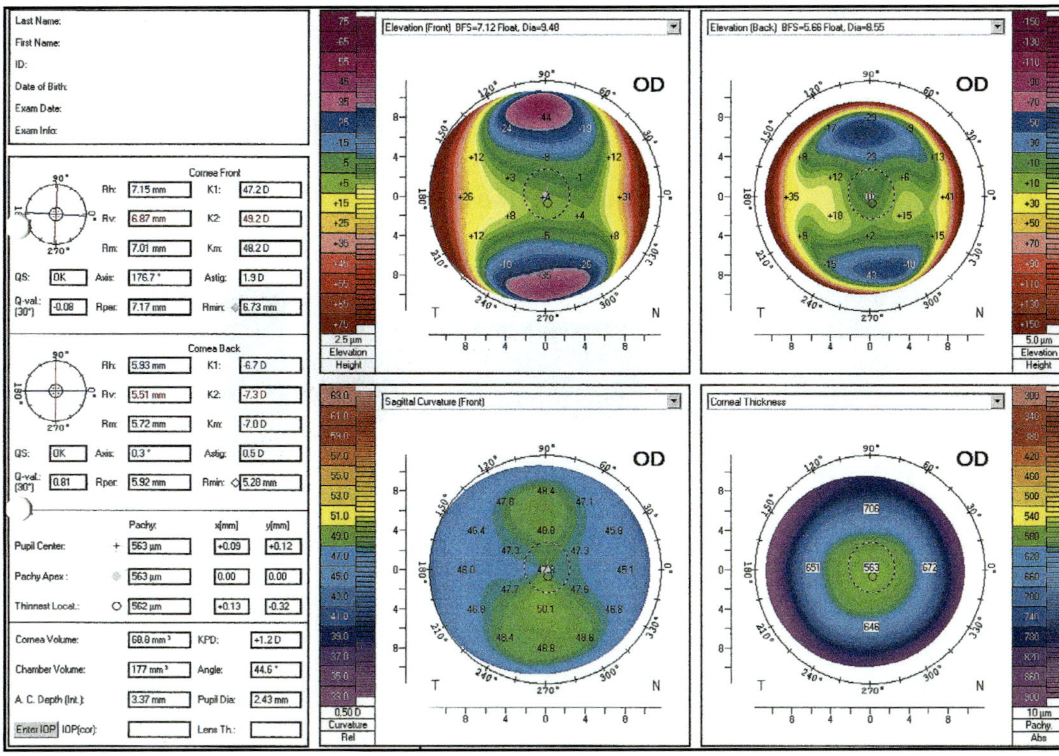
Last Name:
First Name:
ID:
Date of Birth:
Exam Date:
Exam Info:
Cornea Front
Rh: 7.15 mm K1: 47.2 D
Rv: 6.87 mm K2: 49.2 D
Rm: 7.01 mm Km: 48.2 D
QS: OK Axis: 176.7° Astig: 1.9 D
Q-val. (30°): -0.08 Rper: 7.17 mm Rmin: 6.73 mm
Cornea Back
Rh: 5.93 mm K1: -6.7 D
Rv: 5.51 mm K2: -7.3 D
Rm: 5.72 mm Km: -7.0 D
QS: OK Axis: 0.3° Astig: 0.5 D
Q-val. (30°): 0.81 Rper: 5.92 mm Rmin: 5.28 mm
Pachy: x[mm] y[mm]
Pupil Center: + 563 µm +0.09 +0.12
Pachy Apex: 563 µm 0.00 0.00
Thinnest Locat.: 562 µm +0.13 -0.32
Cornea Volume: 60.8 mm³ KPD: +1.2 D
Chamber Volume: 177 mm³ Angle: 44.6°
A. C. Depth (Int.): 3.37 mm Pupil Dia: 2.43 mm
Enter IOP IOP(cor): Lens Th.:
Elevation (Front) BFS=7.12 Float, Dia=9.48
OD
Elevation (Back) BFS=5.66 Float, Dia=8.55
OD
Sagittal Curvature (Front)
OD
Corneal Thickness
OD
2.5 µm Elevation Height
5.0 µm Elevation Height
0.50 D Curvature Rel
10 µm Pachy. Abs

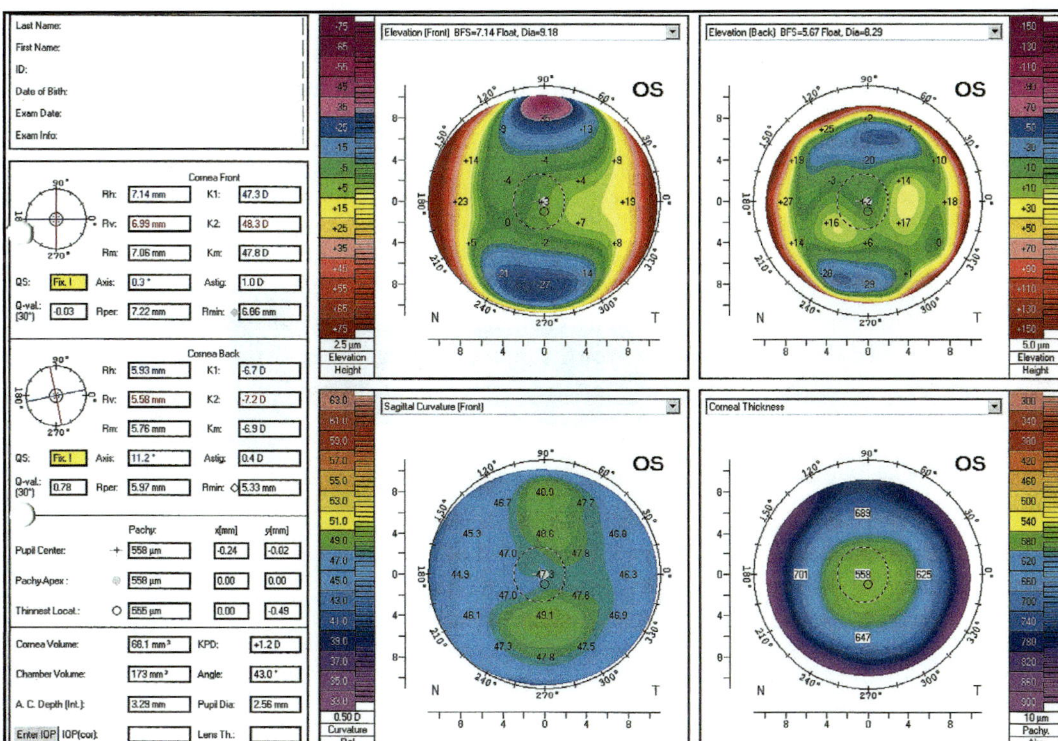
Last Name:
First Name:
ID:
Date of Birth:
Exam Date:
Exam Info:
Cornea Front
Rh: 7.14 mm K1: 47.3 D
Rv: 6.99 mm K2: 48.3 D
Rm: 7.06 mm Km: 47.8 D
QS: Fix. ! Axis: 0.3° Astig: 1.0 D
Q-val. (30°): -0.03 Rper: 7.22 mm Rmin: 6.86 mm
Cornea Back
Rh: 5.93 mm K1: -6.7 D
Rv: 5.58 mm K2: -7.2 D
Rm: 5.76 mm Km: -6.9 D
QS: Fix. ! Axis: 11.2° Astig: 0.4 D
Q-val. (30°): 0.78 Rper: 5.97 mm Rmin: 5.33 mm
Pachy: x[mm] y[mm]
Pupil Center: + 558 µm -0.24 -0.02
Pachy Apex: 558 µm 0.00 0.00
Thinnest Locat.: 555 µm 0.00 -0.49
Cornea Volume: 60.1 mm³ KPD: +1.2 D
Chamber Volume: 173 mm³ Angle: 43.0°
A. C. Depth (Int.): 3.29 mm Pupil Dia: 2.56 mm
Enter IOP IOP(cor): Lens Th.:
Elevation (Front) BFS=7.14 Float, Dia=9.18
OS
Elevation (Back) BFS=5.67 Float, Dia=8.29
OS
Sagittal Curvature (Front)
OS
Corneal Thickness
OS
2.5 µm Elevation Height
5.0 µm Elevation Height
0.50 D Curvature Rel
10 µm Pachy. Abs

—Case 4—
Presbyopia Correction
Monovision

Presbyopia is an inevitable aspect of aging, and a variety of treatments, both surgical and nonsurgical, are available currently. Although maximal visual acuity requires both eyes to function at all distances, many patients have achieved satisfactory near and distance visual acuity through monovision correction (also termed *blended vision*). The success of monovision depends on both the patient's personality and visual demands.

Case Analysis

- Estimated residual stromal bed (RSB) thickness is 385 μm for both eyes.
- Case Figures show normal topographies with symmetric bowtie patterns and good corneal thickness in both eyes.

Pearl: *Beware of patients with mild amblyopia or phorias when considering monovision!*

Questions

1. What special considerations are there for this patient regarding visual acuity outcomes?

   The patient's age and need for near add makes him a candidate for monovision correction; however, his visual demands, for both occupation and hobbies, make bilateral distance visual acuity especially important. If he opts for monovision, he will need to wear spectacles or contact lenses for best distance vision while piloting the helicopter and possibly when golfing. If he opts for full distance correction in both eyes, he will need spectacle aids for near work immediately (or soon) after surgery. This concept may be especially challenging for this myopic patient, who has maintained the ability to see at near through the aging process from his natural myopia.

2. What are the most important factors to use in assisting the patient to make the appropriate decision regarding surgical goals?

   The patient's lifestyle, including occupation and hobbies, is critical to consider. Patients with constant activities requiring functional visual acuity at distance and near, especially in the workplace, may strongly desire monovision. However, other patients with high visual demands at distance, including playing tennis or golf, using firearms, or piloting aircraft, may require best distance visual acuity bilaterally at all times.

3. What are the most likely patient complaints in the early postoperative period for this individual?

   Many patients take some time to adapt to monovision, and, early on, they may feel eyestrain and describe a sense that their eyes are working against one another for clarity at any particular distance. Intermediate distance is especially sensitive to this struggle, as the patient's brain determines which eye to preferentially use at that distance. Night vision complaints may also be greater in these individuals, as one eye is, by design, still myopic.

4. What special considerations are there for this patient regarding potential retreatment for postoperative ametropia?

   Patients with monovision may be particularly sensitive to even low amounts of residual ametropia in the distance-targeted eye. Alternatively, patients may decide that they cannot adapt to monovision. In these circumstances, retreatment of the intended near eye may be necessary to alleviate their symptoms, with detailed explanation that they will be losing their uncorrected near visual acuity.

5. What is the major long-term concern for this patient if he opts for the treatment that provides the broadest available range of visual acuity?

   Rarely, patients with monovision correction experience dissociation of a preexisting phoria, resulting in binocular diplopia. At-risk individuals should be carefully screened for this, and monovision should be reversed if any of these symptoms begin to appear.

Monovision Explained

Monovision correction results in one eye, almost always the dominant eye, that is targeted for best distance visual acuity (plano), and the nondominant eye is targeted for a myopic outcome, frequently based on the patient's age (ie, a target of -0.75 diopters [D] to -1.50 D for patients aged 40 to 50 years and a target of up to -2.50 D for patients aged 50 to 60 years). Ocular dominance can be assessed in a variety of ways, but it is frequently performed by having the patient extend both hands to create a small viewing "window" or hole, through which they site a distant object. The patient is asked to close one eye at a time and determine which eye is being used to fixate the object through the small hole.

Surgery for Presbyopia: Inducing Monovision

When to Consider Monovision

- If the patient is strongly motivated to reduce spectacle independence at all distances.
- If the patient is willing to trade the highest quality visual acuity for enhanced range of vision.
- If no ocular contraindications exist.

Monovision LASIK success rates vary, with more than 90% patient satisfaction reported; however, there is up to 30% retreatment rate, either to improve distance visual acuity in the distance eye or to reverse monovision. Despite advanced technology and newer alternatives, monovision remains the primary surgical approach used for presbyopia. In a 2010 survey, more than 80% of the American Society of Cataract and Refractive Surgery (ASCRS) members surveyed preferred monovision to other forms of presbyopia correction (eg, refractive lens exchange, corneal inlays). However, appropriate patient selection is essential for monovision success.

Throughout the preoperative consultation it should be emphasized to the patient that monovision is a strategy to reduce, not eliminate, the need for visual aids, and the ultimate optimal strategy depends on the patient's lifestyle and activities. Nonsurgical options for near acuity include over-the-counter reading spectacles, monovision contact lenses, and multifocal contact lenses; any of which can be utilized after refractive surgery for distance or monovision correction. Frequently a combination of surgery and ocular devices are necessary for optimal visual acuity at all distances depending on the situation. For example, patients may desire modified monovision for intermediate tasks such as computer use, seeing the dashboard while driving, and being able to read casually without reaching for spectacles, but they need to understand that they will need readers for extended close work or more demanding near visual tasks. Alternatively, patients may opt for full monovision correction but utilize spectacles for best distance visual acuity while driving, watching movies, or other distance-demanding tasks. Alternatively, the patient could use a contact lens to correct the near eye for best distance vision in tasks where binocular visual acuity is more important, such as playing tennis or golf.

Monovision Evaluation

Three distinct patient groups seek monovision based on preoperative refraction: myopes, hyperopes, and plano presbyopes. Because the ablation pattern, the limits of treatment, and the potential tolerance of monovision differ significantly in these groups, the preoperative approach must be tailored to match the refractive group in which the patient falls.

Prior to inducing monovision surgically, all patients should be evaluated to confirm that they can tolerate the visual correction, and they should be screened for any issues that might hinder their outcome. Eliciting a history of successful recent contact lens monovision is most helpful. Some patients may report not tolerating monovision; however, on further questioning it is determined that the patient tolerated the visual acuity well but not the contact lens wear. If a patient has no experience with monovision, an in-office test with trial frames or, more ideally, contact lenses is needed; if the results are equivocal, a short-term home contact lens trial in the patient's daily life situations is beneficial.

Monovision Evaluation: Myopes

Myopic patients are the easiest to evaluate for monovision because there are minimal limitations of treatment, and retreatment to eliminate unsuccessful monovision is relatively easy. The ablation profile is a standard myopic ablation, merely a reduction in the amount treated in one eye. Thus, if retreatment is necessary, it simply requires additional myopic ablation to correct the eye for distance.

Monovision Evaluation: Hyperopes and Plano Presbyopes

A more thorough trial is essential for emmetropic and hyperopic individuals because of the differing ablation profiles needed to induce and reverse monovision in these individuals. It is especially important to determine that the bilateral emmetrope can tolerate monovision and the inevitable reduction in stereoacuity.

Although hyperopic ablations are approved for up to +6.00 D, most refractive surgeons treat less than this, usually recommending only +3.00 to 4.00 D of total hyperopic treatment. Thus, in hyperopes, the necessary treatment needed to induce monovision may exceed the total ablation recommended, when combining the amount of hyperopia needed for plano and the amount needed to induce monovision. It is important to demonstrate monovision that can actually be achieved surgically. For instance, there is no value in using a +7.00-D contact lens to simulate monovision when this cannot be duplicated surgically.

Hyperopic ablation patterns tend to be more sensitive to centration and preoperative keratometry. Hyperopic ablations regress more commonly than myopic ablations; therefore, patients with hyperopic monovision may lose the functional effect quicker as a combined result of aging and regression.

Plano presbyopes also require hyperopic ablation patterns to induce monovision, with many of the aforementioned issues. The amount treated is not great, so total hyperopic ablation is not a concern. However, of greater concern, plano presbyopes usually have excellent bilateral uncorrected distance visual acuity and may have greater difficulty adapting to the loss of it. Therefore, in these individuals, an extended contact lens trial is warranted.

When to Avoid Monovision

When to Avoid Monovision

- Amblyopia
- History of ocular alignment issues
- High visual demands at a particular focal distance

Major visual quality issues with monovision include reduced stereoacuity and, rarely, dissociation of phorias, resulting in diplopia. Monovision is generally not a suitable alternative for patients with moderate amblyopia (corrected acuity 20/30 or worse) as the amblyopic eye frequently does not have the ability to perform sufficiently at any distance without the aid of the nonamblyopic eye.

Patients with a history of strabismus or phoria should be NOT considered for monovision, as the lack of binocularity may dissociate a phoria that leads to manifest diplopia. In rare cases these individuals have required strabismus surgery. A thorough history is required to elicit any history of eye muscle imbalance issues as a child or at any point during adulthood. These include a history of a "lazy eye," patching at any point, or episodes of diplopia in adulthood. Even patients with a history of successful strabismus surgery without diplopia are generally not good candidates for monovision.

Monovision Reversal

If a patient cannot tolerate monovision after a reasonable amount of time postoperatively, usually 6 to 12 weeks or more, then surgical reversal of monovision through LVC retreatment can be performed. Surgical risks are similar to original surgery; however, LASIK retreatment carries an increased risk of epithelial ingrowth, and patients should be counseled about this risk.

For previously emmetropic or hyperopic patients, the original hyperopic ablation pattern used to induce myopia must be counteracted by a new myopic ablation to restore emmetropia. For most individuals, this is still a reasonable option; however, there might be greater potential for irregular astigmatism with this ablation approach.

Surgical Alternatives to Monovision

In the United States, the only current alternatives to monovision with excimer laser surgery are conductive keratoplasty and refractive lens exchange with either a multifocal or pseudoaccommodating IOL. Outside of the United States, a variety of corneal inlays are being used clinically to improve near visual acuity in one eye, and these may be available in the near future. Multifocal corneal ablation is also being performed, although results to date are mixed, and an increased rate of loss of best corrected visual acuity has been reported.

Bibliography

Alarcon A, Anera RG, Villa C, Jimenez del Barco L, Gutierrez R. Visual quality after monovision correction by laser in situ keratomileusis in presbyopic patients. *J Cataract Refract Surg.* 2011;37(9):1629-1635.

Braun EH, Lee J, Steinert RF. Monovision in LASIK. *Ophthalmology.* 2008;115(7):1196-1202.

Farid M, Steinert RF. Patient selection for monovision laser refractive surgery. *Curr Opin Ophthalmol.* 2009;20(4):251-254.

Fawcett SL, Herman WK, Alfieri CD, Castleberry KA, Parks MM, Birch EE. Stereoacuity and foveal fusion in adults with long-standing surgical monovision. *JAAPOS.* 2001;5(6):342-347.

Finkelman YM, Ng JQ, Barrett GD. Patient satisfaction and visual function after pseudophakic monovision. *J Cataract Refract Surg.* 2009;35(6):998-1002.

Garcia-Gonzalez M, Teus MA, Hernandez-Verdejo JL. Visual outcomes of LASIK-induced monovision in myopic patients with presbyopia. *Am J Ophthalmol.* 2010;150(3):381-386.

Ghanem RC, de la Cruz J, Tobaigy FM, Ang LP, Azar DT. LASIK in the presbyopic age group: safety, efficacy, and predictability in 40- to 69-year-old patients. *Ophthalmology.* 2007;114(7):1303-1310.

Goldberg DB. Comparison of myopes and hyperopes after laser in situ keratomileusis monovision. *J Cataract Refract Surg.* 2003;29(9):1695-1701.

Hayashi K, Yoshida M, Manabe S, Hayashi H. Optimal amount of anisometropia for pseudophakic monovision. *J Refract Surg.* 2011;27(5):332-338.

Reilly CD, Lee WB, Alvarenga L, Caspar J, Garcia-Ferrer F, Mannis MJ. Surgical monovision and monovision reversal in LASIK. *Cornea.* 2006;25(2):136-138.

Seijas O, Gomez de Liano P, Gomez de Liano R, Roberts CJ, Piedrahita E, Diaz E. Ocular dominance diagnosis and its influence in monovision. *Am J Ophthalmol.* 2007;144:(2)209-216.

Waring GO IV, Klyce SD. Corneal inlays for the treatment of presbyopia. *Int Ophthalmol Clin.* 2011;51(2):51-62.

Wright KW, Guemes A, Kapadia MS, Wilson SE. Binocular function and patient satisfaction after monovision induced by myopic photorefractive keratectomy. *J Cataract Refract Surg.* 1999;25(2):177-182.

Xiao J, Jiang C, Zhang M. Visual outcomes of LASIK-induced monovision in myopic patients with presbyopia. *Am J Ophthalmol.* 2011;151(3):557; author reply 557-558.

Zhang F, Sugar A, Jacobsen G, Collins M. Visual function and patient satisfaction: Comparison between bilateral diffractive multifocal intraocular lenses and monovision pseudophakia. *J Cataract Refract Surg.* 2011;37(3):446-453.

—CASE 5—

A 43-year-old year old female seeks refractive surgery. Past ocular history is significant for strabismus surgery 10 years ago, with persistent intermittent diplopia, which is longstanding and unchanging over time.

CASE HISTORY		
	Right Eye	**Left Eye**
Present correction	Soft CTL and spectacles	Soft CTL and spectacles
Manifest refraction	-6.00 +0.50 x 121	-5.75 +1.75 x 065
CDVA (current)	20/20	20/20
CNVA (current)	20/20	20/20
Near add	+1.00	+1.00
Cycloplegic refraction	-5.50 +0.50 x 125	-5.00 +1.75 x 065
Dominant eye	Right	
Ocular alignment	Intermittent exotropia (slight)	Intermittent exotropia (slight)
Keratometry		
Flat K	44.9 @ 022	44.2 @ 160
Steep K	46.5 @ 112	47.0 @ 070
Pupil size (bright)	4.5 mm	4.5 mm
Pupil size (dim)	6.5 mm	6.3 mm
Central corneal thickness	524 μm	528 μm
Physical examination	Normal	Normal
Estimated ablation depth	85 μm	85 μm

QUESTIONS

1. What elements of the history and physical examination are the most critical to determine this patient's surgical candidacy and establish the refractive goal?
2. What, if any, additional information would you to like to have before making your surgical decision?
3. What would be your discussion regarding monovision for this patient?
4. What element of the patient's history could you elicit that would make you more comfortable offering the patient a wider variety of refractive surgical goal options?
5. How does the patient's cycloplegic refraction affect your decision and management in this case?

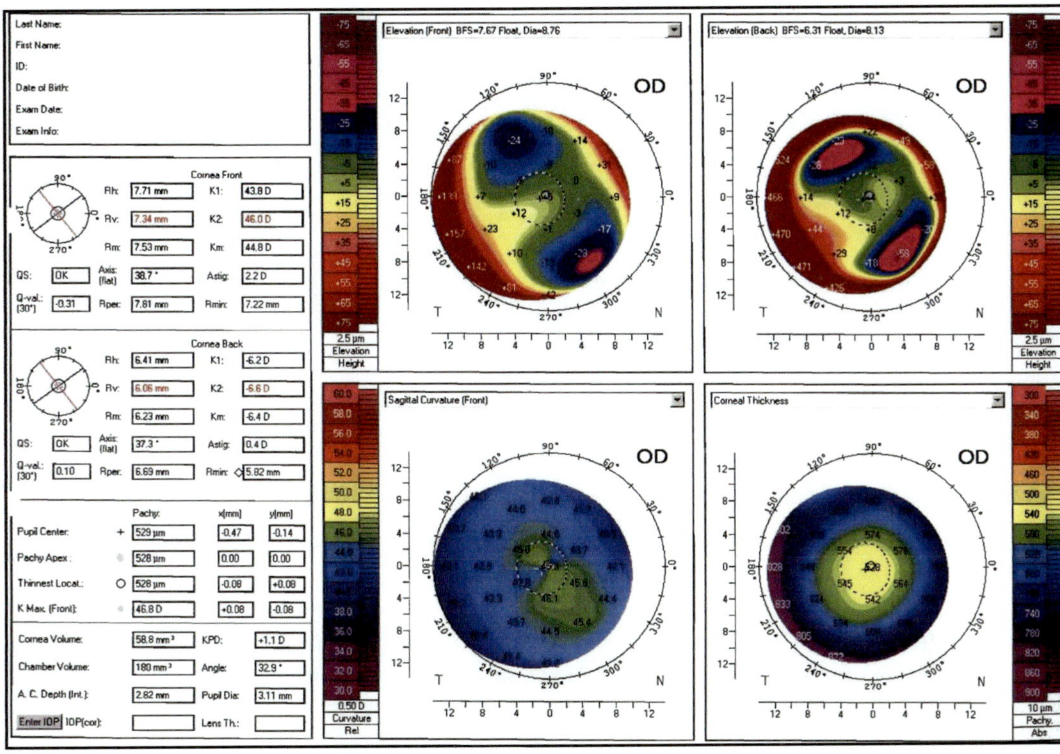
Last Name:
First Name:
ID:
Date of Birth:
Exam Date:
Exam Info:
Cornea Front
Rh: 7.71 mm K1: 43.8 D
Rv: 7.34 mm K2: 46.0 D
Rm: 7.53 mm Km: 44.8 D
QS: OK Axis: (flat) 38.7 ° Astig: 2.2 D
Q-val.: (30°) -0.31 Rper: 7.81 mm Rmin: 7.22 mm
Cornea Back
Rh: 6.41 mm K1: -6.2 D
Rv: 6.06 mm K2: -6.6 D
Rm: 6.23 mm Km: -6.4 D
QS: OK Axis: (flat) 37.3 ° Astig: 0.4 D
Q-val.: (30°) 0.10 Rper: 6.69 mm Rmin: 5.82 mm
Pachy: x[mm] y[mm]
Pupil Center: + 529 µm -0.47 -0.14
Pachy Apex: 528 µm 0.00 0.00
Thinnest Locat.: O 528 µm -0.08 +0.08
K Max. (Front): 46.8 D +0.08 -0.08
Cornea Volume: 58.8 mm³ KPD: +1.1 D
Chamber Volume: 180 mm³ Angle: 32.9 °
A. C. Depth (Int.): 2.82 mm Pupil Dia: 3.11 mm
Enter IOP IOP(cor): Lens Th.:
Elevation (Front) BFS=7.67 Float, Dia=8.76
Elevation (Back) BFS=6.31 Float, Dia=8.13
Sagittal Curvature (Front)
Corneal Thickness
OD
T
N
2.5 µm Elevation Height
0.50 D Curvature Rel
10 µm Pachy. Abs

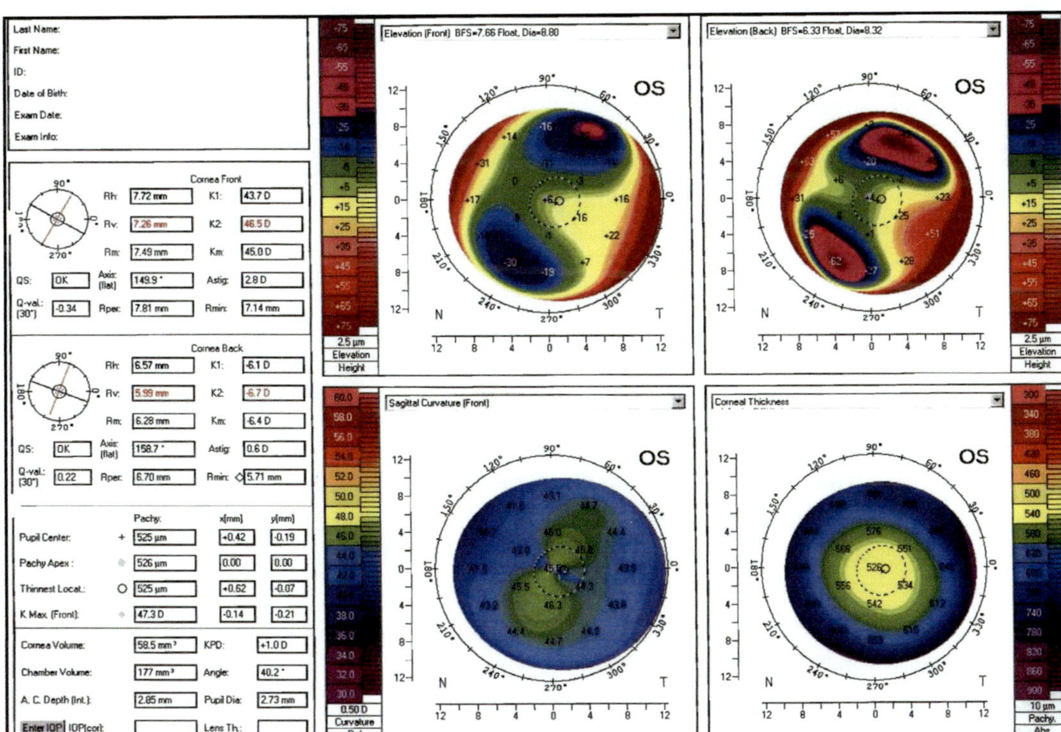
Last Name:
First Name:
ID:
Date of Birth:
Exam Date:
Exam Info:
Cornea Front
Rh: 7.72 mm K1: 43.7 D
Rv: 7.26 mm K2: 46.5 D
Rm: 7.49 mm Km: 45.0 D
QS: OK Axis: (flat) 149.9 ° Astig: 2.8 D
Q-val.: (30°) -0.34 Rper: 7.81 mm Rmin: 7.14 mm
Cornea Back
Rh: 6.57 mm K1: -6.1 D
Rv: 5.99 mm K2: -6.7 D
Rm: 6.28 mm Km: -6.4 D
QS: OK Axis: (flat) 158.7 ° Astig: 0.6 D
Q-val.: (30°) 0.22 Rper: 6.70 mm Rmin: 5.71 mm
Pachy: x[mm] y[mm]
Pupil Center: + 525 µm +0.42 -0.19
Pachy Apex: 526 µm 0.00 0.00
Thinnest Locat.: O 525 µm +0.62 -0.07
K Max. (Front): 47.3 D -0.14 -0.21
Cornea Volume: 58.5 mm³ KPD: +1.0 D
Chamber Volume: 177 mm³ Angle: 40.2 °
A. C. Depth (Int.): 2.85 mm Pupil Dia: 2.73 mm
Enter IOP IOP(cor): Lens Th.:
Elevation (Front) BFS=7.66 Float, Dia=8.80
Elevation (Back) BFS=6.33 Float, Dia=8.32
Sagittal Curvature (Front)
Corneal Thickness
OS
N
T
2.5 µm Elevation Height
0.50 D Curvature Rel
10 µm Pachy. Abs

—CASE 5—
Binocular Diplopia After LASIK

Binocular diplopia is a rare phenomenon after refractive surgery, but it can occasionally manifest in patients with or without a history of strabismus. Issues leading to monocular diplopia are more familiar to most refractive surgeons; however, it is imperative to consider the potential for binocular diplopia after surgery in at-risk individuals.

Case Analysis

- The estimated residual stromal bed (RSB) thickness is 320 to 340 μm for both eyes.
- Case Figures show normal topographies with symmetric bowtie patterns and good corneal thicknesses.

Pearl: *Screen diligently for any history of strabismus or diplopia, even if there is a remote chance of its presence, look for prism in current spectacles, and if any phoria is detected, beware of myopes with exophorias and hyperopes with esophorias wearing spectacles only!*

QUESTIONS

1. What elements of the history and physical examination are the most critical to determine this patient's surgical candidacy and establish the refractive goal?

   The patient has a history of strabismus surgery with persistent, but tolerable, and stable intermittent diplopia.

2. What, if any, additional information would you like to have before making your surgical decision?

   Check for prism in spectacles. Confirm that diplopia is equal with spectacles and contact lenses. Discuss the patient's willingness to wear spectacles for near vision and with prisms as needed postoperatively if diplopia worsens over time.

3. What would be your discussion regarding monovision for this patient?

   This patient is NOT a monovision candidate due to the increased risk of constant diplopia after anisometropic dissociation.

4. What element of the patient's history could you elicit that would make you more comfortable offering the patient a wider variety of refractive surgical goal options?

   If the patient had been a long-term monovision contact lens wearer with no issues, one might consider offering monovision LASIK or surface ablation.

5. How does the patient's cycloplegic refraction affect your decision and management in this case?

   The fact that the manifest and cycloplegic refractions are nearly equivalent means that the current spectacle prescription is not designed specifically to reduce diplopia.

Diplopia After LASIK

Binocular diplopia after LASIK can result from dissociation of previously well-controlled phorias with or without fixation scotomas, alteration of suppression scotomas from unilateral refractive amblyopia surgical correction (potentially inducing aniseikonia by treating significant anisometropia in patients without diplopia), or most commonly, after monovision LASIK, resulting in dissociation in unidentified at-risk individuals.

When screening for individuals at risk for diplopia after refractive surgery, be sure to ascertain a full history of possible symptoms with current corrective methods. Although contact lenses and spectacles should theoretically have the same impact on diplopia, some patients seem to report better strabismic control in spectacles, despite the absence of prisms in them. If patients with slight exophorias are overminused, the resulting increased accommodation required for best visual acuity might also improve ocular alignment. Patients with slight esophorias who are maximally plussed (wearing the maximal tolerated hyperopic correction may benefit from relaxed accommodation). From a refractive surgery perspective, this could prove important for myopes with exophorias and hyperopes with esophorias, where their current refraction may be facilitating strabismus control, in addition to emmetropia. Finally, be careful to screen for prism in current spectacles, as patients may forget to mention this or not be aware if its presence.

If patients with a history of strabismus or a notable phoria/tropia on examination have been successful longstanding contact lens wearers, refractive surgery is unlikely to induce diplopia as long as both eyes are targeted for distance. Monovision is NOT recommended for any individuals with any history of diplopia, strabismus, or a notable phoria on examination unless they have been successful monovision contact lens wearers for a long period of time without difficulty, as the dissociation due to anisometropia may be enough to manifest diplopia in these individuals.

Patients with any suspicion for strabismus risk may be less tolerant of even mild ametropia postoperatively, especially undercorrection of their refractive error. These individuals may require retreatment for the residual errors that are tolerated by other individuals.

The following figure provides a decision tree for determining suitability for LVC in patients at increased risk for diplopia.

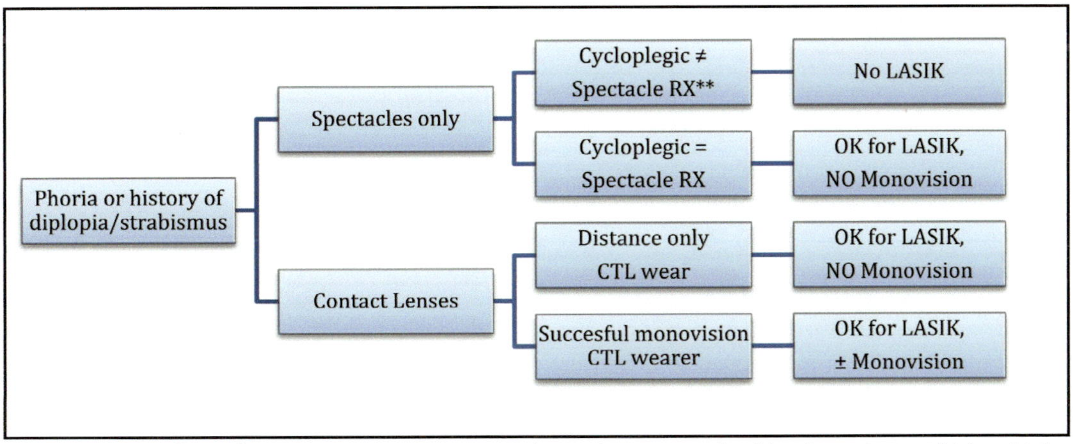

Case Figure 5-1. The evaluation tree represents a screening and treatment algorithm for patients at higher risk for binocular diplopia after corneal refractive surgery. Asterisks denote the cycloplegic examination demonstrating that myopia is overminused or at absolute hyperopia as discussed previously.

Bibliography

Godts D, Tassignon MJ, Gobin L. Binocular vision impairment after refractive surgery. *J Cataract Refract Surg.* 2004;30(1):101-109.

Godts D, Trau R, Tassignon MJ. Effect of refractive surgery on binocular vision and ocular alignment in patients with manifest or intermittent strabismus. *Br J Ophthalmol.* 2006;90(11):1410-1413.

Gunton KB, Armstrong B. Diplopia in adult patients following cataract extraction and refractive surgery. *Curr Opin Ophthalmol.* 2010;21(5):341-344.

Holland D, Amm M, de Decker W. Persisting diplopia after bilateral laser in situ keratomileusis. *J Cataract Refract Surg.* 2000;26(10):1555-1557.

Kirwan C, O'Keefe M, O'Mullane GM, Sheehan C. Refractive surgery in patients with accommodative and non-accommodative strabismus: 1-year prospective follow-up. *Br J Ophthalmol.* 2010;94(7):898-902.

Kowal L. Refractive surgery and diplopia. *Clin Experiment Ophthalmol.* 2000;28(5):344-346.

Kushner BJ, Kowal L. Diplopia after refractive surgery: occurrence and prevention. *Arch Ophthalmol.* 2003;121(3):315-321.

Pollard ZF, Greenberg MF, Bordenca M, Elliott J, Hsu V. Strabismus precipitated by monovision. *Am J Ophthalmol.* 2011;152(3):479-482.

Schuler E, Silverberg M, Beade P, Moadel K. Decompensated strabismus after laser in situ keratomileusis. *J Cataract Refract Surg.* 1999;25(11):1552-1553.

Snir M, Kremer I, Weinberger D, Sherf I, Axer-Siegel R. Decompensation of exodeviation after corneal refractive surgery for moderate to high myopia. *Ophthalmic Surg Lasers Imaging.* 2003;34(5):363-370.

Yildirim R, Oral Y, Uzun A. Exodeviation following monocular myopic regression after laser in situ keratomileusis. *J Cataract Refract Surg.* 2003;29(5):103.

—Case 6—

A 38-year-old female presents for refractive surgical evaluation. She complains that vision in her left eye has been "not good" for as long as she can remember, and she has never felt the vision was "as it should be" with any type of corrective lenses. She does not anticipate getting great vision in her left eye with surgery, but some of her friends have had monovision with contact lenses or surgery, and she is curious if she could have surgery so that her left eye could become her "near" eye for the future.

CASE HISTORY		
	Right Eye	**Left Eye**
UDVA	20/25	20/400
Present correction	None	None
Manifest refraction	-0.75 +0.75 x 150	-5.00 +3.00 x 040
CDVA (current)	20/20	20/40
UNVA	20/20	20/40
Cycloplegic refraction	-0.75 +0.75 x 150	-5.00 +3.00 x 040
Dominant eye	Right	
Ocular alignment	Orthophoric	Orthophoric
Keratometry		
Flat K	42.7 @ 040	41.4 @ 120
Steep K	43.9 @ 130	45.5 @ 030
Pupil size (bright)	4.5 mm	4.3 mm
Pupil size (dim)	7.0 mm	6.8 mm
Central corneal thickness	512 µm	512 µm
Physical examination	Normal	Normal
Estimated ablation depth	15 µm	80 µm

Questions

1. Is this patient a candidate for refractive surgery? If so, what treatment options are available?
2. Considering all factors, what plan would you recommend and why?
3. What are the most significant potential complications for this patient?

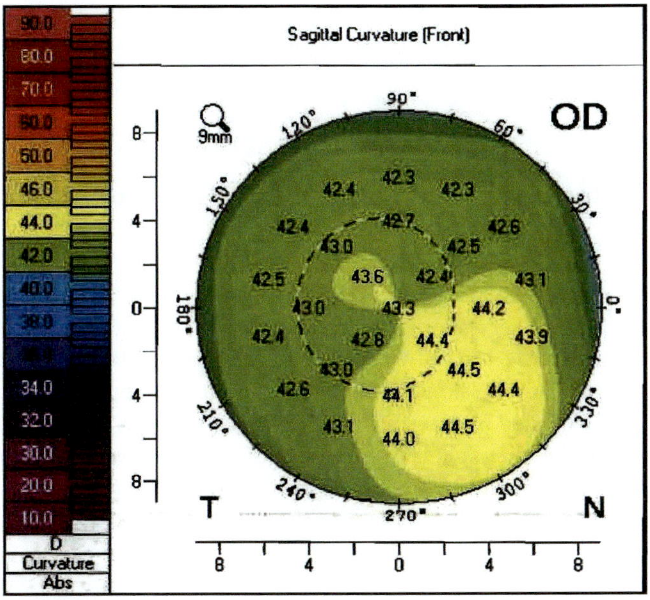
Sagittal Curvature (Front)
OD
9mm
T
N
D
Curvature
Abs

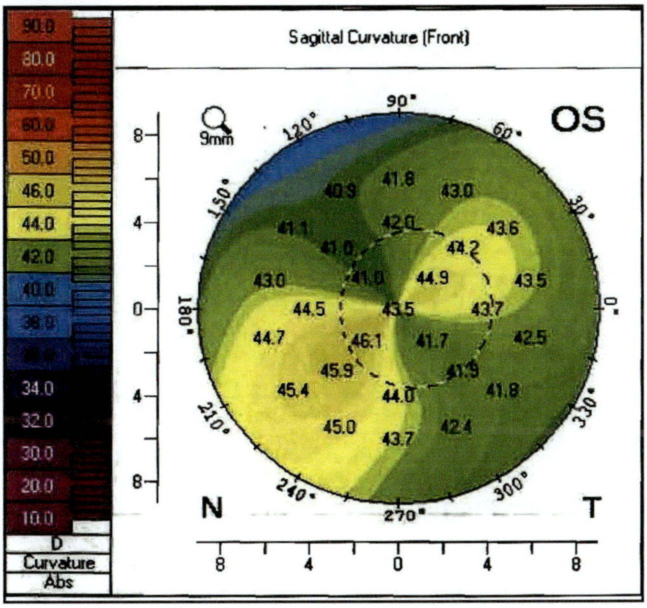
Sagittal Curvature (Front)
OS
9mm
N
T
D
Curvature
Abs

—Case 6—

Amblyopia

Refractive Surgery Considerations

Refractive surgery on adult patients with amblyopia remains controversial. Although conceptually it may seem that surgery should not be offered to any patient with amblyopia, in some situations patients may benefit, from both a functional and safety standpoint, and the decision for surgery is a unique, detailed discussion between the patient and surgeon in these cases. A different screening approach is needed to determine the patient's eligibility for surgery in the amblyopic and nonamblyopic eye, and asthenopia is a major consideration when considering improvement of the amblyopic eye. The degree of amblyopia and the history of refractive correction in the past are major factors in making the determination about surgery.

Case Analysis

- The estimated residual stromal bed (RSB) thickness is 310 to 330 µm in the left eye.
- Case Figures show asymmetric topographies in both eyes, with focal steepening inferonasally in the right eye and oblique asymmetric steepening in the left eye.

Pearl: *Treating patients with significant unilateral amblyopia remains highly controversial, but if you are considering it, beware of induced aniseikonia!*

Questions

1. Is this patient a candidate for refractive surgery? If so, what treatment options are available?

   This patient is technically a candidate for either surface ablation or LASIK, but she is probably not an optimal candidate for either. She has no experience with corrective lenses in her left eye and has amblyopia significant enough that her left eye would not be able to function adequately for monovision.

2. Considering all factors, what plan would you recommend and why?

   If the patient is highly motivated, she should have an extended contact lens trial using various corrective strategies for the left eye (full distance and monovision) to determine how well she tolerates correction and if it provides functional acuity for her.

3. What are the most significant potential complications for this patient?

   If this longstanding refractive error is corrected, the patient may develop diplopia or aniseikonia if she is no longer able to suppress the blurred left eye image.

When to Consider Refractive Surgery in Patients With Amblyopia

Reasons to Operate on Patients With Amblyopia

- Contact lens intolerance
- Anisometropia that is not amenable to spectacle correction
- High corrections with poor functional spectacle visual acuity
- Potential for improved visual acuity
- Patient choice to avoid spectacle wear even when counseled to do so

The surgical correction of ametropia in children with amblyopia is a completely different subject, with different indications, and is beyond the scope of this book. For adults, refractive surgery in patients with amblyopia is a controversial topic. Many studies have found improvement in acuity in the amblyopic eye. In patients with high myopia, improvement may come from functional enlargement of the image on the retina.

Refractive surgery in the nonamblyopic eye is a different issue altogether. Approximately 50% of the American Society of Cataract and Refractive Surgery (ASCRS) surgeons in past surveys have supported operating on the better-seeing eye in an amblyopic patient with 20/50 or worse visual acuity on the amblyopic eye under select circumstances. However, there are relative contraindications to some surgical approaches in these patients, as well as specific complications, to be considered.

Although spectacle wear with polycarbonate lenses remains the safest approach to ametropia correction in amblyopia, in reality, many patients simply refuse to wear spectacles (even when counseled to do so), and in some instances, including significant anisometropia or high corrections, spectacle correction is suboptimal or not feasible. In these instances, both laser vision correction and phakic intraocular implantation may be viable options.

When Not to Consider Refractive Surgery in Patients With Amblyopia

Refractive Surgical Approaches to Avoid in Amblyopic Patients

- Monovision
- Surgical correction that may induce asthenopia or aniseikonia

Monovision correction is a poor choice for amblyopic patients. For most patients, the treatment will be unsuccessful because the amblyopic eye does not have the ability to function adequately at any distance independently, and some patients may develop diplopia from the decreased ability to fuse disparate images or from the loss of blur suppression from the amblyopic eye.

Bibliography

Arruabarrena C, Teus MA, Hernández-Verdejo JL, Cañones R. Visual acuity after laser in situ keratomileusis to correct high astigmatism in adults with meridional amblyopia. *Am J Ophthalmol.* 2011;152(6):964-968.

Barequet IS, Wygnanski-Jaffe T, Hirsh A. Laser in situ keratomileusis improves visual acuity in some adult eyes with amblyopia. *J Refract Surg.* 2004;20(1):25-28.

Holland D, Amm M, de Decker W. Persisting diplopia after bilateral laser in situ keratomileusis. *J Cataract Refract Surg.* 2000;26(10):1555-1557.

Kowal L. Refractive surgery and diplopia. Clin Experiment *Ophthalmol.* 2000;28(5):344-346.

Oruçoğlu-Orucov F, Frucht-Pery J, Landau D, Strasman E, Solomon A. LASIK correction of vision in adults with unilateral amblyopia. *J Refract Surg.* 2011;27(1):18-22.

Paciuc M. Amblyopic adult eyes after LASIK. *J Cataract Refract Surg.* 2005;31(12):2244-2245.

Prakash G, Choudhary V, Sharma N, Titiyal JS. Change in the accommodative convergence per unit of accommodation ratio after bilateral laser in situ keratomileusis for myopia in orthotropic patients: prospective evaluation. *J Cataract Refract Surg.* 2007;33(12):2054-2056.

Sakatani K, Jabbur NS, O'Brien TP. Improvement in best corrected visual acuity in amblyopic adult eyes after laser in situ keratomileusis. *J Cataract Refract Surg.* 2004;30(12):2517-2521.

Vuori E, Tervo TM, Holopainen MV, Holopainen JM. Improvement of visual acuity following refractive surgery for myopia and myopic anisometropia. *J Refract Surg.* 2007;23(5):447-455.

—Case 7—

A 28-year-old female desires refractive surgical correction. She has no significant family, past medical, or ocular history.

CASE HISTORY		
	Right Eye	**Left Eye**
Present correction method	CTL	CTL
Manifest refraction	-6.00 +0.75 x 095	-6.25 +0.50 x 110
CDVA (current)	20/20	20/20
UNVA (current)	20/20	20/20
Dominant eye	Right	
Keratometry		
Flat K	39.2 @ 006	39.6 @ 030
Steep K	40.5 @ 096	40.2 @ 120
Pupil size (bright)	4.1 mm	4.0 mm
Pupil size (dim)	5.8 mm	6.1 mm
Central corneal thickness	558 μm	559 μm
Physical examination	Normal	Normal
Estimated ablation depth	100 μm	100 μm

Questions

1. Is this patient a candidate for refractive surgery? If so, what treatment options are available?
2. Considering all factors, what procedure would you recommend and why?
3. What special considerations are there for this patient regarding the potential quality of vision after surgery?
4. What special considerations are there for this patient regarding the potential retreatment for postoperative ametropia?

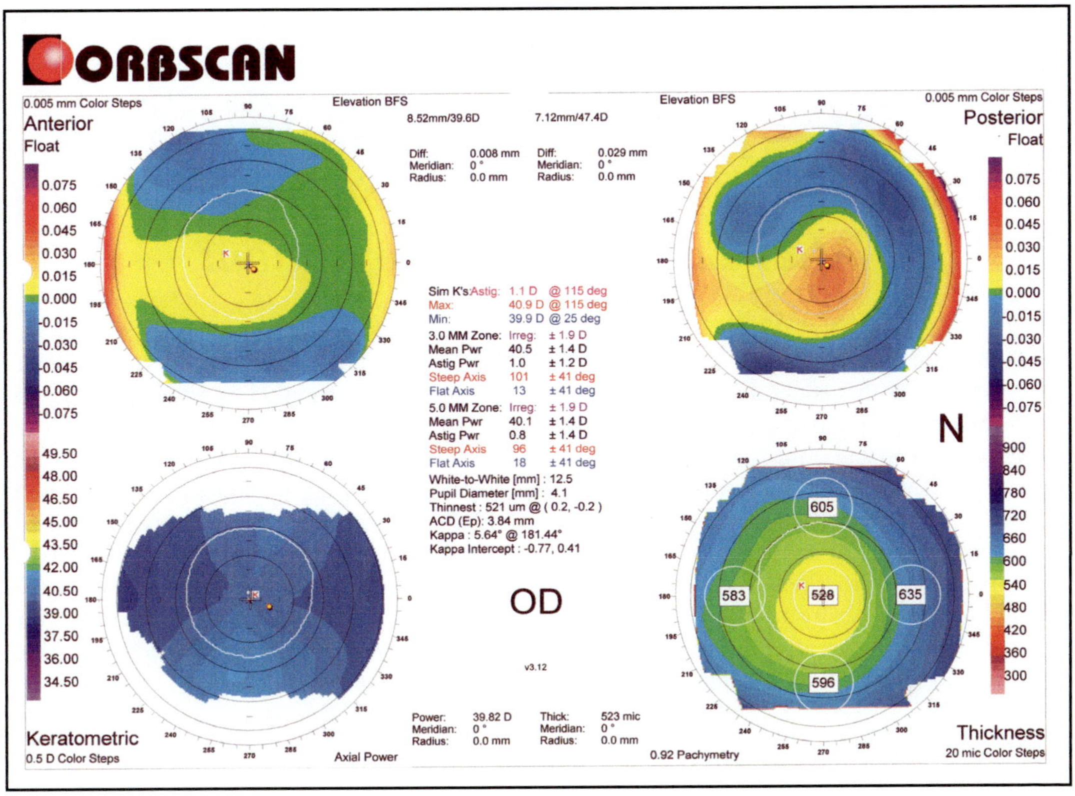
ORBSCAN
0.005 mm Color Steps
Anterior
Float
Elevation BFS
8.52mm/39.6D
7.12mm/47.4D
Diff: 0.008 mm
Meridian: 0 °
Radius: 0.0 mm
Diff: 0.029 mm
Meridian: 0 °
Radius: 0.0 mm
Elevation BFS
0.005 mm Color Steps
Posterior
Float
Sim K's Astig: 1.1 D @ 115 deg
Max: 40.9 D @ 115 deg
Min: 39.9 D @ 25 deg
3.0 MM Zone: Irreg: ± 1.9 D
Mean Pwr 40.5 ± 1.4 D
Astig Pwr 1.0 ± 1.2 D
Steep Axis 101 ± 41 deg
Flat Axis 13 ± 41 deg
5.0 MM Zone: Irreg: ± 1.9 D
Mean Pwr 40.1 ± 1.4 D
Astig Pwr 0.8 ± 1.4 D
Steep Axis 96 ± 41 deg
Flat Axis 18 ± 41 deg
White-to-White [mm] : 12.5
Pupil Diameter [mm] : 4.1
Thinnest : 521 um @ (0.2, -0.2)
ACD (Ep): 3.84 mm
Kappa : 5.64° @ 181.44°
Kappa Intercept : -0.77, 0.41
OD
v3.12
N
605
583
528
635
596
Keratometric
0.5 D Color Steps
Axial Power
Power: 39.82 D
Meridian: 0 °
Radius: 0.0 mm
Thick: 523 mic
Meridian: 0 °
Radius: 0.0 mm
0.92 Pachymetry
Thickness
20 mic Color Steps

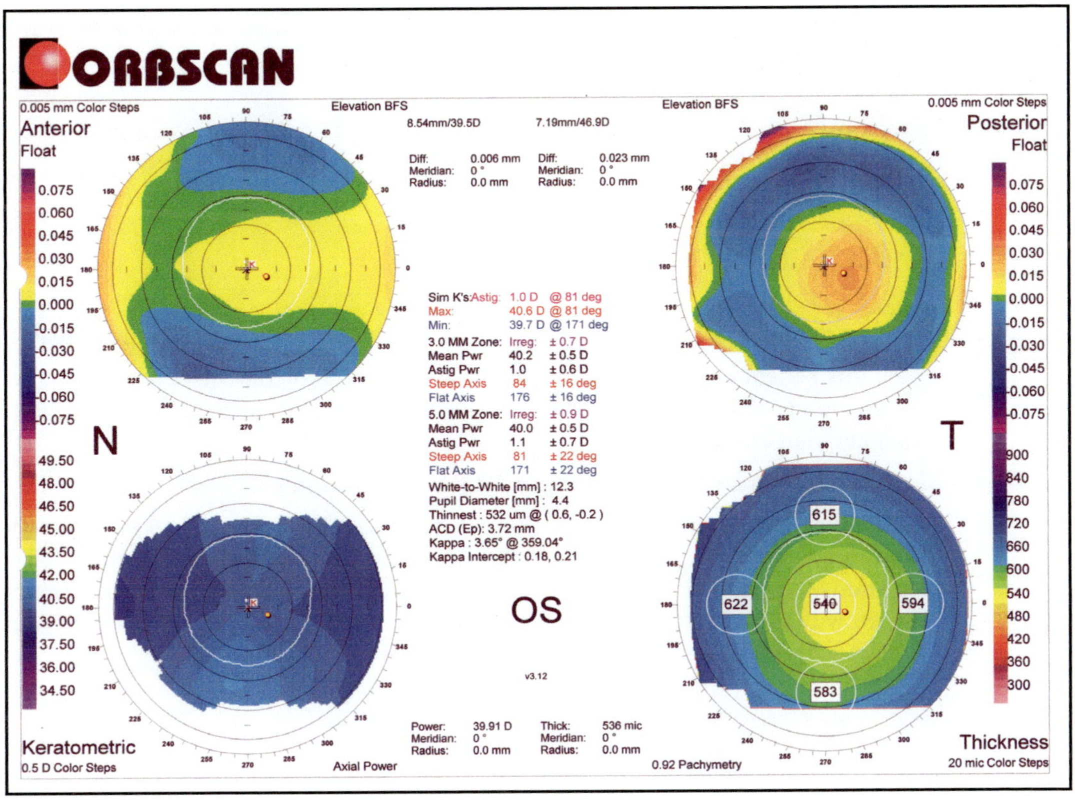
ORBSCAN
0.005 mm Color Steps
Anterior
Float
Elevation BFS
8.54mm/39.5D
7.19mm/46.9D
Diff: 0.006 mm
Meridian: 0 °
Radius: 0.0 mm
Diff: 0.023 mm
Meridian: 0 °
Radius: 0.0 mm
Elevation BFS
0.005 mm Color Steps
Posterior
Float
Sim K's Astig: 1.0 D @ 81 deg
Max: 40.6 D @ 81 deg
Min: 39.7 D @ 171 deg
3.0 MM Zone: Irreg: ± 0.7 D
Mean Pwr 40.2 ± 0.5 D
Astig Pwr 1.0 ± 0.6 D
Steep Axis 84 ± 16 deg
Flat Axis 176 ± 16 deg
5.0 MM Zone: Irreg: ± 0.9 D
Mean Pwr 40.0 ± 0.5 D
Astig Pwr 1.1 ± 0.7 D
Steep Axis 81 ± 22 deg
Flat Axis 171 ± 22 deg
White-to-White [mm] : 12.3
Pupil Diameter [mm] : 4.4
Thinnest : 532 um @ (0.6, -0.2)
ACD (Ep): 3.72 mm
Kappa : 3.65° @ 359.04°
Kappa Intercept : 0.18, 0.21
OS
v3.12
N
T
615
622
540
594
583
Keratometric
0.5 D Color Steps
Axial Power
Power: 39.91 D
Meridian: 0 °
Radius: 0.0 mm
Thick: 536 mic
Meridian: 0 °
Radius: 0.0 mm
0.92 Pachymetry
Thickness
20 mic Color Steps

—CASE 7—

Steep and Flat Corneas

How Flat Is Too Flat and How Steep Is Too Steep After Laser Vision Correction?

Among the many concepts of which to be mindful when screening patients for refractive surgery, any factors that could decrease visual quality postoperatively should be considered. Over the years, much discussion and anecdotal reports have surrounded the topic of final keratometry (K) values and the visual impact of creating a cornea that is "too flat" or "too steep" with laser vision correction (LVC). Many practitioners follow the dogma of keeping postoperative keratometry above 35.00 diopters (D) for myopic treatments and less than 50.00 D for hyperopic treatments; however, there are little scientific data available to support these concepts for myopic corrections. Recently, some researchers have reported a correlation between initial keratometry >44.00 D or worse final visual acuity and patient satisfaction for hyperopic corrections. Thus, perhaps making the cornea "too steep" after hyperopic ablation does reduce visual quality and refractive stability; however, no specific final K value is definitive.

Case Analysis

- The estimated residual stromal bed (RSB) thickness is >330 to 350 µm in both eyes.
- Case Figures show normal topographies in both eyes with a central K ≈40.00 D in both eyes and good corneal thickness in both eyes.

Pearl: *Little clinical evidence exists to support making decisions based on postoperative flat keratometry!*

QUESTIONS

1. Is this patient a candidate for refractive surgery? If so, what treatment options are available?

   Yes, this patient appears to be a reasonable candidate for refractive surgery. In her prescription range, LASIK, surface ablation, and phakic intraocular lens (PIOL) implantation are all options.

2. Considering all factors, what procedure would you recommend and why?

   Given the normal topography, an otherwise normal examination, and her prescription range, all options produce similar results; thus, I would recommend surface ablation or LASIK. The only potential concern for LVC is postoperative keratometry, which will be ≈35.00 D (discussed later in this case). Phakic IOLs avoid change in corneal curvature but carry increased intraocular complication risks.

3. What special considerations are there for this patient regarding the potential quality of vision after surgery?

   There is a purported concern with postoperative corneal curvature less than 35.00 D, which has been proposed to decrease visual quality and contrast sensitivity. However, this concern is debatable.

4. What special considerations are there for this patient regarding the potential retreatment for postoperative ametropia?

   Basic issues surrounding retreatment exist for this patient, but there do not appear to be any special considerations beyond the general risks in this case.

Change in Keratometry After Laser Vision Correction

Change in corneal curvature can be estimated by multiplying the refractive correction in diopters by 0.8. Using this case as an example:

6.00 D of myopia treated x 0.8 ≈4.80 D of central flattening;
Preoperative central K = 39.80 D, postoperative central K ≈35.00 D.

Real and Perceived Concerns When Performing Laser Vision Correction in Flatter Corneas

Intraoperative Risks

When performing LASIK with a mechanical microkeratome, flatter corneas (<40.00 D) increase the risk of creating a free cap. Adjusting the basic flap parameters, such as diameter and hinge width, can mitigate this risk. Keratometry values have minimal impact on flaps created with femtosecond lasers.

Optical Quality Effects

Although primarily theoretical, some surgeons use 35.00 D as a "cutoff" for acceptable postoperative K after myopic LASIK. There are anecdotal reports of reduced visual quality in patients with flatter K values postoperatively; however, in the available literature, these patients also had higher preoperative refractions and frequently had smaller optical zones on older excimer laser platforms with minimal peripheral ablation, both of which are known risks for postoperative glare and halos. Thus, no definitive evidence supports a specific cutoff for corneal flattening after myopic LASIK.

Real and Perceived Concerns When Performing Laser Vision Correction in Steeper Corneas

Intraoperative Risks

When performing LASIK with a mechanical microkeratome, steeper corneas (>48.00 D) increase the risk of creating a buttonhole flap. Adjusting the basic flap parameters, such as diameter and hinge width, can mitigate this risk. Keratometry values have minimal impact on flaps created with femtosecond lasers.

Steep corneas have been debated as a potential marker for keratoconus-suspect corneas. Early studies supported central K > 47.20 D as a discriminating value; however, more recent studies have not supported this specific value. However, although no specific cutoff appears valid, very steep central K values warrant additional attention when screening patients for LASIK.

Optical Quality Effects

Some recent studies have found that treating hyperopia in eyes with preoperative K > 44.00 D increases the risk of less successful visual outcomes and increases the likelihood of refractive regression. Other studies have found a correlation between the amount of hyperopia treated and the final outcomes but found no association with initial or final central steepness. Thus, caution is warranted when evaluating patients with steeper corneas before hyperopic ablation, but no firm cutoff numbers exist.

Bibliography

Ambrósio R Jr, Wilson SE. Complications of laser in situ keratomileusis: etiology, prevention, and treatment. *J Refract Surg.* 2001;17(3):350-379.

Bailey MD, Mitchell GL, Dhaliwal DK, Boxer Wachler BS, Zadnik K. Patient satisfaction and visual symptoms after laser in situ keratomileusis. *Ophthalmology.* 2003;110(7):1371-1378.

Prakash G, Agarwal A, Kumar DA, Chari M, Agarwal A, Jacob S, Srivastava D. Femtosecond sub-bowman keratomileusis: a prospective, long-term, intereye comparison of safety and outcomes of 90- versus 100-μm flaps. *Am J Ophthalmol.* 2011;152(4):582-590.e2.

Varssano D, Waisbourd M, Minkey L, Sela T, Neudorfer M, Binger PS. Visual acuity outcomes in eyes with flat corneas after PRK. *J Refract Surg.* 2013;29(6):384-389.

Williams LB, Dave SB, Moshirfar M. Correlation of visual outcome and patient satisfaction with preoperative keratometry after hyperopic laser in situ keratomileusis. *J Cataract Refract Surg.* 2008;34(7):1083-1088.

Young JJ, Schallhorn SC, Brown MC, Hettinger KA. Effect of keratometry on visual outcomes 1 month after hyperopic LASIK. *J Refract Surg.* 2009;25(7 Suppl):S672-S676.

—Case 8—

A 27-year-old male desires refractive surgical correction. He has no significant family, past medical, or ocular history.

CASE HISTORY		
	Right Eye	**Left Eye**
Present correction method	CTL	CTL
Manifest refraction	-6.25 +0.25 x 100	-7.50 +0.25 x 063
CDVA (current)	20/20	20/20
Dominant eye	Right	
Keratometry		
Flat K	43.25 @ 015	43.50 @ 157
Steep K	44.50 @ 105	44.50 @ 067
Pupil size (bright)	4.1 mm	4.0 mm
Pupil size (dim)	8.4 mm	8.0 mm
Central corneal thickness	559 µm	568 µm
Physical examination	Normal	Normal
Estimated ablation depth	100 µm	100 µm

Questions

1. Is this patient a candidate for refractive surgery? If so, what treatment options are available?
2. What unique aspects of this patient's examination warrant further discussion prior to surgery?
3. Considering all factors, what procedure would you recommend and why?
4. How might any special concerns be best avoided for this individual?

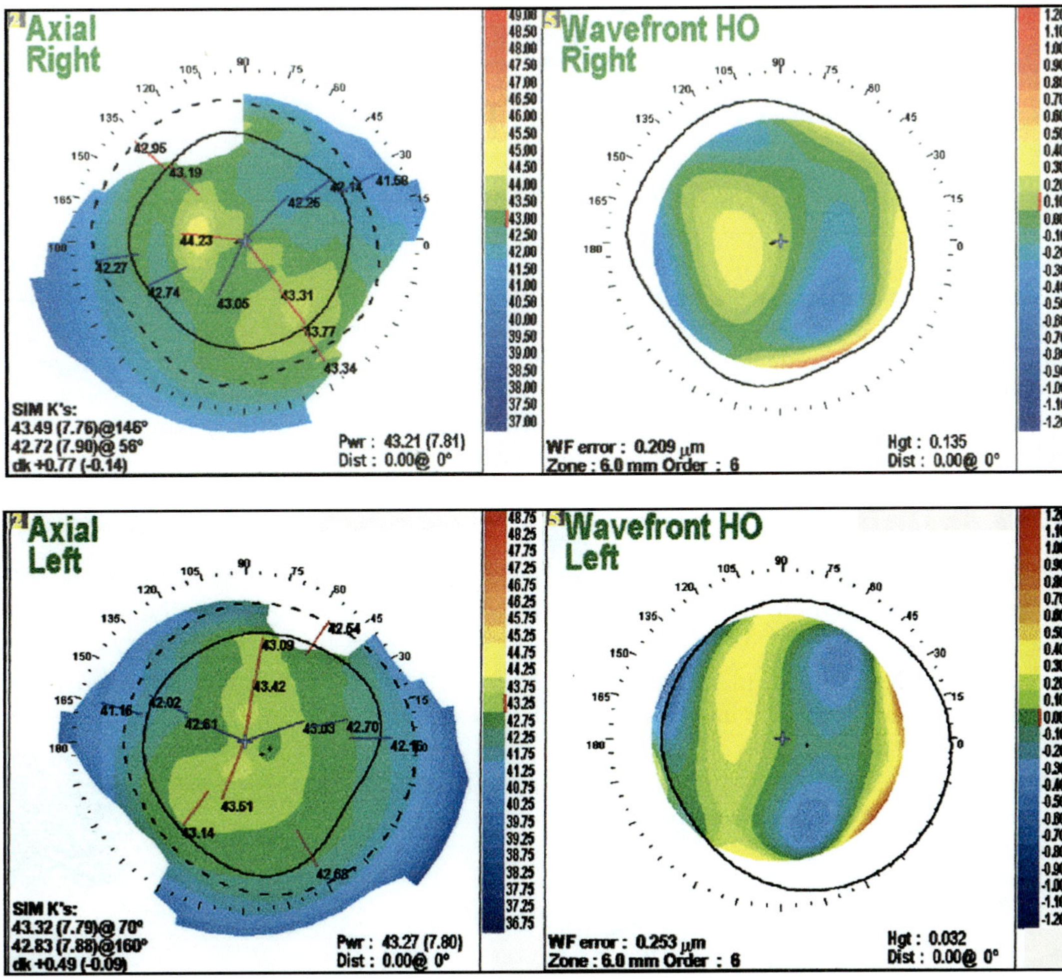
Axial
Right
SIM K's:
43.49 (7.76)@146°
42.72 (7.90)@ 56°
dk +0.77 (-0.14)
Pwr : 43.21 (7.81)
Dist : 0.00@ 0°
Wavefront HO
Right
WF error : 0.209 μm
Zone : 6.0 mm Order : 6
Hgt : 0.135
Dist : 0.00@ 0°
Axial
Left
SIM K's:
43.32 (7.79)@ 70°
42.83 (7.88)@160°
dk +0.49 (-0.09)
Pwr : 43.27 (7.80)
Dist : 0.00@ 0°
Wavefront HO
Left
WF error : 0.253 μm
Zone : 6.0 mm Order : 6
Hgt : 0.032
Dist : 0.00@ 0°

—Case 8—

Patients With Large Pupils

Special Considerations

Postoperative glare and halos have been a major potential complaint for patients undergoing both laser vision correction (LVC) and phakic intraocular lens (PIOL) implantation since the inception of these procedures. Although the incidence has reduced dramatically over the past decade with newer ablation patterns, glare and halos, generically termed as *night vision complaints* (NVC), still affect a small percentage of patients after surgery and can be highly symptomatic. The role of pupil size in this complaint has been the source of great debate and controversy.

Case Analysis

- The estimated residual stromal bed (RSB) thickness is approximately 330 to 350 μm in both eyes for a 6.5-mm optical zone (OZ) and approximately 310 to 330 μm in both eyes for a 7.0-mm OZ.
- Case Figures show normal topographies (left eye) with symmetric bowtie patterns (left image). Total HOA (right image) are between 0.20 and 0.25 μm in both eyes.

Pearl: *NVC can occur after LVC; however, to date, no clinical data support a relationship between large pupil size and NVC after LVC!*

Questions

1. Is this patient a candidate for refractive surgery? If so, what treatment options are available?

   Yes, this patient appears to be a reasonable candidate for refractive surgery. In his prescription range, LASIK, surface ablation, and phakic intraocular lens (PIOL) implantation are all options.

2. What unique aspects of this patient's examination warrant further discussion prior to surgery?

   The patient's pupils are larger than average and warrant specific discussion with regard to NVC after surgery. Although there is no evidence to support a relationship between pupil size and NVC, there is a common perception that large pupils portend an increased risk for these complaints.

3. Considering all factors, what procedure would you recommend and why?

   LASIK, surface ablation, and PIOL implantation are all options for this individual. Unless the patient had some specific motivation for photorefractive keratectomy, I would opt for LASIK. Although PIOL implantation might otherwise be a reasonable option for the patient's myopia, his dark-adapted pupil size will be larger than the IOL optic, potentiating the risk for glare and halo.

4. How might any special concerns be best avoided for this individual?

Excimer laser ablation performed with wavefront-optimized or wavefront-guided profiles will provide significantly better peripheral ablation profiles compared with conventional ablations. Further, although unproven, a larger planned optical zone (7.0 mm) may provide added benefit for this individual to minimize the potential for NVC. Larger optical zones create deeper ablations; therefore, RSB should be determined accordingly.

Night Vision Complaints After Laser Vision Correction

NVC encompass a range of reported unwanted visual phenomena such as glare, halos, starburst, and problems with night driving. Although it is quite common to notice these phenomena in the first days to weeks after LVC, with modern laser ablation profiles, they now rarely persist in the long term. Approximately 1% to 5% of patients note night vision symptoms after wavefront-optimized or wavefront-guided platforms, and a much smaller percentage note significant visual disturbances. However, these symptoms can be functionally debilitating in affected individuals.

Pupil Size and Night Vision Complaints

There may be no more controversial topic discussed in this book than the relationship, or lack thereof, between pupil size and NVC. The US Food and Drug Administration includes pupil size on their "LASIK Checklist" and cautions that large pupils can cause glare, halos, and other NVC after LASIK. However, to date, there are no well-controlled studies that have found direct associations between large pupil size and NVC after LASIK or surface ablation.

Problems with pupil size and NVC were much more common when standard excimer laser optical zones were small (approximately 5.0 mm) and had no "blend" zone, or peripheral treatment, applied outside of the optical zone. Those issues have been mitigated with wavefront-optimized and wavefront-guided ablation profiles. Multiple, well-designed studies have addressed this topic, and none have found a relationship between large pupils and NVC; some have even found an inverse relationship. Despite this, there persists an assumed association in many people's minds, including some surgeons and legal experts; therefore, the topic warrants discussion prior to surgery with patients who have larger-than-average pupils (approximately >7.0-mm dark-adapted, depending on measurement device).

Pupil size can play a role with symptoms after PIOL implantation if the dark-adapted pupil is larger than the lens optic; however, for most patients, PIOLs induce less NVC than excimer laser ablation.

Risk Factors for Night Vision Complaints After Laser Vision Correction

Known risk factors for NVC after excimer laser ablation include the high preoperative myopic error treated, residual refractive error, and small treatment optical zones (<6.0 mm). HOA also have been associated with increased NVC, especially spherical and coma aberrations.

Ablation Profiles and Night Vision Complaints

Multiple unique excimer laser ablation platforms exist today. These can be generally classified as conventional, wavefront-optimized or wavefront-guided. Conventional LASIK treatments are based on lower-order aberrations only (sphere and cylinder) and have no blend zone beyond the programmed optical zone. Wavefront-guided treatments customize ablation patterns based on higher- and lower-order aberration profiles that are unique to the eye being treated. Wavefront-optimized treatments use preprogrammed peripheral ablation profiles based on population analysis to minimize postoperative spherical aberration. Wavefront-guided treatments are designed to reduce preoperative HOAs, whereas wavefront-optimized treatments theoretically minimize the induction of postoperative HOAs. Both modalities induce significantly less postoperative HOAs compared with conventional laser ablations, which increase most HOAs. For most patients, the difference between wavefront-guided and wavefront-optimized outcomes appears minimal in patients with normal preoperative HOA profiles (< 0.3 μm).

Bibliography

Bühren J, Kühne C, Kohnen T. Influence of pupil and optical zone diameter on higher-order aberrations after wavefront-guided myopic LASIK. *J Cataract Refract Surg.* 2005;31(12):2272-2280.

Chalita MR, Chavala S, Xu M, Krueger RR. Wavefront analysis in post-LASIK eyes and its correlation with visual symptoms, refraction, and topography. *Ophthalmology.* 2004;111(3):447-453.

Chan A, Manche EE. Effect of preoperative pupil size on quality of vision after wavefront-guided LASIK. *Ophthalmology.* 2011;118(4):736-741.

Jabbur NS, Sakatani K, O'Brien TP. Survey of complications and recommendations for management in dissatisfied patients seeking a consultation after refractive surgery. *J Cataract Refract Surg.* 2004;30(9):1867-1874.

Mok KH, Lee VW. Effect of optical zone ablation diameter on LASIK-induced higher order optical aberrations. *J Refract Surg.* 2005;21(2):141-143.

Myung D, Schallhorn S, Manche EE. Pupil size and LASIK: a review. *J Refract Surg.* 2013;29(11):734-741

Padmanabhan P, Mrochen M, Basuthkar S, Viswanathan D, Joseph R. Wavefront-guided versus wavefront-optimized laser in situ keratomileusis: contralateral comparative study. *J Cataract Refract Surg.* 2008;34(3):389-397.

Perez-Straziota CE, Randleman JB, Stulting RD. Visual acuity and higher order aberrations with wavefront-guided and wavefront-optimized laser in situ keratomileusis. *J Cataract Refract Surg.* 2010;36(3):437-441.

Pop M, Payette Y. Risk factors for night vision complaints after LASIK for myopia. *Ophthalmology.* 2004;111(1):3-10.

Queirós A, Villa-Collar C, González-Méijome JM, Jorge J, Gutiérrez AR. Effect of pupil size on corneal aberrations before and after standard laser in situ keratomileusis, custom laser in situ keratomileusis, and corneal refractive therapy. *Am J Ophthalmol.* 2010;150(1):97-109.e1.

Randleman JB, Hu MH, Loft ES, Perez-Straziota CE, White AJ, Stulting RD. High order aberrations after wavefront-optimized advanced surface ablation and laser in situ keratomileusis. *J Cataract Refract Surg.* 2009;35(2):260-264.

Schallhorn S, Tanzer D, Sanders DR, Sanders M, Brown M, Kaupp SE. Night driving simulation in a randomized prospective comparison of Visian toric implantable collamer lens and conventional PRK for moderate to high myopic astigmatism. *J Refract Surg.* 2010;26(5):321-326.

Schallhorn SC, Kaupp SE, Tanzer DJ, Tidwell J, Laurent J, Bourque LB. Pupil size and quality of vision after LASIK. *Ophthalmology.* 2003;110(8):1606-1614.

Schallhorn SC, Tanzer DJ, Kaupp SE, Brown M, Malady SE. Comparison of night driving performance after wavefront-guided and conventional LASIK for moderate myopia. *Ophthalmology.* 2009;116(4):702-709.

Sharma M, Wachler BS, Chan CC. Higher order aberrations and relative risk of symptoms after LASIK. *J Refract Surg.* 2007;23(3):252-256.

Stonecipher KG, Kezirian GM. Wavefront-optimized versus wavefront-guided LASIK for myopic astigmatism with the ALLEGRETTO WAVE: three-month results of a prospective FDA trial. *J Refract Surg.* 2008;24(4):S424-S430.

—Case 9—

A 39-year-old female presents for refractive surgery evaluation. She has no significant family or past medical history. She reports 22 years of full-time soft contact lens wear, but she has experienced a significant decrease in wear time over the past year due to discomfort.

CASE HISTORY		
	Right Eye	**Left Eye**
Present correction method	Spectacles	Spectacles
Manifest refraction	-8.50 +0.50 x 100	-8.75 +0.75 x 100
CDVA (current)	$20/15^{-2}$	20/20
UNVA (current)	20/20	20/20
Near add	0	0
Dominant eye	Right	
Keratometry		
Flat K	45.25 @ 174	45.25 @ 173
Steep K	46.50 @ 084	46.75 @ 083
Pupil size (bright)	4.9 mm	4.7 mm
Pupil size (dim)	6.6 mm	6.4 mm
Central corneal thickness	523 µm	532 µm
Physical examination	See Figure	See Figure (symmetrical appearance)
Estimated ablation depth	125 µm	125 µm

Questions

1. What, if any, notable findings are present in the slit-lamp image?
2. Is this patient a candidate for refractive surgery? If so, what treatment options are available?
3. Considering all factors, what procedure would you recommend and why?

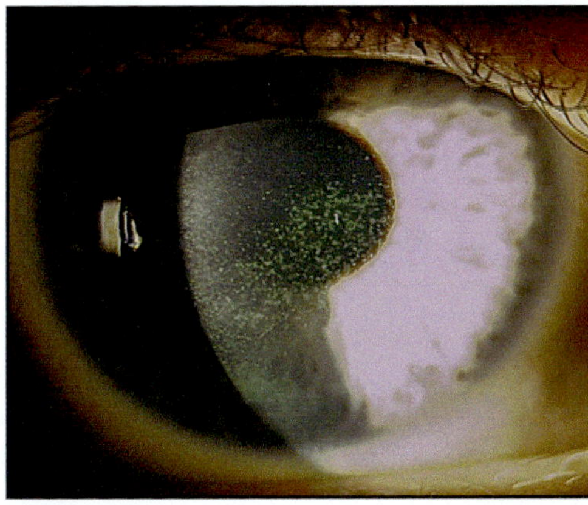

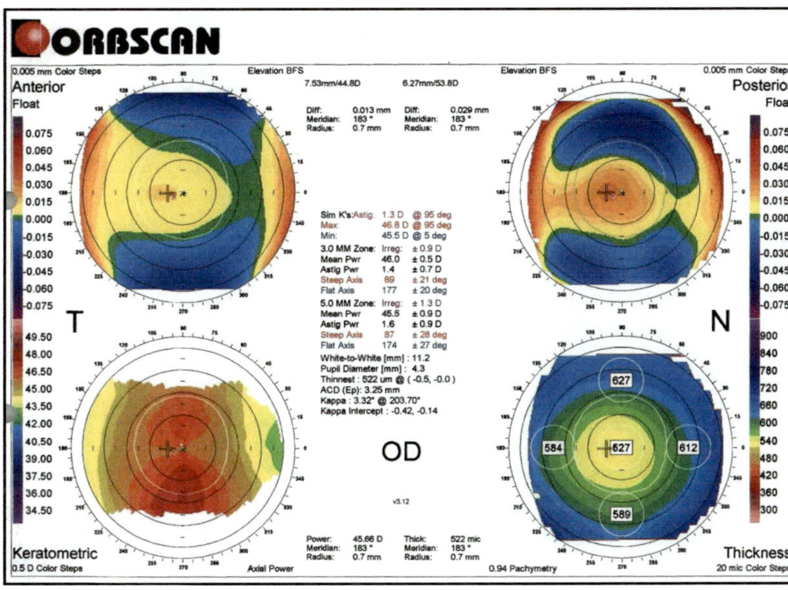
ORBSCAN
0.005 mm Color Steps
Anterior
Float
Elevation BFS
7.53mm/44.8D
6.27mm/53.8D
Diff: 0.013 mm
Meridian: 183 °
Radius: 0.7 mm
Diff: 0.029 mm
Meridian: 183 °
Radius: 0.7 mm
Posterior
Float
Sim K's:Astig: 1.3 D @ 95 deg
Max: 46.8 D @ 95 deg
Min: 45.5 D @ 5 deg
3.0 MM Zone: Irreg: ± 0.9 D
Mean Pwr 46.0 ± 0.5 D
Astig Pwr 1.4 ± 0.7 D
Steep Axis 89 ± 21 deg
Flat Axis 177 ± 20 deg
5.0 MM Zone: Irreg: ± 1.3 D
Mean Pwr 45.5 ± 0.9 D
Astig Pwr 1.6 ± 0.9 D
Steep Axis 87 ± 28 deg
Flat Axis 174 ± 27 deg
White-to-White [mm] : 11.2
Pupil Diameter [mm] : 4.3
Thinnest : 522 um @ (-0.5, -0.0)
ACD (Ep): 3.25 mm
Kappa : 3.32° @ 203.70°
Kappa Intercept : -0.42, -0.14
T
N
OD
627
584
627
612
589
v3.12
Power: 45.66 D
Meridian: 183 °
Radius: 0.7 mm
Thick: 522 mic
Meridian: 183 °
Radius: 0.7 mm
Keratometric
0.5 D Color Steps
Axial Power
0.94 Pachymetry
Thickness
20 mic Color Steps

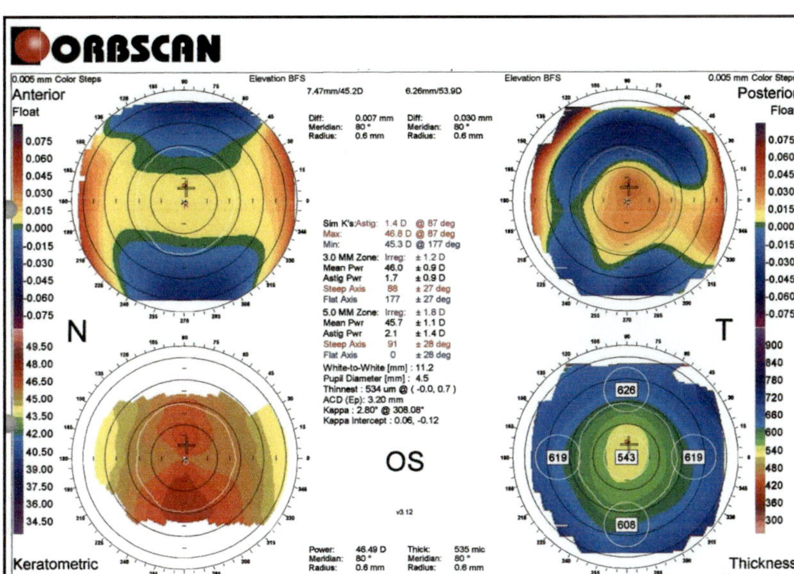
ORBSCAN
0.005 mm Color Steps
Anterior
Float
Elevation BFS
7.47mm/45.2D
6.26mm/53.9D
Diff: 0.007 mm
Meridian: 80 °
Radius: 0.6 mm
Diff: 0.030 mm
Meridian: 80 °
Radius: 0.6 mm
Posterior
Float
Sim K's:Astig: 1.4 D @ 87 deg
Max: 46.8 D @ 87 deg
Min: 45.3 D @ 177 deg
3.0 MM Zone: Irreg: ± 1.2 D
Mean Pwr 46.0 ± 0.9 D
Astig Pwr 1.7 ± 0.9 D
Steep Axis 88 ± 27 deg
Flat Axis 177 ± 27 deg
5.0 MM Zone: Irreg: ± 1.8 D
Mean Pwr 45.7 ± 1.1 D
Astig Pwr 2.1 ± 1.4 D
Steep Axis 91 ± 28 deg
Flat Axis 0 ± 28 deg
White-to-White [mm] : 11.2
Pupil Diameter [mm] : 4.5
Thinnest : 534 um @ (-0.0, 0.7)
ACD (Ep): 3.20 mm
Kappa : 2.80° @ 308.08°
Kappa Intercept : 0.06, -0.12
N
T
OS
626
619
543
619
608
v3.12
Power: 46.49 D
Meridian: 80 °
Radius: 0.6 mm
Thick: 535 mic
Meridian: 80 °
Radius: 0.6 mm
Keratometric
0.5 D Color Steps
Axial Power
0.94 Pachymetry
Thickness
20 mic Color Steps

—CASE 9—
Laser Vision Correction in Patients With Dry Eye

Dry eye symptoms are one of the most commonly reported side effects of laser vision correction (LVC) in the early postoperative period. However, the incidence of chronic dry eye induced by surgery is low in patients without significant dry eye symptoms before surgery. Appropriate screening for patients with significant dry eye is critical, as preoperative management can alleviate early postoperative complications from dry eye.

Case Analysis

- The estimated residual stromal bed (RSB) thickness is approximately 280 to 300 µm in both eyes with LASIK and is approximately 330 to 350 µm in both eyes with surface ablation.
- Case Figures show topography (Orbscan II; Bausch & Lomb) images for the right and left eyes demonstrating mild asymmetric bowtie patterns in both eyes, which are common in dry eye, but they are otherwise unremarkable. The slit lamp image is notable for significant corneal staining and punctate epitheliopathy, consistent with dry eye.

Pearl: *Always optimize the patient's ocular surface before laser vision correction when issues arise in screening!*

QUESTIONS

1. What, if any, notable findings are present in the slit-lamp image?

   The slit-lamp image demonstrates significant, diffuse punctate epithelial keratopathy (PEK).

2. Is this patient a candidate for refractive surgery? If so, what treatment options are available?

   The patient is not an ideal candidate for LVC at this time due to poorly controlled dry eye. She is a candidate for phakic intraocular lens (PIOL) implantation, but she may be a candidate for LVC with appropriate preoperative treatment.

3. Considering all factors, what procedure would you recommend and why?

   I would recommend no surgery at this time. The patient would benefit from treatment of dry eye and reevaluation at a later date.

—Case 9 (Part 2)—

The patient, who has been using topical cyclosporine drops routinely, returns for reevaluation 6 weeks after the initial evaluation. She reports improved stable visual acuity and improved ocular comfort and tearing, and she is highly motivated to pursue corneal refractive surgery. Slit-lamp examination is now unremarkable in both eyes, with no corneal staining in either eye.

CASE HISTORY		
	Right Eye	**Left Eye**
Present correction method	Spectacles	Spectacles
Manifest refraction	-8.50 +0.50 x 100	-8.75 +0.75 x 100
CDVA (current)	20/15	20/20
UNVA (current)	20/20	20/20
Keratometry		
Flat K	45.25 @ 174	45.25 @ 173
Steep K	46.50 @ 084	46.75 @ 083
Central corneal thickness	523 μm	532 μm
Schirmer's test with anesthesia (five minutes)	12 mm	15 mm
Estimated ablation depth	125 μm	125 μm

Questions

1. Is this patient now a candidate for refractive surgery?
2. Considering all factors, what procedure would you recommend, based on this examination, and why?
3. What unique aspects of this patient's examination warrant further discussion prior to surgery?
4. How might more likely complications be minimized for this individual?

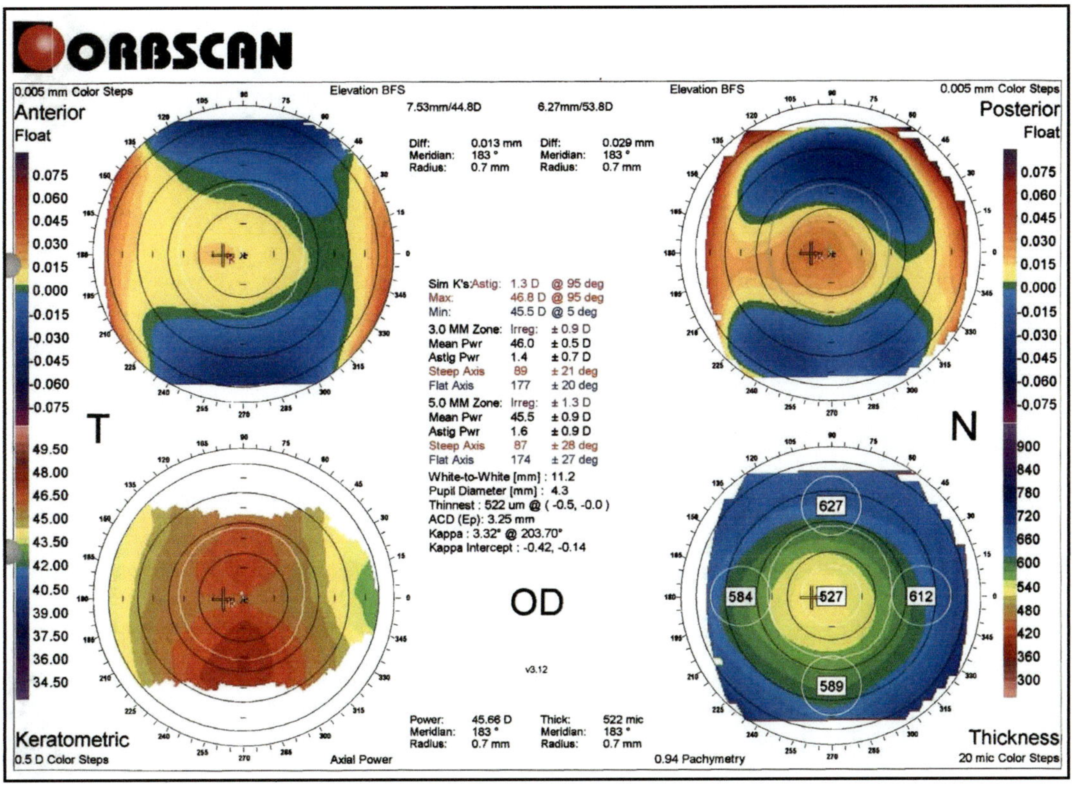
ORBSCAN
0.005 mm Color Steps
Anterior
Float
Elevation BFS
7.53mm/44.8D
6.27mm/53.8D
Elevation BFS
0.005 mm Color Steps
Posterior
Float
Diff: 0.013 mm
Meridian: 183 °
Radius: 0.7 mm
Diff: 0.029 mm
Meridian: 183 °
Radius: 0.7 mm
Sim K's:Astig: 1.3 D @ 95 deg
Max: 46.8 D @ 95 deg
Min: 45.5 D @ 5 deg
3.0 MM Zone: Irreg: ± 0.9 D
Mean Pwr 46.0 ± 0.5 D
Astig Pwr 1.4 ± 0.7 D
Steep Axis 89 ± 21 deg
Flat Axis 177 ± 20 deg
5.0 MM Zone: Irreg: ± 1.3 D
Mean Pwr 45.5 ± 0.9 D
Astig Pwr 1.6 ± 0.9 D
Steep Axis 87 ± 28 deg
Flat Axis 174 ± 27 deg
White-to-White [mm] : 11.2
Pupil Diameter [mm] : 4.3
Thinnest : 522 um @ (-0.5, -0.0)
ACD (Ep): 3.25 mm
Kappa : 3.32° @ 203.70°
Kappa Intercept : -0.42, -0.14
T
N
OD
v3.12
627
584
527
612
589
Power: 45.66 D
Meridian: 183 °
Radius: 0.7 mm
Thick: 522 mic
Meridian: 183 °
Radius: 0.7 mm
Keratometric
0.5 D Color Steps
Axial Power
0.94 Pachymetry
Thickness
20 mic Color Steps

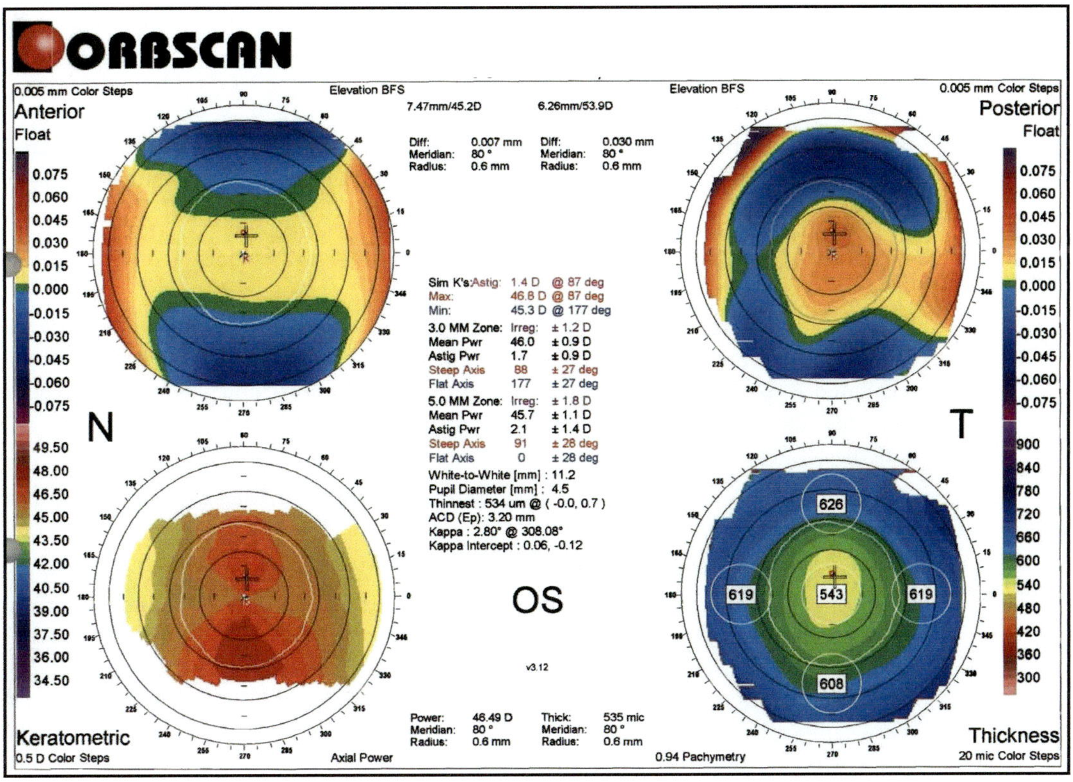
ORBSCAN
0.005 mm Color Steps
Anterior
Float
Elevation BFS
7.47mm/45.2D
6.26mm/53.9D
Elevation BFS
0.005 mm Color Steps
Posterior
Float
Diff: 0.007 mm
Meridian: 80 °
Radius: 0.6 mm
Diff: 0.030 mm
Meridian: 80 °
Radius: 0.6 mm
Sim K's:Astig: 1.4 D @ 87 deg
Max: 46.8 D @ 87 deg
Min: 45.3 D @ 177 deg
3.0 MM Zone: Irreg: ± 1.2 D
Mean Pwr 46.0 ± 0.9 D
Astig Pwr 1.7 ± 0.9 D
Steep Axis 88 ± 27 deg
Flat Axis 177 ± 27 deg
5.0 MM Zone: Irreg: ± 1.8 D
Mean Pwr 45.7 ± 1.1 D
Astig Pwr 2.1 ± 1.4 D
Steep Axis 91 ± 28 deg
Flat Axis 0 ± 28 deg
White-to-White [mm] : 11.2
Pupil Diameter [mm] : 4.5
Thinnest : 534 um @ (-0.0, 0.7)
ACD (Ep): 3.20 mm
Kappa : 2.80° @ 308.08°
Kappa Intercept : 0.06, -0.12
N
T
OS
v3.12
626
619
543
619
608
Power: 46.49 D
Meridian: 80 °
Radius: 0.6 mm
Thick: 535 mic
Meridian: 80 °
Radius: 0.6 mm
Keratometric
0.5 D Color Steps
Axial Power
0.94 Pachymetry
Thickness
20 mic Color Steps

—Case 9 (Part 2)—
Laser Vision Correction in Patients With Dry Eye

With appropriate treatment, most patients with mild-to-moderate dry eye may be reasonable candidates for corneal refractive surgery (LASIK or surface ablation). Patients who do not respond to treatment or who have worse symptoms may be better candidates for other surgical options or no surgery at all.

Case Analysis

- The estimated RSB is approximately 280 to 300 μm in both eyes with LASIK and is approximately 330 to 350 μm in both eyes with surface ablation.
- Case Figures show topography images for the right and left eyes that are essentially unchanged from initial visit.

Pearl: *Dry eye is not an absolute contraindication for laser vision correction; however, diligent preoperative screening and management is required to maximize outcomes in surgical candidates and will exclude patients who are not good candidates!*

Questions

1. Is this patient now a candidate for refractive surgery?

   Yes, the patient had a good treatment response to topical cyclosporine, with stable visual acuity and improved symptoms, and is otherwise now a good surgical candidate.

2. Considering all factors, what procedure would you recommend, based on this examination, and why?

   Although the patient is a candidate for LASIK, photorefractive keratectomy, or PIOL implantation, she is motivated to pursue corneal refractive surgery. Due to the estimated RSB thickness, I would opt for surface ablation, which is at least as good as LASIK for patients with dry eye and will have biomechanical advantages for this patient.

3. What unique aspects of this patient's examination warrant further discussion prior to surgery?

   This patient should be counseled that although she has seen improvement in her symptoms with treatment, her dry eye is not "cured," and she will likely continue to experience symptoms, at least intermittently, with or without surgery. Further, although most patients experience some dry eye symptoms after surgery, she is likely to experience more significant symptoms than average initially and will likely have these symptoms for a longer time period than average. She must also know that LVC can worsen her dry eye symptoms.

4. How more likely might complications be minimized for this individual?

   This patient will likely need aggressive postoperative management of dry eye, including frequent use of artificial tears; continuing use of topical cyclosporine, at least through the early postoperative period; and she may benefit from adjunctive measures such as punctual plug placement.

Dry Eye and LASIK

Dry eye is another controversial topic in LVC, and the relationship between dry eye and LASIK has been the focus of countless studies and discussions. The US Food and Drug Administration's website contains information for patients about dry eye worsening after surgery and indicates there is the potential to develop chronic dry eye after LASIK "as a result of surgery." However, well-controlled clinical trials have determined that the risk of developing chronic dry eye is low for patients without significant preoperative dry eye. Recent meta-analyses have determined that, although at least mild dry eye is relatively common after LASIK and presents in up to 35% of patients, 32% had dry eye before LASIK. Therefore, appropriate patient screening and counseling is critical in this respect.

The risk of dry eye has been thought to be lower after surface ablation than after LASIK due to less disruption of the corneal nerve plexus with more superficial ablations. However, thinner flaps appear to have mitigated this difference to some extent.

Dry Eye Evaluation Before Laser Vision Correction

A variety of tests are available to evaluate patients during refractive surgical evaluation. These include tear production tests, tear break-up time evaluation, and vital dyes to assess staining patterns. Lissamine green and fluorescein staining are useful to identify significant dry eye findings. Other more advanced testing modalities are now available, including tear osmolarity and functional tear film evaluation. No method for optimal tear film evaluation has yet been established, but a thorough examination based on clinical experience is necessary, especially for higher risk patients who include women, patients above age 40 years, and individuals who have already developed dry eye symptoms.

Dry Eye: Differences Between Surface Ablation, LASIK, and Phakic Intraocular Lens Implantation

The mechanism for dry eye symptoms after excimer laser ablation is not completely understood. Some authors have proposed that post-LASIK dry eye more closely resembles a neurotrophic response, rather than reduced tear production. Corneal nerve fiber disruption at the time of surgery stimulates some of the symptoms; however, because symptoms are highly variable between patients, other underlying processes must be involved.

In the past, dry eye was more common after LASIK than after surface ablation, and many patients with dry eye were counseled to undergo surface ablation instead of LASIK. The likely source of this difference was more significant corneal nerve interruption with LASIK flap creation in the deeper corneal stroma, which affects more corneal nerves and results in longer nerve regeneration time. Recent studies have found significantly less difference between surface ablation and LASIK with thinner corneal flaps. Past studies also have found a difference between nasally and superiorly hinged flaps; however, recent studies have found no differences based on flap location.

Phakic IOLs induce minimal changes in the ocular surface, and whereas their use is not as wide spread as corneal refractive procedures, these may be an excellent option for patients who are less than ideal candidates for corneal surgery.

Bibliography

Ambrósio R Jr, Tervo T, Wilson SE. LASIK-associated dry eye and neurotrophic epitheliopathy: pathophysiology and strategies for prevention and treatment. *J Refract Surg.* 2008;24(4):396-407.

Barequet IS, Hirsh A, Levinger S. Effect of thin femtosecond LASIK flaps on corneal sensitivity and tear function. *J Refract Surg.* 2008;24(9):897-902.

De Paiva CS, Chen Z, Koch DD, et al. The incidence and risk factors for developing dry eye after myopic LASIK. *Am J Ophthalmol.* 2006;141(3):438-445.

Dooley I, D'Arcy F, O'Keefe M. Comparison of dry-eye disease severity after laser in situ keratomileusis and laser-assisted subepithelial keratectomy. *J Cataract Refract Surg.* 2012;38(6):1058-1064.

Konomi K, Chen LL, Tarko RS, et al. Preoperative characteristics and a potential mechanism of chronic dry eye after LASIK. *Invest Ophthalmol Vis Sci.* 2008;49(1):168-174.

Mian SI, Li AY, Dutta S, Musch DC, Shtein RM. Dry eyes and corneal sensation after laser in situ keratomileusis with femtosecond laser flap creation. Effect of hinge position, hinge angle, and flap thickness. *J Cataract Refract Surg.* 2009;35(12):2092-2098.

Nettune GR, Pflugfelder SC. Post-LASIK tear dysfunction and dysesthesia. *Ocul Surf.* 2010;8(3):135-145.

Rosenfeld SI. Evaluation and management of post-LASIK dry eye syndrome. *Int Ophthalmol Clin.* 2010;50(3):191-199.

Salomão MQ, Ambrósio R Jr, Wilson SE. Dry eye associated with laser in situ keratomileusis: mechanical microkeratome versus femtosecond laser. *J Cataract Refract Surg.* 2009;35(10):1756-1760.

Slade SG, Durrie DS, Binder PS. A prospective, contralateral eye study comparing thin-flap LASIK (sub-Bowman keratomileusis) with photorefractive keratectomy. *Ophthalmology.* 2009;116(6):1075-1082.

Ursea R, Purcell TL, Tan BU, Nalgirkar A, Lovaton ME, Ehrenhaus MR, Schanzlin DJ. The effect of cyclosporine A (Restasis) on recovery of visual acuity following LASIK. *J Refract Surg.* 2008;24(5):473-476.

Vroman DT, Sandoval HP, Fernández de Castro LE, Kasper TJ, Holzer MP, Solomon KD. Effect of hinge location on corneal sensation and dry eye after laser in situ keratomileusis for myopia. *J Cataract Refract Surg.* 2005;31(10):1881-1887.

—Case 10—

A 24-year-old female desires refractive surgical correction. She has no significant family, past medical, or ocular history.

CASE HISTORY		
	Right Eye	**Left Eye**
Present correction method	CTL	CTL
Manifest refraction	-4.25 +1.50 x 070	-4.75 +2.00 x 095
CDVA (current)	20/20	20/20
Ocular alignment	Orthophoric	Orthophoric
Keratometry		
Flat K	46.3 @ 175	45.7 @ 005
Steep K	47.9 @ 085	48.4 @ 095
Pupil size (bright)	4.7 mm	4.0 mm
Pupil size (dim)	6.8 mm	6.9 mm
Central corneal thickness	510 µm	520 µm
Physical examination	See figure	See figure
Estimated ablation depth	75 µm	75 µm

Questions

1. Is this patient a candidate for refractive surgery? If so, what treatment options are available?
2. Considering all factors, what procedure would you recommend and why?
3. What are the most likely patient complaints in the postoperative period for this individual for each of the potential treatment options?
4. What are the most significant potential complications for each procedure available for this patient based on her examination?

A

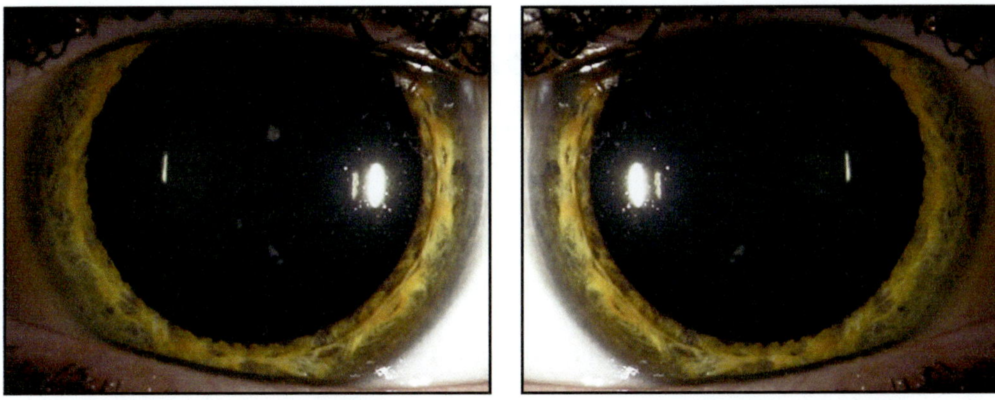

B

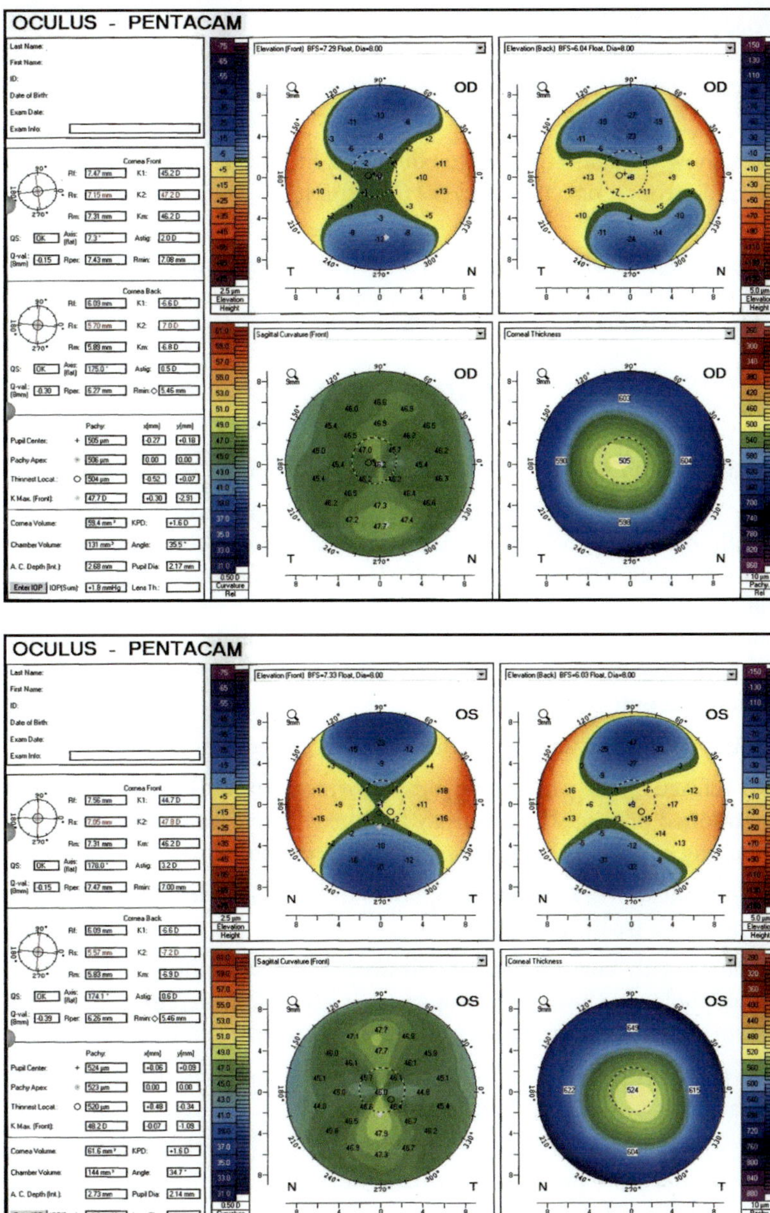

—Case 10—

Refractive Surgery in Patients With Corneal Dystrophies

Patients with subtle corneal dystrophies may present for refractive surgical evaluation. In these cases, careful slit-lamp examination is necessary to accurately diagnose the specific dystrophy present, which will direct management options. Laser vision correction is contraindicated in most, but not all, stromal and endothelial dystrophies.

Case Analysis

- The estimated residual stromal bed (RSB) thickness is approximately 310 to 350 µm in both eyes.
- Case Figures show (A) slit-lamp photos of the right and left eyes, exhibiting multiple, scattered, focal mid-stromal opacities and (B) topographies are unremarkable.

Pearl: *Perform a diligent slit-lamp examination on all patients, and do NOT perform laser vision correction for patients with most corneal stromal dystrophies!*

Questions

1. Is this patient a candidate for refractive surgery? If so, what treatment options are available?

   No, this patient exhibits findings of a stromal corneal dystrophy (granular or Avellino variants), which are contraindications to laser vision correction (LVC). The patient's astigmatism precludes her from having a successful outcome after phakic intraocular lens (PIOL) implantation until a toric version is available. At that point, she may be a candidate for PIOL implantation, albeit at the lower end of the approved range; however, the likely progression of her corneal findings may limit her long-term functional outcomes.

2. Considering all factors, what procedure would you recommend and why?

   No refractive surgery should be performed. In addition to the risks with surgery mentioned previously, there may be a benefit to contact lens wear, as the ultraviolet blocking effect may delay dystrophy progression.

3. What are the most likely patient complaints in the postoperative period for this individual for each potential treatment option?

   Patients with corneal stromal dystrophies who undergo LVC often present with photophobia in the early postoperative period, followed by gradual reduction in both uncorrected and corrected visual acuity as the dystrophy progresses.

4. What are the most significant potential complications for each procedure that is available for this patient based on her examination?

   The most significant complication is exacerbation of her underlying stromal dystrophy, with a more pronounced worsening of her condition and visual acuity than she would otherwise have without surgery.

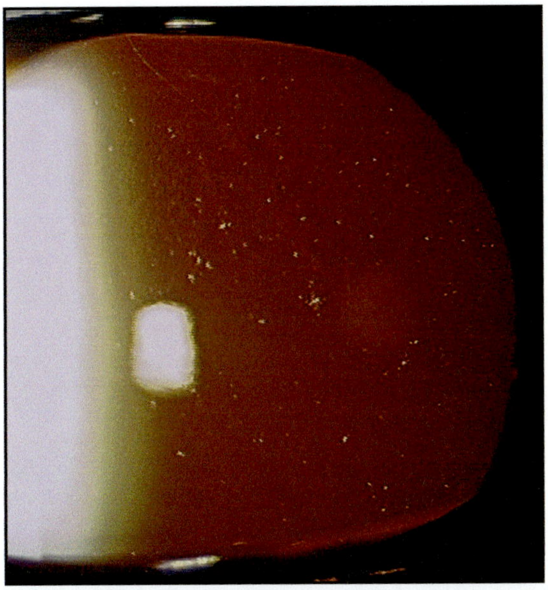

Case Figure 10-1. Fleck corneal dystrophy. Note the multiple, fine, scattered deposits visible in retroillumination. Fleck dystrophy is not a contraindication to laser vision correction.

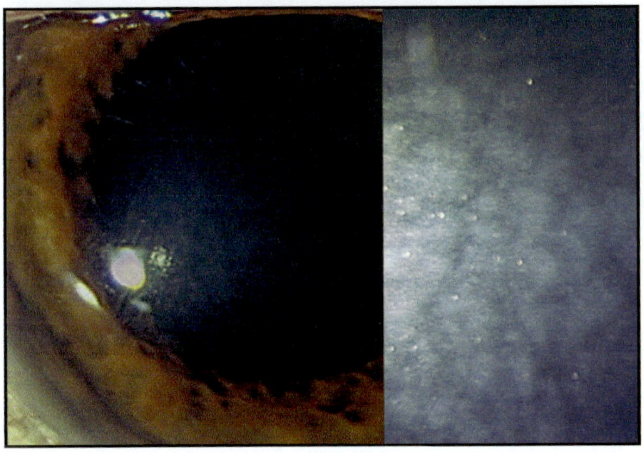

Case Figure 10-2. Posterior shagreen. Note the polygonal, deep stromal opacified regions in the central cornea arranged in a mosaic pattern, with regions of opacification that is interrupted with clear, crack-like lines. Posterior shagreen is not a contraindication to laser vision correction.

Laser Vision Correction and Stromal Dystrophies

Laser vision correction is contraindicated in patients with most corneal stromal dystrophies. These dystrophies, including granular and Avellino types (among others), have undergone changes in nomenclature over the years as more definitive genotypic information has been determined, which complicates literature review, as the same entity may have different names over different time periods. However, there is no functional distinction between these entities with regard to refractive surgery evaluation, so these entities will be discussed together.

The BIGH3 dystrophies are exacerbated by the excimer laser's ultraviolet light energy, mediated through increased transforming growth factor beta (TGF-β) activity, which results in activation of the BIGH3 gene and subsequent overexpression of the gene product, keratoepithelin. TGF-β is upregulated by corneal injury, as well as ultraviolet light, which explains why dystrophy exacerbation is more severe after LASIK, with additional flap creation, than after surface ablation.

Other less common, nonprogressive stromal dystrophies, including fleck dystrophy (Case Figure 10-1) and posterior shagreen (or central cloudy dystrophy) (Case Figure 10-2), arise

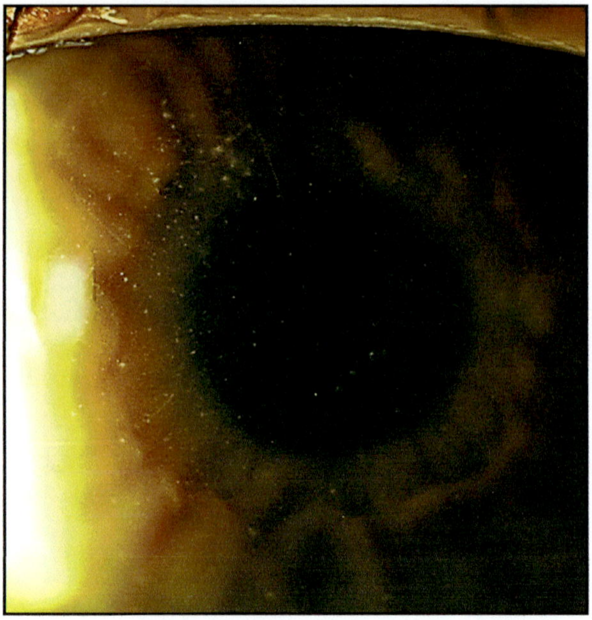

Case Figure 10-3. Shows likely anterior stromal dystrophy. There are multiple, fine, scattered deposits localized to the subepithelial and anterior stromal region. The appearance is not classic for any of the BIGH3 stromal dystrophies. Genetic testing ruled out any of the traditional stromal dystrophy mutations, but it failed to lead to a conclusive diagnosis. The patient ultimately had uneventful surface ablation with a good outcome and an unremarkable postoperative course.

from different mutations and mechanisms and do not progress after laser vision correction; thus, they are not contraindications for surgery. For more information see Chapter 2.

In cases with indeterminate anterior stromal opacities that appear consistent with a corneal dystrophy but do not follow a clearly identifiable pattern (Case Figure 10-3), the best course of action remains to be determined. Surface ablation may be acceptable in some cases, but patients must be counseled that their condition may progress after any laser vision correction. Genetic testing is appropriate in these cases to rule out known progressive stromal dystrophies.

Laser Vision Correction and Endothelial Dystrophies

LASIK does not cause worsening but is nonetheless contraindicated in Fuchs' corneal dystrophy. Flap adherence is dependent on endothelial pump function, and early flap slippage may result in patients with even mild corneal findings, including central guttae without edema. Later, corneal decompensation may occur, and a notable fluid cleft can arise within the LASIK interface. The safety of surface ablation has not been thoroughly evaluated, and there are reports of successful photorefractive keratectomy after endothelial keratoplasty; however, the most conservative approach is to avoid elective laser vision correction in these patients. Phakic IOL implantation is specifically contraindicated in any patient with suboptimal endothelial cell function.

In contrast, both LASIK and surface ablation can be safely performed in patients with posterior polymorphous corneal dystrophy (PPMD).

Bibliography

Banning CB, Kim WC, Randleman JB, Kim EK, Stulting RD. Exacerbation of Avellino Corneal Dystrophy after LASIK in North America. *Cornea*. 2006;25(4):482-484.

Banning CS, Larson PM, Randleman JB. Outcome of LASIK in fleck corneal dystrophy. *Cornea*. 2006;25(10):1262-1264.

Bower KS, Trudo EW, Ryan DS, et al. Photorefractive keratectomy in posterior polymorphous dystrophy with vesicular and band subtypes. *J Cataract Refract Surg.* 2011;37(6):1101-1108.

Dastjerdi MH, Sugar A. Corneal decompensation after laser in situ keratomileusis in Fuchs' endothelial dystrophy. *Cornea.* 2003;22(4):379-381.

Jun RM, Tchah H, Kim T, et al. Avellino corneal dystrophy after LASIK. *Ophthalmology.* 2004;111(3):463-468.

Kim TI, Kim T, Kim SW, Kim EK. Comparison of corneal deposits after LASIK and PRK in eyes with granular corneal dystrophy type II. *J Refract Surg.* 2008;24(4):392-395.

Lee ES, Kim EK. Surgical do's and don'ts of corneal dystrophies. *Curr Opin Ophthalmol.* 2003;14(4):186-191.

Moshirfar M, Barsam CA, Tanner MC. Laser in situ keratomileusis in patients with posterior polymorphous dystrophy. *Cornea.* 2005;24(2):230-232.

Moshirfar M, Feiz V, Feilmeier MR, Kang PC. Laser in situ keratomileusis in patients with corneal guttata and family history of Fuchs' endothelial dystrophy. *J Cataract Refract Surg.* 2005;31(12):2281-2286.

Vroman DT, Solomon KD, Holzer MP, Peng Q, Apple DJ, Bowie EM. Endothelial decompensation after laser in situ keratomileusis. *J Cataract Refract Surg.* 2002;28(11):2045-2049.

Woodward M, Randleman JB, Larson PM. In vivo confocal microscopy of polymorphic amyloid degeneration and posterior crocodile shagreen. *Cornea.* 2007;26(1):98-101.

Zaidi A, McLeod SD. Laser in situ keratomileusis in a patient with presumed central cloudy corneal dystrophy of Francois. *Am J Ophthalmol.* 2005;139(2):376-377.

—Case 11—

A 52-year-old male desires refractive surgical correction. He has noted blurred vision in both eyes for many years, even with correction. He has not had any change in refraction, and does not feel the blur has been progressively worsening. He has no significant family, past medical, or ocular history.

CASE HISTORY		
	Right Eye	**Left Eye**
Present correction method	Spectacles	Spectacles
Manifest refraction	-5.75 +2.25 x 110	-3.75 +1.00 x 017
CDVA (current)	20/30	20/25
CNVA (current)	20/30	20/20
Near add	+2.25	+2.25
Dominant eye	Right	
Keratometry		
Flat K	44.50 @ 015	44.25 @ 138
Steep K	46.50 @ 115	45.00 @ 048
Pupil size (bright)	3.4 mm	4.1 mm
Pupil size (dim)	5.8 mm	5.8 mm
Central corneal thickness	568 µm	564 µm
Physical examination	See Figure	See Figure
Estimated ablation depth	95 µm	65 µm

Questions

1. Is this patient a candidate for refractive surgery? If so, what treatment options are available?
2. Considering all factors, what procedure would you recommend and why?
3. What additional information could be of particular utility in evaluating this patient for surgery?
4. What are the most significant potential complications for each procedure available for this patient, based on his examination?
5. What additional steps might one take preoperatively to maximize the final postoperative refractive outcome in this patient?

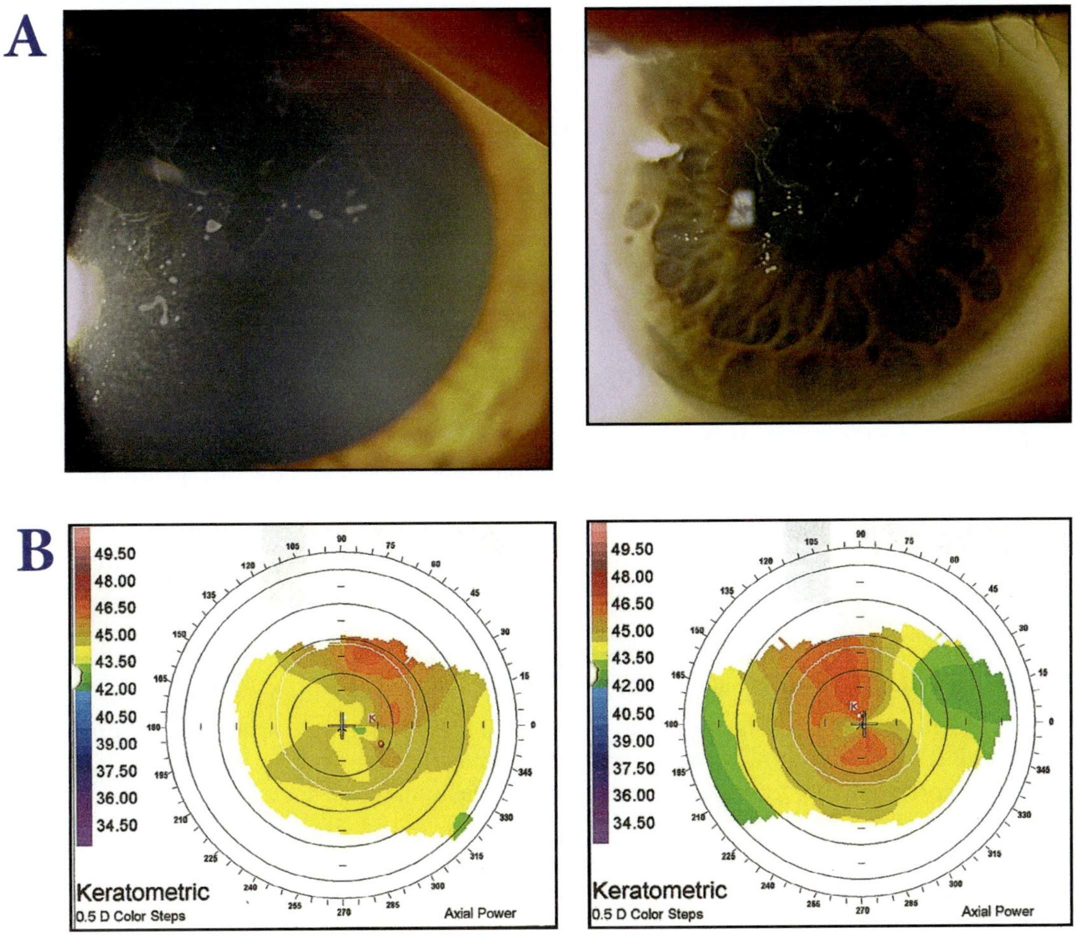
A
B
49.50
48.00
46.50
45.00
43.50
42.00
40.50
39.00
37.50
36.00
34.50
Keratometric
0.5 D Color Steps
Axial Power
49.50
48.00
46.50
45.00
43.50
42.00
40.50
39.00
37.50
36.00
34.50
Keratometric
0.5 D Color Steps
Axial Power

—CASE 11—

Epithelial Basement Membrane Dystrophy

Considerations for Laser Vision Correction

Epithelial basement membrane dystrophy (EBMD), also termed *anterior basement membrane dystrophy* (ABMD), *basement membrane degeneration* (rather than dystrophy), *map-dot fingerprint dystrophy*, and *Cogan's dystrophy*, can significantly complicate LASIK cases intraoperatively or in the postoperative period. Surface ablation, on the other hand, can be a therapeutic, as well as refractive, procedure in these eyes. Careful history and slit-lamp examination is necessary for accurate diagnosis and surgical planning.

Case Analysis

- The estimated residual stromal bed (RSB) thickness is approximately 350 to 370 μm in the right eye, and approximately 400 μm in the left eye.
- Case Figures show (A) slit-lamp images depicting the "map-dot" line opacities that are typical in EBMD, and (B) corresponding topographic images demonstrating irregular astigmatic patterns corresponding to the areas of irregular epithelium.

Pearl: *Avoid LASIK and opt for surface ablation in patients with EBMD!*

QUESTIONS

1. Is this patient a candidate for refractive surgery? If so, what treatment options are available for this patient?

   Yes, this patient has EBMD; however, he is still a reasonable candidate for refractive surgery. The most appropriate procedure for this patient is surface ablation.

2. Considering all factors, what procedure would you recommend and why?

   In patients with EBMD, surface ablation procedures may be therapeutic as well as refractive. LASIK, on the other hand, can cause intraoperative epithelial defects and predispose the patient to complications, including recurrent erosions postoperatively.

3. What additional information could be of particular utility in evaluating this patient for surgery?

   Although the patient's decreased best-corrected visual acuity is most likely reduced from corneal irregularity induced by EBMD, it is important to rule out other likely causes for decreased acuity in his demographic, including early cataract formation or a macular or optic nerve disorder.

4. What are the most significant potential complications for each procedure available for this patient, based on his examination?

   With EBMD, the patient is at risk for developing recurrent erosion syndrome (RES) with or without surgery. Surface ablation reduces but does not eliminate this risk, and LASIK exacerbates the likelihood of RES developing postoperatively. Further, intraoperative epithelial defects during LASIK predispose patients to develop interface inflammation or diffuse lamellar keratitis, infectious keratitis, epithelial ingrowth, or scarring.

5. What additional steps might one take preoperatively to maximize the final postoperative refractive outcome in this patient?

   In patients with severe EBMD, it may not be possible to obtain accurate refractive and topographic measurements. Although it is ideal to perform epithelial removal as part of the surface ablation procedure, in some cases it may be necessary to first perform epithelial scraping to normalize the surface prior to laser ablation.

Refractive Surgery in Patients With Epithelial Basement Membrane Dystrophy

With EBMD, epithelial adhesions to Bowman's layer are compromised. The mechanical forces applied to the epithelium during LASIK with a mechanical microkeratome, and, to a much lesser extent, with the femtosecond laser, can cause intraoperative epithelial defects (ED) and related postoperative complications.

Intraoperative Complications

LASIK with a mechanical microkeratome has a higher rate of ED creation than femtosecond lasers for all eyes, and eyes with EBMD have a significantly higher rate of ED formation. Potentially severe epithelial sloughing can occur. If a significant ED occurs in the first eye of a planned immediately sequential case, the second-eye procedure should be postponed.

Postoperative Complications

Epithelial defects can occur in the early postoperative period in patients with clinical or subclinical EBMD. When an ED develops, the risk of interface inflammation also increases significantly. Postoperative ED also predisposes to infection. Recurrent erosions after LASIK can occur in eyes with EBMD. These may also result in recurrent interface inflammation (Case Figure 11-1).

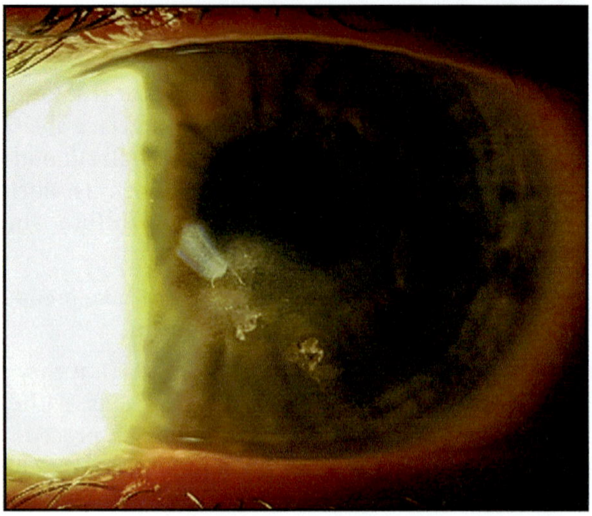

Case Figure 11-1. Slit-lamp image from a patient 3 months after LASIK. The patient had undiagnosed EBMD preoperatively and developed an ED intraoperatively, with repeat recurrent erosions with accompanying interface inflammation at the site of the ED.

Bibliography

Brilakis HS, Holland EJ. Anterior stromal puncture in the treatment of loose epithelium after LASIK. *J Refract Surg.* 2006;22(1):103-105.

Chen S, Feng Y, Stojanovic A, Jankov MR II, Wang Q. IntraLase femtosecond laser vs mechanical microkeratomes in LASIK for myopia: a systematic review and meta-analysis. *J Refract Surg.* 2012;28(1):15-24.

Dastgheib KA, Clinch TE, Manche EE, Hersh P, Ramsey J. Sloughing of corneal epithelium and wound healing complications associated with laser in situ keratomileusis in patients with epithelial basement membrane dystrophy. *Am J Ophthalmol.* 2000;130(3):297-303.

Elderkin SJ, Epstein RJ, Seldomridge DL. Successful treatment of recurrent epithelial ingrowth associated with interface fluid syndrome, flap necrosis, and epithelial defects following LASIK. *J Refract Surg.* 2011;27(1):70-73.

Esquenazi S, Bui V. Long-term refractive results of myopic LASIK complicated with intraoperative epithelial defects. *J Refract Surg.* 2006;22(1):54-60.

Faktorovich EG, Nosova E. Epithelial removal and phototherapeutic keratectomy for residual refractive error following LASIK in eyes with corneal epithelial basement membrane degeneration. *J Refract Surg.* 2009;25(8):723-729.

Jin GJ, Lyle WA, Merkley KH. Late-onset idiopathic diffuse lamellar keratitis after laser in situ keratomileusis. *J Cataract Refract Surg.* 2005;31(2):435-437.

Kenyon KR, Paz H, Greiner JV, Gipson IK. Corneal epithelial adhesion abnormalities associated with LASIK. *Ophthalmology.* 2004;111(1):11-17.

Kohnen T, Terzi E, Mirshahi A, Bühren J. Intraindividual comparison of epithelial defects during laser in situ keratomileusis using standard and zero-compression Hansatome microkeratome heads. *J Cataract Refract Surg.* 2004;30(1):123-126.

Kymionis GD, Diakonis VF, Bouzoukis DI, Yoo SH, Pallikaris IG. Photorefractive keratectomy in a patient with epithelial basement membrane dystrophy. *Semin Ophthalmol.* 2007;22(1):59-61.

Mirshahi A, Bühren J, Kohnen T. Clinical course of severe central epithelial defects in laser in situ keratomileusis. *J Cataract Refract Surg.* 2004;30(8):1636-1641.

Moshirfar M, Gardiner JP, Schliesser JA. Laser in situ keratomileusis flap complications using mechanical microkeratome versus femtosecond laser: retrospective comparison. *J Cataract Refract Surg.* 2010;36(11):1925-1933.

Oliva MS, Ambrósio Júnior R, Wilson SE. Influence of intraoperative epithelial defects on outcomes in LASIK for myopia. *Am J Ophthalmol.* 2004;137(2):244-249.

Pérez-Santonja JJ, Galal A, Cardona C, Artola A, Ruíz-Moreno JM, Alió JL. Severe corneal epithelial sloughing during laser in situ keratomileusis as a presenting sign for silent epithelial basement membrane dystrophy. *J Cataract Refract Surg.* 2005;31(10):1932-1937.

Polk EE, Wexler SA, Kymes S. Incidence of corneal epithelial defects with the standard and zero-compression Hansatome microkeratomes. *J Refract Surg.* 2005;21(4):359-364.

Rezende RA, Uchoa UC, Cohen EJ, Laibson PR, Rapuano CJ. Complications associated with anterior basement membrane dystrophy after laser in situ keratomileusis. *J Cataract Refract Surg.* 2004;30(11):2328-2331.

—Case 12—

A 30-year-old female desires refractive surgical correction. The patient reports a history of extended contact lens wear, with increasing difficulties of decreased wear time and increasing discomfort over the past year. The patient has been prescribed topical cyclosporine drops (Restasis) twice daily in both eyes, but she reports poor compliance.

CASE HISTORY		
	Right Eye	**Left Eye**
Present correction method	CTL	CTL
Manifest refraction	-6.50 +0.50 x 092	-6.75 sphere
CDVA (current)	20/50	20/50
UNVA (current)	20/40	20/40
Dominant eye	Right	
Ocular alignment	Orthophoric	Orthophoric
Keratometry		
Flat K	43.75 @ 010	43.75 @ 180
Steep K	46.50 @ 100	46.00 @ 90
Pupil size (bright)	4.9 mm	4.4 mm
Pupil size (dim)	5.9 mm	5.6 mm
Central corneal thickness	537 µm	542 µm
Schirmer's test with anesthesia	27 mm	35 mm
Physical examination	Similar to left eye	See Figure
Estimated ablation depth	105 µm	105 µm

Questions

1. Is this patient a candidate for refractive surgery? If so, what treatment options are available?
2. What is in your differential diagnosis for the slit-lamp and topographic findings?
3. Considering all factors, what would you recommend, based on this examination, and why?

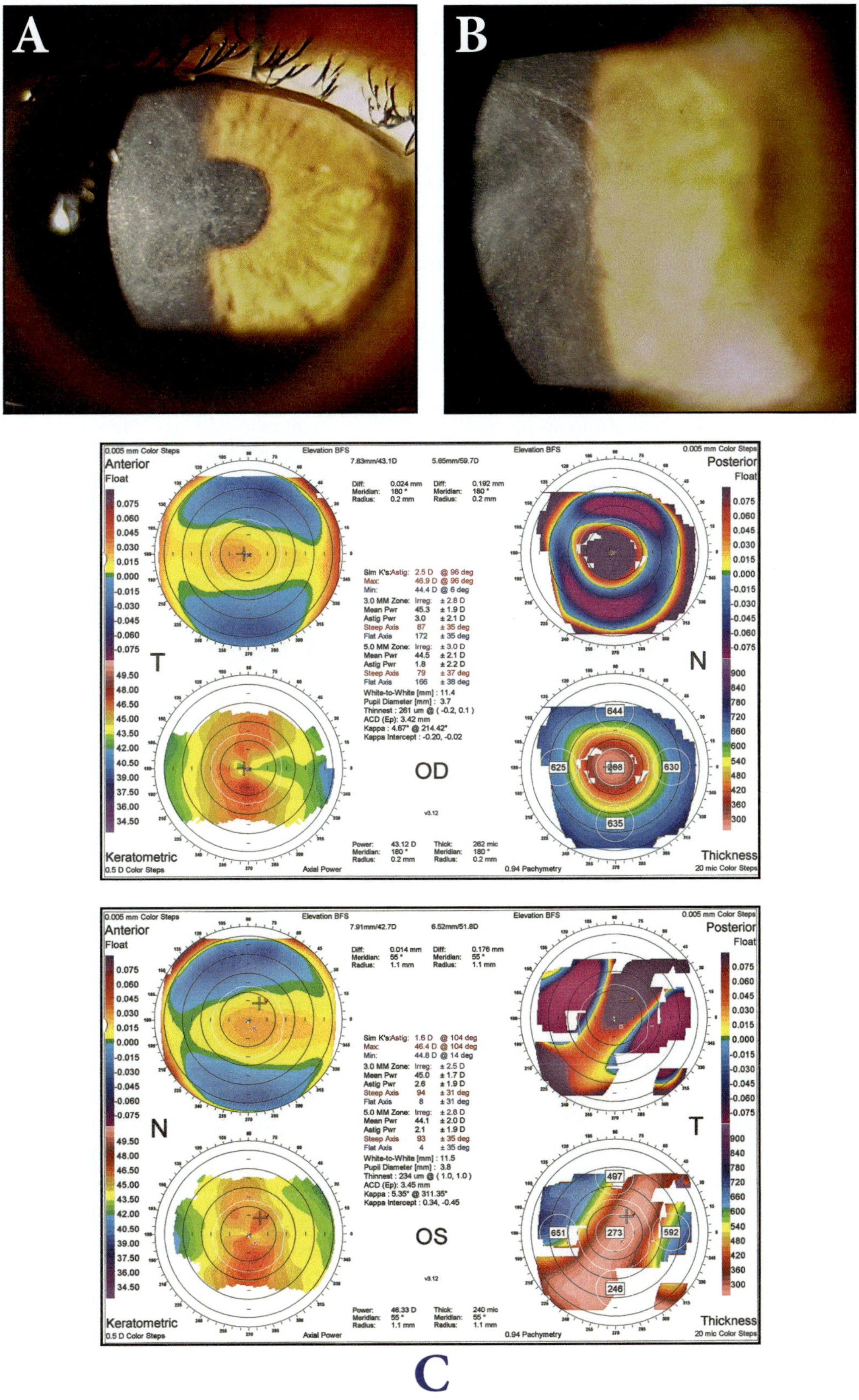
A
B
0.005 mm Color Steps
Anterior
Float
Elevation BFS
7.83mm/43.1D
5.65mm/59.7D
Diff: 0.024 mm Meridian: 180 ° Radius: 0.2 mm
Diff: 0.192 mm Meridian: 180 ° Radius: 0.2 mm
Posterior
Float
0.075 0.060 0.045 0.030 0.015 0.000 -0.015 -0.030 -0.045 -0.060 -0.075
T
N
Sim K's:Astig: 2.5 D @ 96 deg
Max: 46.9 D @ 96 deg
Min: 44.4 D @ 6 deg
3.0 MM Zone: Irreg: ± 2.8 D
Mean Pwr 45.3 ± 1.9 D
Astig Pwr 3.0 ± 2.1 D
Steep Axis 87 ± 35 deg
Flat Axis 172 ± 35 deg
5.0 MM Zone: Irreg: ± 3.0 D
Mean Pwr 44.5 ± 2.1 D
Astig Pwr 1.8 ± 2.2 D
Steep Axis 79 ± 37 deg
Flat Axis 166 ± 38 deg
White-to-White [mm] : 11.4
Pupil Diameter [mm] : 3.7
Thinnest : 261 um @ (-0.2, 0.1)
ACD (Ep): 3.42 mm
Kappa : 4.67° @ 214.42°
Kappa Intercept : -0.20, -0.02
OD
v3.12
49.50 48.00 46.50 45.00 43.50 42.00 40.50 39.00 37.50 36.00 34.50
900 840 780 720 660 600 540 480 420 360 300
644
625
268
630
635
Power: 43.12 D Meridian: 180 ° Radius: 0.2 mm
Thick: 262 mic Meridian: 180 ° Radius: 0.2 mm
Keratometric
0.5 D Color Steps
Axial Power
0.94 Pachymetry
Thickness
20 mic Color Steps
0.005 mm Color Steps
Anterior
Float
Elevation BFS
7.91mm/42.7D
6.52mm/51.8D
Diff: 0.014 mm Meridian: 55 ° Radius: 1.1 mm
Diff: 0.176 mm Meridian: 55 ° Radius: 1.1 mm
Posterior
Float
N
T
Sim K's:Astig: 1.6 D @ 104 deg
Max: 46.4 D @ 104 deg
Min: 44.8 D @ 14 deg
3.0 MM Zone: Irreg: ± 2.5 D
Mean Pwr 45.0 ± 1.7 D
Astig Pwr 2.6 ± 1.9 D
Steep Axis 94 ± 31 deg
Flat Axis 8 ± 31 deg
5.0 MM Zone: Irreg: ± 2.8 D
Mean Pwr 44.1 ± 2.0 D
Astig Pwr 2.1 ± 1.9 D
Steep Axis 93 ± 35 deg
Flat Axis 4 ± 35 deg
White-to-White [mm] : 11.5
Pupil Diameter [mm] : 3.8
Thinnest : 234 um @ (1.0, 1.0)
ACD (Ep): 3.45 mm
Kappa : 5.35° @ 311.35°
Kappa Intercept : 0.34, -0.45
OS
v3.12
497
651
273
592
246
Power: 46.33 D Meridian: 55 ° Radius: 1.1 mm
Thick: 240 mic Meridian: 55 ° Radius: 1.1 mm
Keratometric
0.5 D Color Steps
Axial Power
0.94 Pachymetry
Thickness
20 mic Color Steps
C

—Case 12—

Irregular Astigmatism From Ocular Surface Issues: Blepharitis

Corneal topographic patterns can be irregular for a variety of reasons, including disruption of the ocular surface through a variety of mechanisms.

Case Analysis

- The estimated residual stromal bed (RSB) thickness is approximately 315 to 335 µm in both eyes.
- Case Figures show (A) slit-lamp image of the left cornea showing diffuse, dense epitheliopathy. (B) Close up image of the left cornea demonstrating the whorl-like epitheliopathy. (C) Irregular keratometric maps demonstrating significant anterior curvature irregularity. The significant epitheliopathy prevents the Orbscan II (Bausch & Lomb) from attaining accurate thickness measurements; thus, significant topographic artifacts are visible in the thickness and elevation maps.

Pearl: *Some patients need a longer period of being out of contact lenses, and they may not be happy initially, but both you and the patient will ultimately benefit from the additional time and testing prior to surgery!*

Questions

1. Is this patient a candidate for refractive surgery? If so, what treatment options are available for this patient?

   No, not at this time. Given the patient's slit-lamp appearance and irregular corneal topography, she is currently not a candidate for laser vision correction (LVC). This may be temporary or permanent, but it cannot be determined from this evaluation alone.

2. What is in your differential diagnosis for the slit-lamp and topographic findings?

   The patient's physical examination findings could be consistent with significant dry eye disorder, contact lens over-wear, or a remote process resulting in significant corneal scarring. The latter is unlikely, given the patient's history, and dry eye is less likely to be causing all of the findings because the patient has good tear production, making contact lens over-wear the most likely cause for the majority of the findings.

3. Considering all factors, what would you recommend, based on this examination, and why?

   An extended trial out of contact lenses is warranted to reevaluate the corneal clarity, refractive status, and topographic pattern assessment. The patient will most likely benefit from topical cyclosporine, so consistent use should be stressed.

—Case 12 (Part 2)—

The patient returns for reevaluation 12 weeks after the initial evaluation, and she has been out of contact lenses during this time period. She reports improved visual acuity and ocular comfort, and she is now regularly using topical cyclosporine drops (Restasis, Allergan) twice daily in both eyes.

Case History		
	Right Eye	**Left Eye**
Present correction method	Spectacles	Spectacles
Manifest refraction	-6.50 sphere	-6.75 sphere
CDVA (current)	20/20	20/20
UNVA (current)	20/20	20/20
Keratometry		
Flat K	44.25 @ 176	43.50 @ 005
Steep K	46.25 @ 086	45.50 @ 095
Schirmer's test with anesthesia	35 mm	25 mm
Physical examination	Similar to the left eye	See Figure
Estimated ablation depth	105 μm	105 μm

Questions

1. Is this patient now a candidate for refractive surgery? If so, what treatment options are available?
2. Considering all factors, what procedure would you recommend, based on this examination, and why?
3. With the added evaluation 12 weeks following the initial evaluation, what is the most likely diagnosis for this patient's physical and topographic findings?

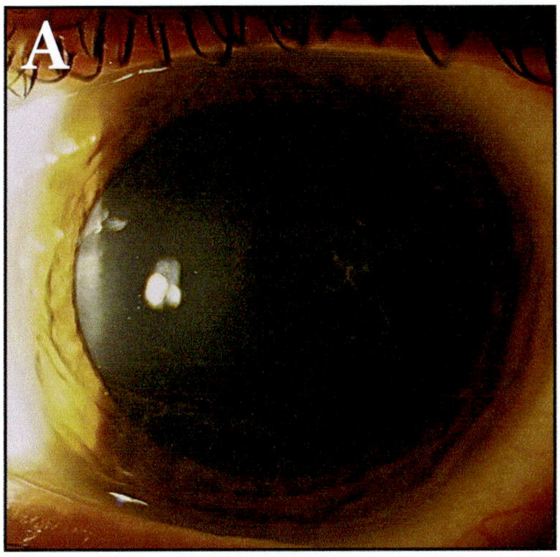
A

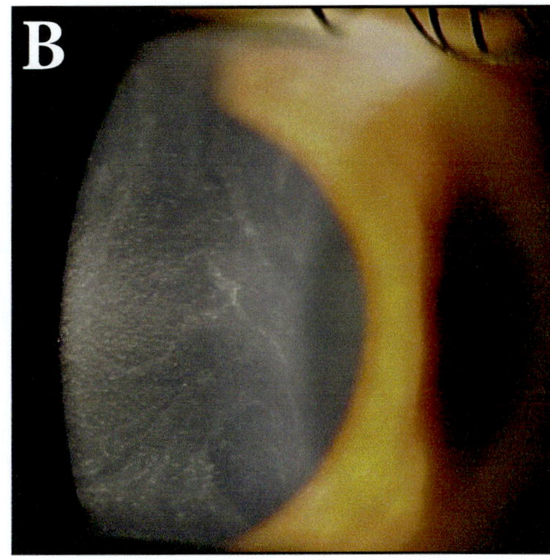
B

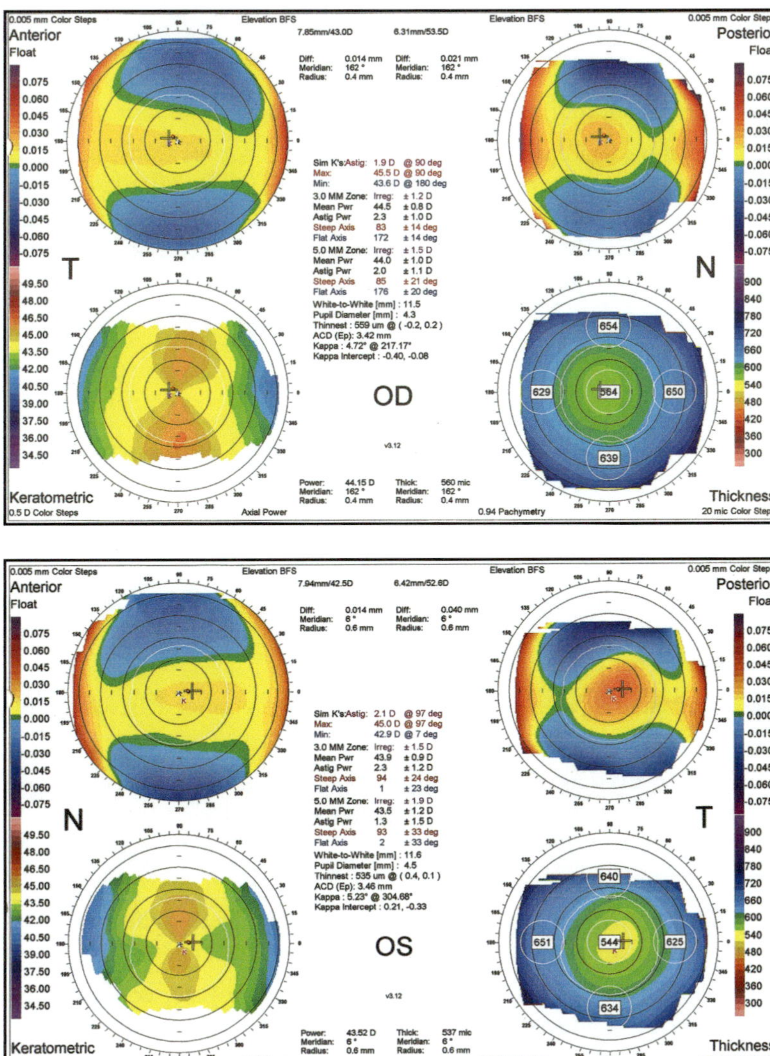
0.005 mm Color Steps
Anterior
Float
0.075
0.060
0.045
0.030
0.015
0.000
-0.015
-0.030
-0.045
-0.060
-0.075
Elevation BFS
7.85mm/43.0D
6.31mm/53.5D
Elevation BFS
0.005 mm Color Steps
Posterior
Float
Diff: 0.014 mm
Meridian: 162 °
Radius: 0.4 mm
Diff: 0.021 mm
Meridian: 162 °
Radius: 0.4 mm
Sim K's:Astig: 1.9 D @ 90 deg
Max: 45.5 D @ 90 deg
Min: 43.6 D @ 180 deg
3.0 MM Zone: Irreg: ± 1.2 D
Mean Pwr 44.5 ± 0.8 D
Astig Pwr 2.3 ± 1.0 D
Steep Axis 83 ± 14 deg
Flat Axis 172 ± 14 deg
5.0 MM Zone: Irreg: ± 1.5 D
Mean Pwr 44.0 ± 1.0 D
Astig Pwr 2.0 ± 1.1 D
Steep Axis 85 ± 21 deg
Flat Axis 176 ± 20 deg
White-to-White [mm] : 11.5
Pupil Diameter [mm] : 4.3
Thinnest : 559 um @ (-0.2, 0.2)
ACD (Ep): 3.42 mm
Kappa : 4.72° @ 217.17°
Kappa Intercept : -0.40, -0.08
OD
v3.12
T
N
49.50
48.00
46.50
45.00
43.50
42.00
40.50
39.00
37.50
36.00
34.50
900
840
780
720
660
600
540
480
420
360
300
654
629
564
650
639
Power: 44.15 D
Meridian: 162 °
Radius: 0.4 mm
Thick: 560 mic
Meridian: 162 °
Radius: 0.4 mm
Keratometric
0.5 D Color Steps
Axial Power
0.94 Pachymetry
Thickness
20 mic Color Steps
0.005 mm Color Steps
Anterior
Float
Elevation BFS
7.94mm/42.5D
6.42mm/52.6D
Elevation BFS
0.005 mm Color Steps
Posterior
Float
Diff: 0.014 mm
Meridian: 6 °
Radius: 0.6 mm
Diff: 0.040 mm
Meridian: 6 °
Radius: 0.6 mm
Sim K's:Astig: 2.1 D @ 97 deg
Max: 45.0 D @ 97 deg
Min: 42.9 D @ 7 deg
3.0 MM Zone: Irreg: ± 1.5 D
Mean Pwr 43.9 ± 0.9 D
Astig Pwr 2.3 ± 1.2 D
Steep Axis 94 ± 24 deg
Flat Axis 1 ± 23 deg
5.0 MM Zone: Irreg: ± 1.9 D
Mean Pwr 43.5 ± 1.2 D
Astig Pwr 1.3 ± 1.5 D
Steep Axis 93 ± 33 deg
Flat Axis 2 ± 33 deg
White-to-White [mm] : 11.6
Pupil Diameter [mm] : 4.5
Thinnest : 535 um @ (0.4, 0.1)
ACD (Ep): 3.46 mm
Kappa : 5.23° @ 304.68°
Kappa Intercept : 0.21, -0.33
OS
v3.12
N
T
640
651
544
625
634
Power: 43.52 D
Meridian: 6 °
Radius: 0.6 mm
Thick: 537 mic
Meridian: 6 °
Radius: 0.6 mm
Keratometric
0.5 D Color Steps
Axial Power
0.94 Pachymetry
Thickness
20 mic Color Steps

C

—Case 12 (Part 2)—

Irregular Astigmatism From Ocular Surface Issues

Contact Lens-Related Irregular Topography

Contact lens wear can induce significant epitheliopathy, especially in patients who wear their lenses inappropriately, either by wearing them for an extended fashion with insufficient breaks or by utilizing poor cleaning and storage processes. These patients frequently present with abnormal corneal and topographic examinations and require an extended period of time without contact lens wear to assess surgical candidacy and to assure accurate measurements.

Case Analysis

- The estimated RSB is approximately 315 to 335 μm in both eyes.
- The Case Figures show (A-B) slit-lamp images of the left cornea showing significant improvement in epitheliopathy, with reduced haze and scarring. (C) Regular keratometric maps demonstrating symmetric bowtie patterns. The improved ocular surface now allows for regular measurements of corneal thickness and float maps without significant artifact.

Pearl: *If ocular surface issues resolve, LVC is appropriate; if they persist, consider phakic intraocular lens implantation for eligible patients!*

Questions

1. Is this patient a candidate for refractive surgery? If so, what treatment options are available for this patient?

   Yes, based on the improvement in corneal clarity, topographic findings, and visual acuity, along with an otherwise consistent refractive examination, this patient is now a candidate for surgery.

2. Considering all factors, what procedure would you recommend, based on this examination, and why?

   Due to the residual epitheliopathy, surface ablation is the best surgical approach. Surface ablation may be partially therapeutic as well as refractive, whereas LASIK carries increased risk of epithelial sloughing intraoperatively or in the early postoperative period.

3. With the added evaluation 12 weeks following the initial evaluation, what is the most likely diagnosis for this patient's physical and topographic findings?

   The improvements in the patient's examination further confirm the initial thought of contact lens-induced corneal irregularity.

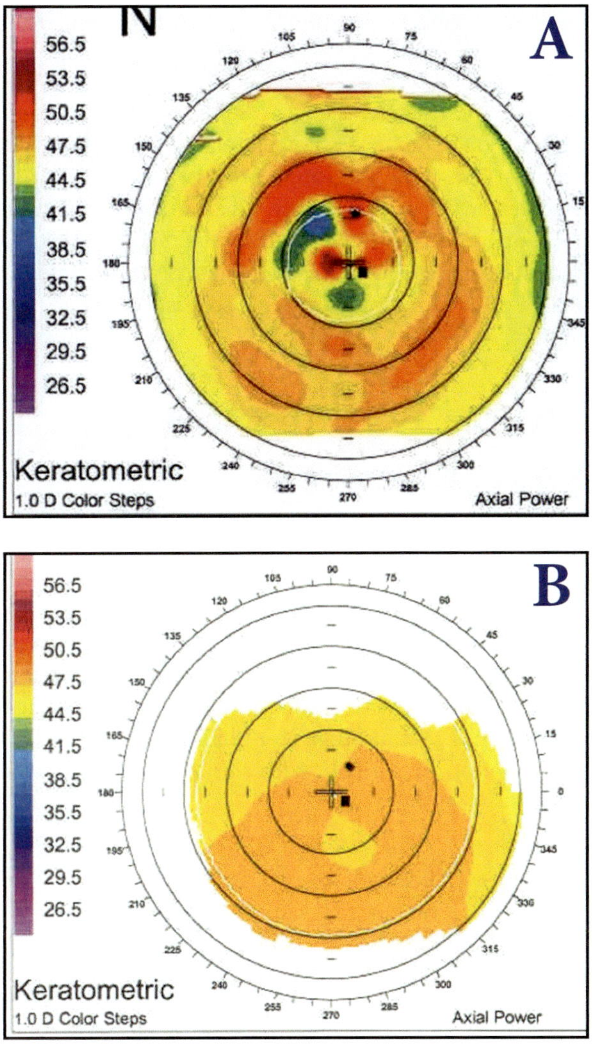

Case Figure 12-1. (A) Irregular astigmatism from tear deficiency that has (B) resolved after a short course of artificial tear use.

Irregular Astigmatism From Ocular Surface Disorders

Topographic evaluation is the centerpiece of refractive surgical evaluations; however, ocular surface disorders may create suspicious topographic findings in otherwise biomechanically normal corneas. Thus, the root cause for the irregularity must be determined and corrected prior to making a surgical decision.

The case presented herein is an extreme example of contact lens-induced topographic and ocular surface changes. More subtle abnormalities may actually be harder to appreciate clinically, especially the effects of decreased tear production that presents as irregular astigmatism without physical findings (Case Figure 12-1). Placido imaging is most sensitive to tear film abnormalities, making it a good technology to pick up subtle ocular surface issues but prone to artifact when the tear film is compromised. In theory, Placido imaging should be more susceptible to testing artifact, and Scheimpflug imaging should be less affected by surface issues; however, in practice, all imaging devices currently available may generate artifactual maps if ocular surface abnormalities are significant.

In cases with irregular topographic or tomographic images, it is reasonable to treat the suspected cause and repeat corneal mapping at a later date. Surface changes related to contact lens wear require an extended time period out of contact lens wear. Although most practices require a minimum of a few days to 2 to 3 weeks of contact lens wear cessation prior to an initial evaluation, patients with extended contact lens wear history, or more significant issues, may require weeks to months out of contact lenses to obtain an accurate evaluation. Many patients express distress at this notion, but it is critical to obtain accurate data prior to making any final surgical decision. For more information on approval ranges see Chapter 2.

Refractive Surgery for Patients With Ocular Surface Disorders

The best surgical procedure for patients with ocular surface abnormalities ultimately depends on the severity of these issues and their response to treatment prior to surgery. Patients with isolated topographic abnormalities from any of the aforementioned issues that resolve relatively quickly are usually reasonable candidates for both surface ablation or LASIK, whereas patients with more normalized test results, but persistent clinical findings, are likely better suited for surface ablation. LASIK is more likely to induce epithelial defects in patients with a compromised ocular surface. Depending on the level of myopia, these individuals may be candidates for phakic intraocular lens implantation, and this is an especially attractive option in patients with significantly decreased tear production.

Bibliography

Arita R, Itoh K, Inoue K, Kuchiba A, Yamaguchi T, Amano S. Contact lens wear is associated with decrease of meibomian glands. *Ophthalmology.* 2009;116(3):379 384.

de Paiva CS, Harris LD, Pflugfelder SC. Keratoconus-like topographic changes in keratoconjunctivitis sicca. *Cornea.* 2003;22(1):22-24.

Lebow KA, Grohe RM. Differentiating contact lens induced warpage from true keratoconus using corneal topography. *CLAO J.* 1999;25(2):114-122.

Liu Z, Pflugfelder SC. Corneal surface regularity and the effect of artificial tears in aqueous tear deficiency. *Ophthalmology.* 1999;106(5):939-943.

Németh J, Erdélyi B, Csákány B. Corneal topography changes after a 15 second pause in blinking. *J Cataract Refract Surg.* 2001;27(4):589-592.

Tseng SS, Hsiao JC, Chang DC. Mistaken diagnosis of keratoconus because of corneal warpage induced by hydrogel lens wear. *Cornea.* 2007;26(9):1153-1155.

—Case 13—

A 35-year-old male desires refractive surgical correction. The patient notes moderate irritation with contact lens wear. He has no significant family or past medical history.

CASE HISTORY		
	Right Eye	**Left Eye**
Present correction method	CTL	CTL
Manifest refraction	-3.00 sphere	-3.25 sphere
CDVA (current)	20/25	20/20
UNVA (current)	20/20	20/20
Dominant eye		Left
Ocular alignment	Orthophoric	Orthophoric
Keratometry		
Flat K	45.2 @ 154	45.2 @ 020
Steep K	45.6 @ 064	45.7 @ 110
Pupil size (bright)	3.9 mm	4.3 mm
Pupil size (dim)	7.0 mm	7.3 mm
Central corneal thickness	579 μm	586 μm
Physical examination	See figure	See figure
Estimated ablation depth	55 μm	55 μm

Questions

1. Is this patient a candidate for refractive surgery? If so, what treatment options are available?
2. What is the most likely cause for the topographic findings?
3. Considering all factors, what would you recommend, based on this examination, and why?

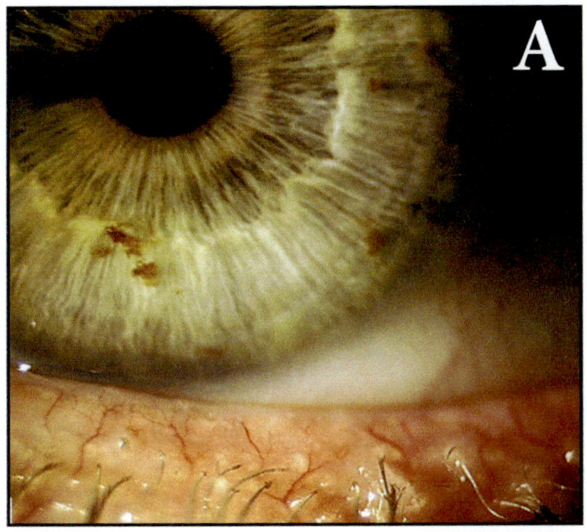
A

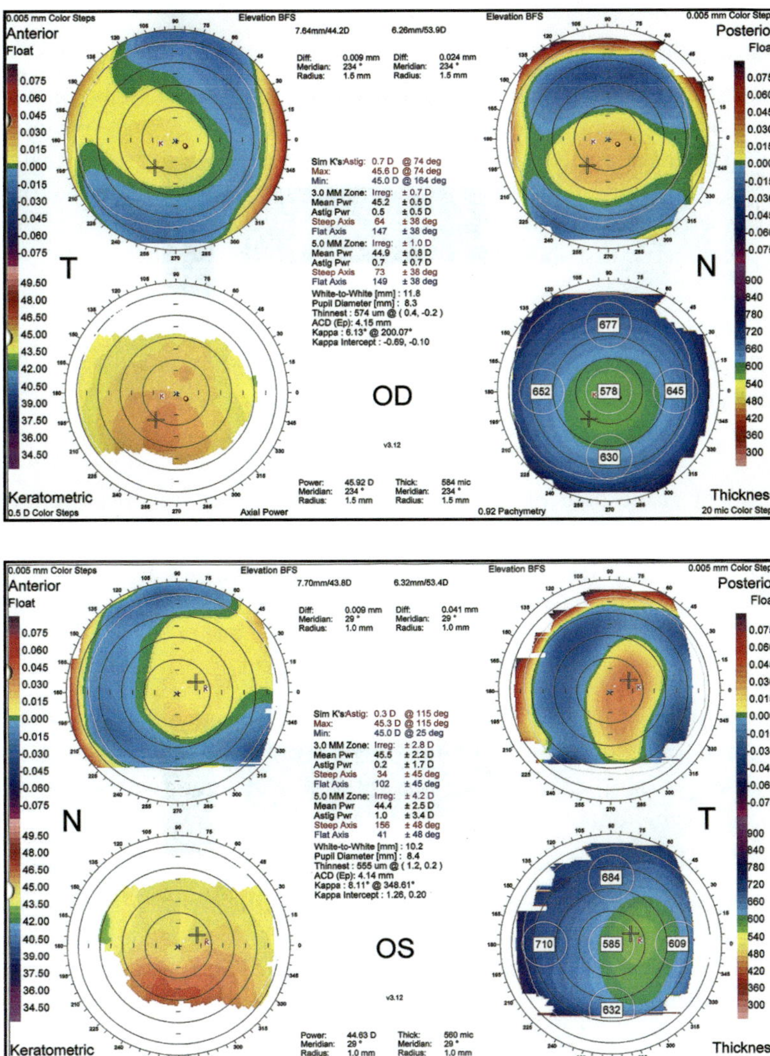
0.005 mm Color Steps
Elevation BFS
Anterior
Float
7.64mm/44.2D
6.26mm/53.9D
Posterior
Float
Diff: 0.009 mm
Meridian: 234 °
Radius: 1.5 mm
Diff: 0.024 mm
Meridian: 234 °
Radius: 1.5 mm
T
N
Sim K's:Astig: 0.7 D @ 74 deg
Max: 45.6 D @ 74 deg
Min: 45.0 D @ 164 deg
3.0 MM Zone: Irreg: ± 0.7 D
Mean Pwr 45.2 ± 0.5 D
Astig Pwr 0.5 ± 0.5 D
Steep Axis 64 ± 38 deg
Flat Axis 147 ± 38 deg
5.0 MM Zone: Irreg: ± 1.0 D
Mean Pwr 44.9 ± 0.8 D
Astig Pwr 0.7 ± 0.7 D
Steep Axis 73 ± 38 deg
Flat Axis 149 ± 38 deg
White-to-White [mm] : 11.8
Pupil Diameter [mm] : 8.3
Thinnest : 574 um @ (0.4, -0.2)
ACD (Ep): 4.15 mm
Kappa : 6.13° @ 200.07°
Kappa Intercept : -0.69, -0.10
OD
677
652
578
645
630
Keratometric
0.5 D Color Steps
Axial Power
Power: 45.92 D
Meridian: 234 °
Radius: 1.5 mm
Thick: 584 mic
Meridian: 234 °
Radius: 1.5 mm
0.92 Pachymetry
Thickness
20 mic Color Steps
0.005 mm Color Steps
Elevation BFS
Anterior
Float
7.70mm/43.8D
6.32mm/53.4D
Posterior
Float
Diff: 0.009 mm
Meridian: 29 °
Radius: 1.0 mm
Diff: 0.041 mm
Meridian: 29 °
Radius: 1.0 mm
N
T
Sim K's:Astig: 0.3 D @ 115 deg
Max: 45.3 D @ 115 deg
Min: 45.0 D @ 25 deg
3.0 MM Zone: Irreg: ± 2.8 D
Mean Pwr 45.5 ± 2.2 D
Astig Pwr 0.2 ± 1.7 D
Steep Axis 34 ± 45 deg
Flat Axis 102 ± 45 deg
5.0 MM Zone: Irreg: ± 4.2 D
Mean Pwr 44.4 ± 2.5 D
Astig Pwr 1.0 ± 3.4 D
Steep Axis 156 ± 48 deg
Flat Axis 41 ± 48 deg
White-to-White [mm] : 10.2
Pupil Diameter [mm] : 8.4
Thinnest : 555 um @ (1.2, 0.2)
ACD (Ep): 4.14 mm
Kappa : 8.11° @ 348.61°
Kappa Intercept : 1.26, 0.20
OS
684
710
585
609
632
Keratometric
0.5 D Color Steps
Axial Power
Power: 44.63 D
Meridian: 29 °
Radius: 1.0 mm
Thick: 560 mic
Meridian: 29 °
Radius: 1.0 mm
0.92 Pachymetry
Thickness
20 mic Color Steps

B

—Case 13—

Irregular Astigmatism From Ocular Surface Issues

Blepharitis

Corneal topographic patterns can be irregular for a variety of reasons, including disruption of the ocular surface through a variety of mechanisms.

Case Analysis

- The estimated residual stromal bed (RSB) thickness is > 400 µm in both eyes.
- Case Figures show (A) slit-lamp image demonstrating significant meibomian gland dysfunction with telangiectasias on the eyelid margin. The cornea is clear. (B) Irregular keratometric maps demonstrating significant inferior steepening in the left eye greater than right. Relative pachymetry appears normal in the right eye, without any significant anterior or posterior float changes. The left eye (B) demonstrates a displaced thinnest corneal point temporally, with abnormal pachymetric distribution and increased posterior elevation.

Pearl: *Blepharitis is equally important and impactful as dry eye, so do not overlook it!*

Questions

1. Is this patient a candidate for refractive surgery? If so, what treatment options are available for this patient?

   No, not at this time. Although the topographic images are likely artifact caused by blepharitis, this must be confirmed by reevaluation after the meibomian gland dysfunction is treated.

2. What is the most likely cause for the topographic findings?

   The patient's physical examination findings are most consistent with blepharitis, although dry eye disorder and contact lens over-wear are also possible. Blepharitis can cause significant fluctuations in Placido imaging with or without significant patient symptoms.

3. Considering all factors, what would you recommend based on this examination and why?

   Treatment of meibomian gland dysfunction with eyelid hygiene and a short course of topical azithromycin or oral doxycycline, along with contact lens wear cessation, is warranted prior to reevaluation of his refractive status and topographic pattern assessment.

—Case 13 (Part 2)—

The patient returned for reevaluation 8 weeks after the initial evaluation and has not worn contact lenses since that time. He reports improved ocular comfort and good compliance with eyelid hygiene, and he has completed a course of topical azithromycin.

CASE HISTORY		
	Right Eye	**Left Eye**
Present correction method	Spectacles	Spectacles
Manifest refraction	-3.00 sphere	-3.00 sphere
CDVA (current)	20/20	20/15
UNVA (current)	20/20	20/20
Physical examination	Improved eyelid appearance	Improved eyelid appearance

Questions

1. Is this patient now a candidate for refractive surgery? If so, what treatment options are available?
2. Considering all factors, what procedure would you recommend, based on this examination, and why?
3. What additional complications is this patient at risk for, given his history?

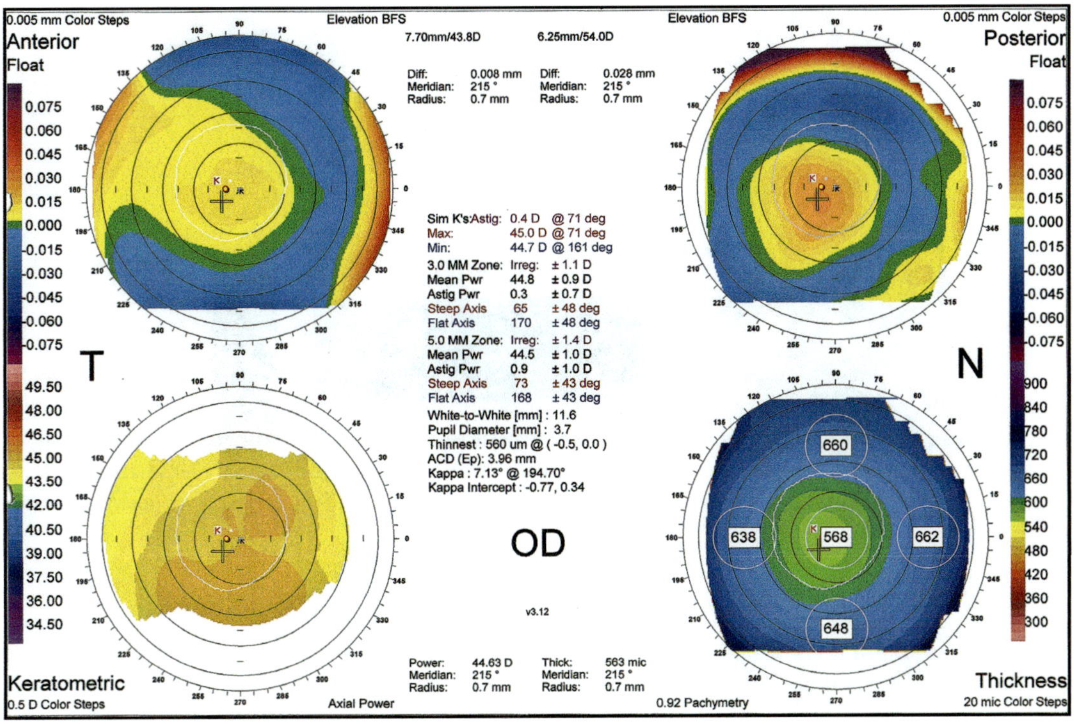
0.005 mm Color Steps
Elevation BFS
Anterior
Float
7.70mm/43.8D
6.25mm/54.0D
Diff: 0.008 mm
Meridian: 215 °
Radius: 0.7 mm
Diff: 0.028 mm
Meridian: 215 °
Radius: 0.7 mm
Elevation BFS
0.005 mm Color Steps
Posterior
Float
0.075
0.060
0.045
0.030
0.015
0.000
-0.015
-0.030
-0.045
-0.060
-0.075
T
N
Sim K's Astig: 0.4 D @ 71 deg
Max: 45.0 D @ 71 deg
Min: 44.7 D @ 161 deg
3.0 MM Zone: Irreg: ± 1.1 D
Mean Pwr 44.8 ± 0.9 D
Astig Pwr 0.3 ± 0.7 D
Steep Axis 65 ± 48 deg
Flat Axis 170 ± 48 deg
5.0 MM Zone: Irreg: ± 1.4 D
Mean Pwr 44.5 ± 1.0 D
Astig Pwr 0.9 ± 1.0 D
Steep Axis 73 ± 43 deg
Flat Axis 168 ± 43 deg
White-to-White [mm] : 11.6
Pupil Diameter [mm] : 3.7
Thinnest : 560 um @ (-0.5, 0.0)
ACD (Ep): 3.96 mm
Kappa : 7.13° @ 194.70°
Kappa Intercept : -0.77, 0.34
OD
v3.12
49.50
48.00
46.50
45.00
43.50
42.00
40.50
39.00
37.50
36.00
34.50
900
840
780
720
660
600
540
480
420
360
300
660
638
568
662
648
Power: 44.63 D
Meridian: 215 °
Radius: 0.7 mm
Thick: 563 mic
Meridian: 215 °
Radius: 0.7 mm
Keratometric
0.5 D Color Steps
Axial Power
0.92 Pachymetry
Thickness
20 mic Color Steps

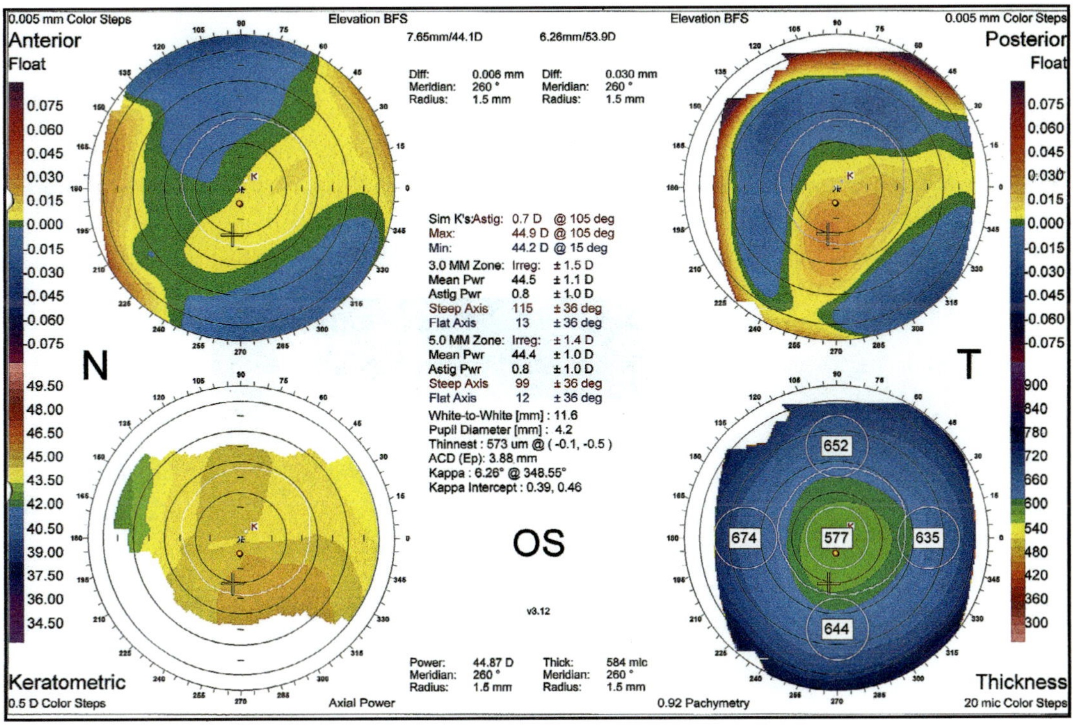
0.005 mm Color Steps
Elevation BFS
Anterior
Float
7.65mm/44.1D
6.26mm/53.9D
Diff: 0.006 mm
Meridian: 260 °
Radius: 1.5 mm
Diff: 0.030 mm
Meridian: 260 °
Radius: 1.5 mm
Elevation BFS
0.005 mm Color Steps
Posterior
Float
0.075
0.060
0.045
0.030
0.015
0.000
-0.015
-0.030
-0.045
-0.060
-0.075
N
T
Sim K's Astig: 0.7 D @ 105 deg
Max: 44.9 D @ 105 deg
Min: 44.2 D @ 15 deg
3.0 MM Zone: Irreg: ± 1.5 D
Mean Pwr 44.5 ± 1.1 D
Astig Pwr 0.8 ± 1.0 D
Steep Axis 115 ± 36 deg
Flat Axis 13 ± 36 deg
5.0 MM Zone: Irreg: ± 1.4 D
Mean Pwr 44.4 ± 1.0 D
Astig Pwr 0.8 ± 1.0 D
Steep Axis 99 ± 36 deg
Flat Axis 12 ± 36 deg
White-to-White [mm] : 11.6
Pupil Diameter [mm] : 4.2
Thinnest : 573 um @ (-0.1, -0.5)
ACD (Ep): 3.88 mm
Kappa : 6.26° @ 348.55°
Kappa Intercept : 0.39, 0.46
OS
v3.12
49.50
48.00
46.50
45.00
43.50
42.00
40.50
39.00
37.50
36.00
34.50
900
840
780
720
660
600
540
480
420
360
300
652
674
577
635
644
Power: 44.87 D
Meridian: 260 °
Radius: 1.5 mm
Thick: 584 mic
Meridian: 260 °
Radius: 1.5 mm
Keratometric
0.5 D Color Steps
Axial Power
0.92 Pachymetry
Thickness
20 mic Color Steps

—Case 13 (Part 2)—
Irregular Astigmatism From Ocular Surface Issues
Blepharitis-Related Irregular Topography

Blepharitis is an underappreciated factor impacting topographic patterns, especially Placido imaging, and can create irregular patterns as dramatic as tear deficiency or contact lens warpage. In patients with significant blepharitis, treatment to maximize eyelid gland function may be necessary before an accurate assessment of surgical candidacy can be made. Blepharitis is also a leading cause of contact lens intolerance, and thus is a common finding in patients seeking refractive surgery.

Case Analysis

- The Case Figures show normal topographies with only mild asymmetric bowtie patterns and otherwise normal pachymetric distributions and float values.

Pearl: *For best results, manage blepharitis aggressively before AND after laser vision correction!*

Questions

1. Is this patient now a candidate for refractive surgery? If so, what treatment options are available for this patient?

    Yes, based on the improvement in topographic patterns, slightly improved visual acuity, and an otherwise stable refractive examination, this patient is now a candidate for surgery. The patient is potentially a candidate for surface ablation or LASIK.

2. Considering all factors, what procedure would you recommend, based on this examination, and why?

    This patient is a reasonable candidate for surface ablation or LASIK. Given the potential increased risk of infection from blepharitis and no biomechanical concerns, LASIK is likely the best option.

3. What additional complications is this patient at risk for, given his history?

    In addition to increased infection risk with surface ablation, patients with significant blepharitis have an increased risk for interface debris at the time of LASIK and diffuse lamellar keratitis or peripheral keratitis postoperatively.

Irregular Astigmatism From Ocular Surface Disorders

Placido imaging is most sensitive to tear film abnormalities, making it a good technology to identify subtle ocular surface issues, but it is more likely to generate artifacts. As demonstrated by the topographic figures in this case, scanning-slit technology is not immune to artifact when the tear film is compromised. Scheimpflug imaging appears to be less sensitive to tear film anomalies than other imaging technologies in most cases (Case Figure 13-1).

Pretreating Patients With Blepharitis to Maximize Laser Vision Correction Outcomes

Meibomian gland dysfunction may be improved with eyelid hygiene and a short course of topical azithromycin or oral doxycycline. Both of these antibiotic treatment protocols are "off-label" use. Macrolide antibiotics improve meibomian gland lipid composition and flow, thereby reducing bacterial overgrowth.

Beyond improving screening evaluation, reducing meibomian gland dysfunction can improve early refractive outcomes by improving tear film quantity and quality and reduce the risk of infection or interface complications, such as DLK. For more information on approval ranges, see Chapter 2.

Refractive Surgery for Patients With Blepharitis

The best surgical procedure for patients with ocular surface abnormalities ultimately depends on the severity of these issues and their response to treatment prior to surgery. For patients with severe blepharitis that is refractory to treatment, laser vision correction is not recommended. However, most patients respond well to straightforward treatment plans and are surgical candidates. Patients should be counseled that neither the treatment used for their blepharitis nor laser vision correction will eliminate their underlying condition and that the foreign body sensation symptoms they have attributed to contact lens wear may or may not improve after surgery.

Due to the increased risk of infection from significant blepharitis, these patients are often better suited for LASIK than surface ablation. Peripheral infiltrates, either infectious or sterile, are still possible and should be managed aggressively (Case Figure 13-2). Further, patients with blepharitis may be more likely to develop diffuse lamellar keratitis, and they should be watched closely for this.

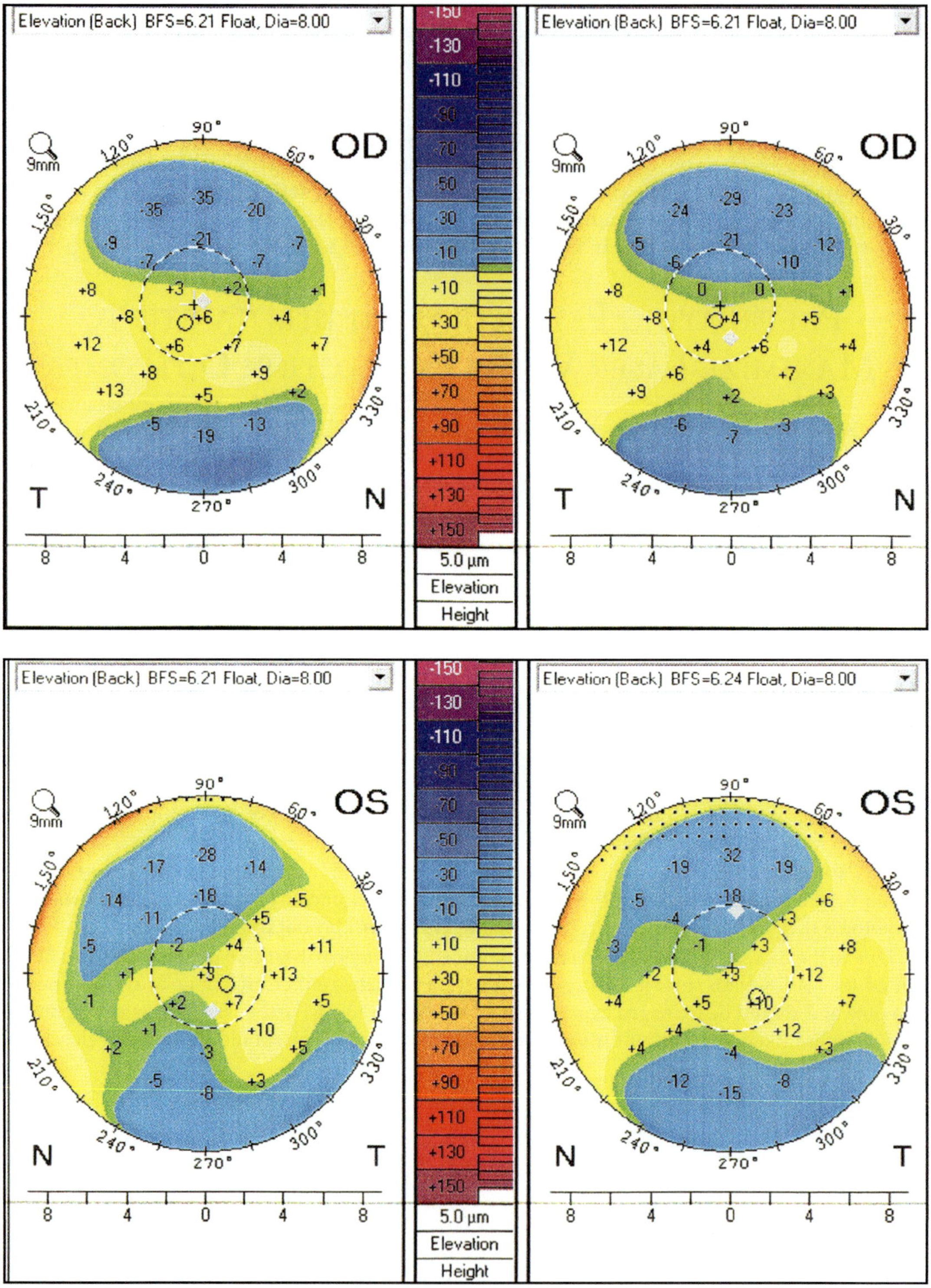

Case Figure 13-1. Pentacam (OCULUS Optikgerate GmbH) posterior elevation maps before (left) and after (right) a short course of treatment for blepharitis. Note that, compared with the dramatic changes observed in Placido and scanning-slit beam imaging, there is relatively little change in the "before" and "after" images.

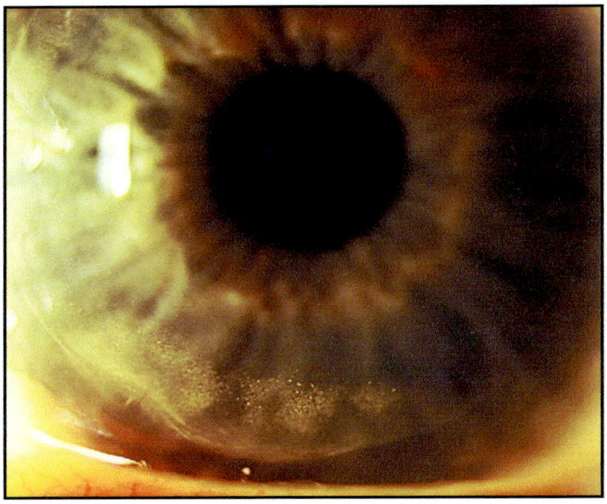

Case Figure 13-2. Slit-lamp image of a patient with blepharitis who developed significant inflammation at the flap edge after LASIK.

Bibliography

Ambrósio R Jr, Periman LM, Netto MV, Wilson SE. Bilateral marginal sterile infiltrates and diffuse lamellar keratitis after laser in situ keratomileusis. *J Refract Surg*. 2003;19(2):154-158.

Dursun D, Piniella AM, Pflugfelder SC. Pseudokeratoconus caused by rosacea. *Cornea*. 2001;20(6):668-669.

Foulks GN, Borchman D, Yappert M, Kim SH, McKay JW. Topical azithromycin therapy for meibomian gland dysfunction: clinical response and lipid alterations. *Cornea*. 2010;29(7):781-788.

Haque RM, Torkildsen GL, Brubaker K, et al. Multicenter open-label study evaluating the efficacy of azithromycin ophthalmic solution 1% on the signs and symptoms of subjects with blepharitis. *Cornea*. 2010;29(8):871-877.

Igami TZ, Holzchuh R, Osaki TH, Santo RM, Kara-Jose N, Hida RY. Oral azithromycin for treatment of posterior blepharitis. *Cornea*. 2011;30(10):1145-1149.

Joffre C, Souchier M, Grégoire S, et al. Differences in meibomian fatty acid composition in patients with meibomian gland dysfunction and aqueous-deficient dry eye. *Br J Ophthalmol*. 2008;92(1):116-119.

Karimian F, Baradaran-Rafii A, Javadi MA, Nazari R, Rabei HM, Jafarinasab MR. Bilateral bacterial keratitis in three patients following photorefractive keratectomy. *J Refract Surg*. 2007;23(7):312-315.

Lahners WJ, Hardten DR, Lindstrom RL. Peripheral keratitis following laser in situ keratomileusis. *J Refract Surg*. 2003;19(6):671-675.

Levinson BA, Rapuano CJ, Cohen EJ, Hammersmith KM, Ayres BD, Laibson PR. Referrals to the Wills Eye Institute Cornea Service after laser in situ keratomileusis: reasons for patient dissatisfaction. *J Cataract Refract Surg*. 2008 Jan;34(1):32-39.

Markomanolakis MM, Kymionis GD, Aslanides IM, Astyrakakis N, Pallikaris IG. Induced videokeratography alterations in patients with excessive meibomian secretions. *Cornea*. 2005;24:16-19.

Matsumoto Y, Dogru M, Goto E, et al. Efficacy of a new warm moist air device on tear functions of patients with simple meibomian gland dysfunction. *Cornea*. 2006;25(6):644-650.

Pinna A, Piccinini P, Carta F. Effect of oral linoleic and gamma-linolenic acid on meibomian gland dysfunction. *Cornea*. 2007;26(3):260-264.

Souchier M, Joffre C, Grégoire S, et al. Changes in meibomian fatty acids and clinical signs in patients with meibomian gland dysfunction after minocycline treatment. *Br J Ophthalmol*. 2008;92(6):819-822.

Veldman P, Colby K. Current evidence for topical azithromycin 1% ophthalmic solution in the treatment of blepharitis and blepharitis-associated ocular dryness. *Int Ophthalmol Clin*. 2011;51(4):43-52.

—Case 14—

A 35-year-old female desires refractive surgical correction. She has no significant family, past medical, or ocular history.

CASE HISTORY		
	Right Eye	**Left Eye**
Present correction method	CTL	CTL
Manifest refraction	-4.00 +0.50 x 087	-3.75 +0.50 x 065
CDVA (current)	20/20	20/20
Dominant eye	Right	
Ocular alignment	Orthophoric	Orthophoric
Keratometry		
Flat K	44.0 @ 140	44.0 @ 030
Steep K	44.5 @ 050	44.5 @ 120
Pupil size (bright)	4.6 mm	4.4 mm
Pupil size (dim)	6.2 mm	5.9 mm
Central corneal thickness	478 µm	479 µm
Physical examination	Normal	Normal
Estimated ablation depth	65 µm	65 µm

Questions

1. Is this patient a candidate for refractive surgery? If so, what treatment options are available?
2. Considering all factors, what procedure would you recommend and why?
3. What additional information could be of particular utility in evaluating this patient for surgery?
4. What are the most significant potential complications for each procedure available for this patient, based on her examination?
5. What special considerations are there for this patient regarding potential retreatment for postoperative ametropia?

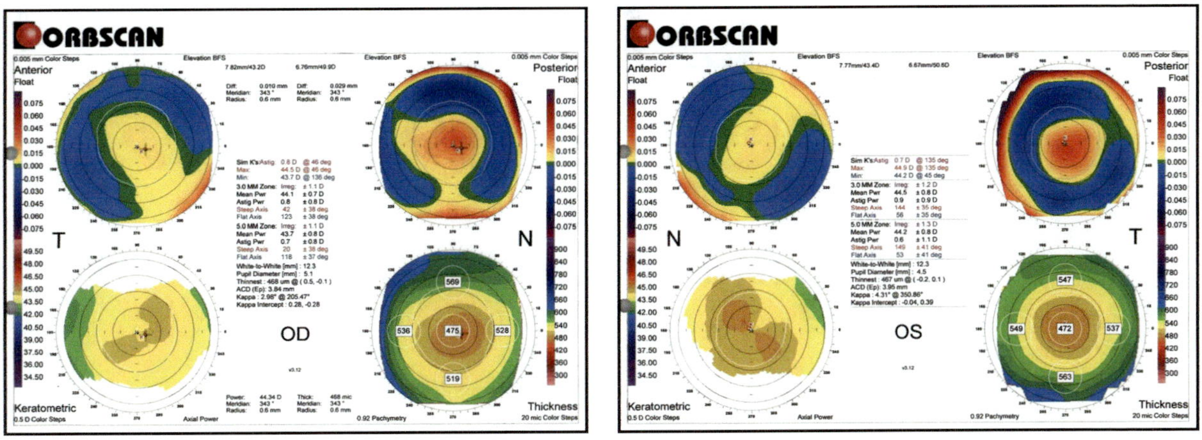
ORBSCAN
Anterior
Float
Posterior
Float
T
N
OD
Keratometric
Thickness
ORBSCAN
Anterior
Float
Posterior
Float
N
T
OS
Keratometric
Thickness

A

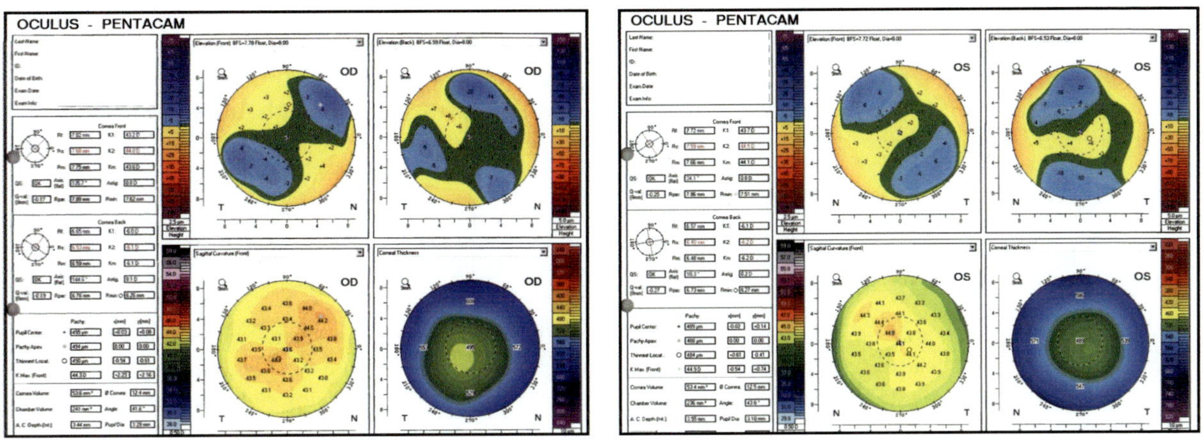
OCULUS - PENTACAM
OD
OCULUS - PENTACAM
OS

B

—Case 14—

Laser Vision Correction in Thin Corneas

How Thin Is Too Thin for LASIK?

Laser vision correction (LVC) screening for patients with thin corneas remains a hot topic of debate; specifically, the appropriate screening strategies to differentiate "normal" thin corneas from "ectasia-susceptible" thin corneas. Corneal ectatic disorders are associated with reduced corneal thickness, and keratoconic populations have significantly thinner corneas, on average, than normal patient populations; however, significant overlap exists. This does not mean that thin corneas are abnormal; it merely means that additional screening, consideration of multiple treatment options, and a full informed discussion is warranted in these patients. Although many anecdotal reports use 500 µm as the "cutoff" value for LASIK, no evidence exists to support this.

Case Analysis

- The estimated residual stromal bed (RSB) thickness is approximately 295 to 315 µm in both eyes
- Case Figures show normal topographic patterns in both eyes mild asymmetry with normal tomographic features. Ultrasonic and Scheimpflug pachymetry data correspond relatively well in this patient, and there is no significant focal anterior or posterior elevation in either eye in either scanning-slit or Scheimplfug imaging.

Pearl: *Thin, but otherwise normal, corneas do not appear to incur additional postoperative risk, but what constitutes "normal" is still heavily debated!*

Questions

1. Is this patient a candidate for refractive surgery? If so, what treatment options are available?

    Yes, this patient appears to be a reasonable candidate for refractive surgery. In her prescription range, LASIK and surface ablation are both possible options.

2. Considering all factors, what procedure would you recommend and why?

    Given this normal topography and an otherwise normal examination, in her prescription range both options produce ultimately similar visual results. Anticipated RSB thickness is reasonable for LASIK and excellent for surface ablation, so either approach is reasonable. This case requires a thorough discussion with the patient regarding risks and benefits unique to her situation to allow her to make an informed decision.

3. What additional information could be of particular utility in evaluating this patient for surgery?

   Given the patient's normal topography, age, and relatively low refraction, the amount of data available is likely sufficient for both surgeon and patient to make an informed decision.

4. What are the most significant potential complications for each procedure available for this patient, based on her examination?

   Routine concerns for surface ablation and LASIK; these risks are likely no higher than with any other patient.

5. What special considerations are there for this patient regarding potential retreatment for postoperative ametropia?

   Due to the patient's preoperative corneal thickness, if she undergoes LASIK and subsequently needs retreatment, it may be best to offer surface ablation (depending on actual measured intraoperative RSB, rather than estimated preoperative values). If the patient initially has surface ablation, then repeat surface ablation would be the best retreatment option.

Laser Vision Correction in Thin Corneas

Multiple studies have found that long-term visual quality is equivalent between surface ablation and LASIK for routine patients. However, LASIK has advantages in the early postoperative period, and many patients are motivated to undergo LASIK instead of surface ablation. Multiple considerations for LASIK in thin corneas include: the accuracy of thickness measurements, flap thickness, biomechanical evaluation, and surgical outcomes.

Measuring Corneal Thickness

In this case, ultrasound central pachymetry values are comparable to those determined by scanning slit-beam and Scheimpflug imaging. Ultrasound pachymetry is still considered the gold standard for thickness evaluation, but other techniques, especially optical coherence tomography and Scheimpflug imaging, provide accurate central and regional thickness measurements. Scanning slit-beam imaging (Orbscan II; Bausch & Lomb) has traditionally been less accurate than ultrasound; however, with correction factors, the Orbscan II presents a reasonable representation of corneal thickness. Still, variations among technologies for individual eyes continue to occur, and they do not appear to be clearly interchangeable.

LASIK Flap Thickness

Thin-flap LASIK produces visual results equivalent to thicker flaps while imparting biomechanical advantages to these corneas by functionally removing less corneal tissue. Flap thickness reproducibility is critical when considering LASIK in patients with thin corneas. Some modern microkeratomes and most femtosecond lasers are able to create thin reproducible flap thickness with standard deviations ±10 µm. However, there may be a limit to how thin corneal flaps can be reasonably made due to the reported increased risk of haze formation in ultra-thin flaps (< 90 µm).

Residual Stromal Bed Thickness Calculations

Using this case as an example, estimated RSB thickness approximately 295 µm or thicker in both eyes for thin-flap LASIK by utilizing 120 µm as a safe estimated flap thickness (2 standard deviations above the 100-µm settings). A thinner RSB thickness could occur, but it should happen in less than 1% of eyes. Although no specific RSB thickness cutoff has been established, 250 µm has been used for years as the lowest value recommended, despite a lack of supportive empiric data. In practice, most surgeons use ≈250 to 300 µm, but this number has been gradually increasing, rather than decreasing, over the past few years.

Estimated RSB thickness is just that—a prediction based on average flap thicknesses and ablation depths. Many surgeons advocate measuring intraoperative pachymetry routinely. In this specific case measured intraoperative pachymetry, after the flap has been created and lifted but before stromal ablation, is critical. Estimated RSB thickness values are invaluable for surgical planning, but actual values should be obtained for any borderline cases to ensure that a thick flap did not occur.

Ectasia Risk for Thin Corneas

The critical consideration for patients with thin corneas is their risk for developing postoperative ectasia. Multiple case-control studies have found corneal thickness to be an independent risk factor for postoperative ectasia, even in patients with normal preoperative topography; in every controlled population study to date, corneas that developed ectasia were thinner than the control eyes. However, there are also numerous reports of corneas < 500 µm that undergo uneventful LASIK without developing ectasia. Thus, detailed biomechanical evaluation can be helpful in assessing suspicious corneas.

Given the variables of age, topography and tomography, and ablation depth in the patient presented, there does not appear to be additional cause for concern with thin-flap LASIK, especially when considering the "big picture" of balancing the ectasia risk with LASIK against the infection risk with surface ablation procedures. For more information, see the section on Postoperative Corneal Ectasia in Chapter 5.

Bibliography

Azar DT, Ghanem RC, de la Cruz J, et al. Thin-flap (sub-Bowman keratomileusis) versus thick-flap laser in situ keratomileusis for moderate to high myopia: case-control analysis. *J Cataract Refract Surg.* 2008;34(12):2073-2078.

Bansal A, Doherty T, Randleman JB, Stulting RD. Influence of flap thickness on visual and refractive outcomes after laser in situ keratomileusis performed with a mechanical microkeratome. *J Cataract Refract Surg* .2010;36(5):810-813.

Barequet IS, Hirsh A, Levinger S. Effect of thin femtosecond LASIK flaps on corneal sensitivity and tear function. *J Refract Surg.* 2008;24(9):897-902.

Binder PS, Trattler WB. Evaluation of a risk factor scoring system for corneal ectasia after LASIK in eyes with normal topography. *J Refract Surg.* 2010;26(4):241-250.

Caster AI, Friess DW, Potvin RJ. Absence of keratectasia after LASIK in eyes with preoperative central corneal thickness of 450 to 500 microns. *J Refract Surg.* 2007;23(8):782-788.

Cheng AC, Tang E, Mohamed S, Lam DS. Correction factor in Orbscan II in the assessment of corneal pachymetry. *Cornea.* 2006;25(10):1158-1161.

de Benito-Llopis L, Teus MA, Sánchez-Pina JM. Comparison between LASEK with mitomycin C and LASIK for the correction of myopia of -7.00 to -13.75 D. *J Refract Surg.* 2008;24(5):516-523.

Hafezi F, Seiler T. Persistent subepithelial haze in thin-flap LASIK. *J Refract Surg.* 2010;26(3):222-225.

Kymionis GD, Bouzoukis D, Diakonis V, et al. Long-term results of thin corneas after refractive laser surgery. *Am J Ophthalmol.* 2007;144(2):181-185.

Kymionis GD, Portaliou DM, Tsiklis NS, Panagopoulou SI, Pallikaris IG. Thin LASIK flap creation using the SCHWIND Carriazo-Pendular microkeratome. *J Refract Surg.* 2009;25(1):33-36.

Moshirfar M, Hatch BB, Chang JC, Kurz CJ, Eugarrios MF, Mifflin MD. Prospective, contralateral comparison of 120-μm and 90-μm LASIK flaps using the IntraLase FS60 femtosecond laser. *J Refract Surg.* 2011;27(4):251-259.

Randleman JB, Loft ES, Banning CS, Lynn MJ, Stulting RD. Outcomes of wavefront-optimized surface ablation. *Ophthalmology.* 2007;114(5):983-988.

Randleman JB, Trattler WB, Stulting RD. Validation of the Ectasia Risk Score System for preoperative laser in situ keratomileusis screening. *Am J Ophthalmol.* 2008;145(5):813-818.

Randleman JB, Woodward M, Lynn MJ, Stulting RD. Risk assessment for ectasia after corneal refractive surgery. *Ophthalmology.* 2008;115(1):37-50.

Rocha KM, Kagan R, Smith SD, Krueger RR. Thresholds for interface haze formation after thin-flap femtosecond laser in situ keratomileusis for myopia. *Am J Ophthalmol.* 2009;147(6):966-972, 972.e1.

Rocha KM, Randleman JB, Stulting RD. Analysis of microkeratome thin flap architecture using Fourier-domain optical coherence tomography. *J Refract Surg.* 2011;27(10):759-763.

Salz JJ, Binder PS. Is there a "magic number" to reduce the risk of ectasia after laser in situ keratomileusis and photorefractive keratectomy? *Am J Ophthalmol.* 2007;144(2):284-285.

Stahl JE, Durrie DS, Schwendeman FJ, Boghossian AJ. Anterior segment OCT analysis of thin IntraLase femtosecond flaps. *J Refract Surg.* 2007;23(6):555-558.

Vaddavalli PK, Yoo SH. Femtosecond laser in-situ keratomileusis flap configurations. *Curr Opin Ophthalmol.* 2011;22(4):245-250.

—Case 15—

A 34-year-old male desires refractive surgical correction. He has no significant family, past medical, or ocular history.

CASE HISTORY		
	Right Eye	**Left Eye**
Present correction method	CTL	CTL
Manifest refraction	-4.50 +1.50 x 095	-5.75 +1.00 x 095
CDVA (current)	20/20	20/20
Dominant eye	Right	
Ocular alignment	Orthophoric	Orthophoric
Keratometry		
Flat K	44.0 @ 180	44.0 @ 180
Steep K	46.0 @ 090	45.5 @ 090
Pupil size (bright)	3.1 mm	3.0 mm
Pupil size (dim)	5.6 mm	5.6 mm
Central corneal thickness	471 μm	480 μm
Physical examination	Normal	Normal
Estimated ablation depth	70 μm	90 μm

Questions

1. Is this patient a candidate for refractive surgery? If so, what treatment options are available?
2. Considering all factors, what procedure would you recommend and why?
3. What additional information could be of particular utility in evaluating this patient for surgery?
4. What are the most significant potential complications for each procedure available for this patient, based on his examination?
5. What special considerations are there for this patient regarding potential retreatment for postoperative ametropia?

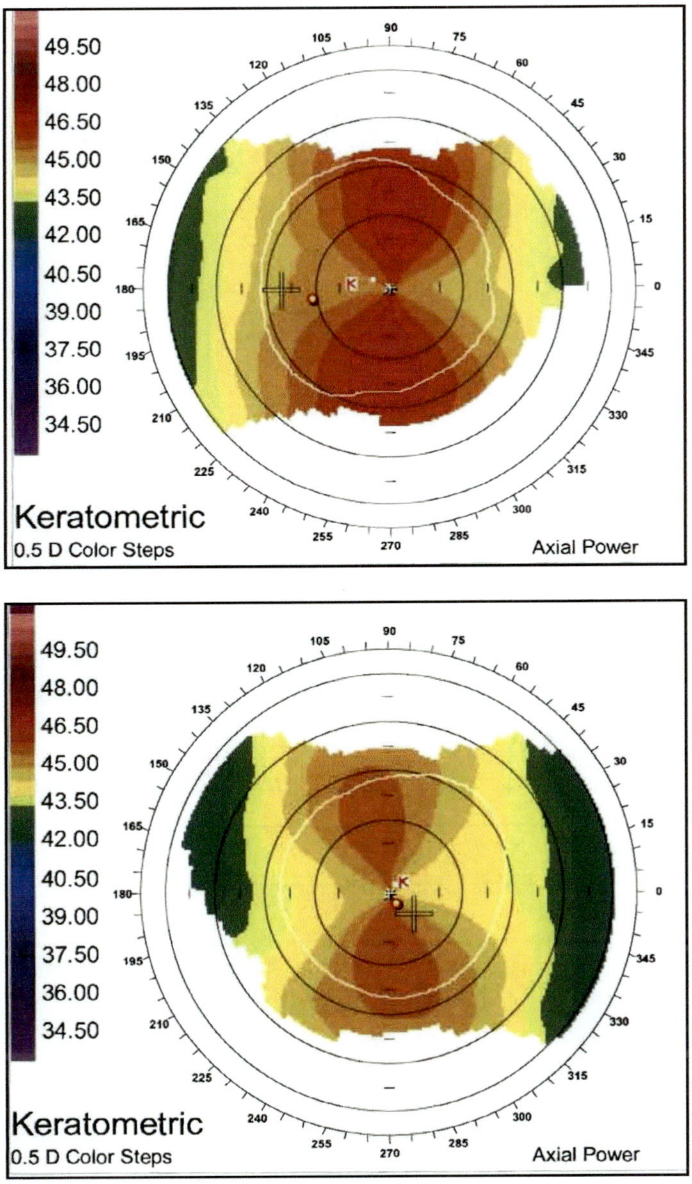
49.50
48.00
46.50
45.00
43.50
42.00
40.50
39.00
37.50
36.00
34.50
Keratometric
0.5 D Color Steps
Axial Power
49.50
48.00
46.50
45.00
43.50
42.00
40.50
39.00
37.50
36.00
34.50
Keratometric
0.5 D Color Steps
Axial Power

A

B

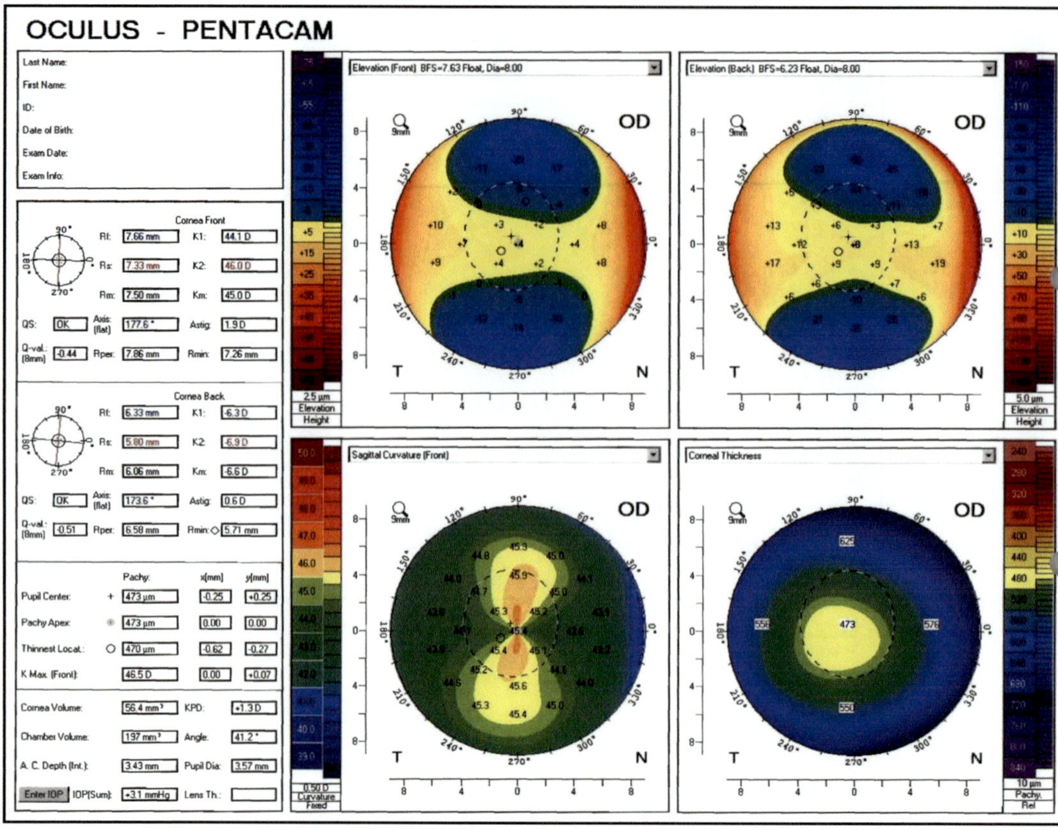
OCULUS - PENTACAM
Last Name:
First Name:
ID:
Date of Birth:
Exam Date:
Exam Info:
Cornea Front
Rf: 7.66 mm K1: 44.1 D
Rs: 7.33 mm K2: 46.0 D
Rm: 7.50 mm Km: 45.0 D
QS: OK Axis (flat): 177.6° Astig: 1.9 D
Q-val. (8mm): -0.44 Rper: 7.86 mm Rmin: 7.26 mm
Cornea Back
Rf: 6.33 mm K1: -6.3 D
Rs: 5.80 mm K2: -6.9 D
Rm: 6.06 mm Km: -6.6 D
QS: OK Axis (flat): 173.6° Astig: 0.6 D
Q-val. (8mm): -0.51 Rper: 6.58 mm Rmin: 5.71 mm
Pachy x[mm] y[mm]
Pupil Center: + 473 µm -0.25 +0.25
Pachy Apex: 473 µm 0.00 0.00
Thinnest Locat.: ○ 470 µm -0.62 -0.27
K Max. (Front): 46.5 D 0.00 +0.07
Cornea Volume: 56.4 mm³ KPD: +1.3 D
Chamber Volume: 197 mm³ Angle: 41.2°
A. C. Depth (Int.): 3.43 mm Pupil Dia: 3.57 mm
Enter IOP IOP(Sum): +3.1 mmHg Lens Th.:
Elevation (Front) BFS=7.63 Float, Dia=8.00
Elevation (Back) BFS=6.23 Float, Dia=8.00
Sagittal Curvature (Front)
Corneal Thickness
OD
T N
2.5 µm Elevation Height
5.0 µm Elevation Height
0.50 D Curvature Fixed
10 µm Pachy. Rel
473
625
556
576
550

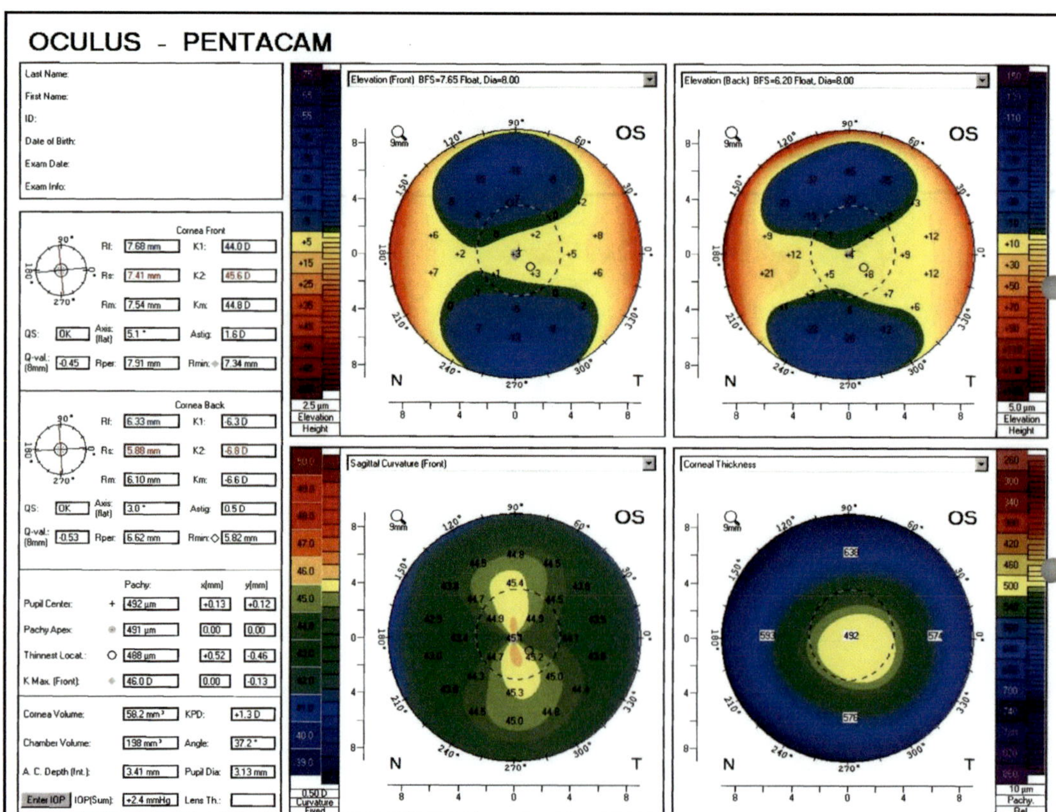
OCULUS - PENTACAM
Last Name:
First Name:
ID:
Date of Birth:
Exam Date:
Exam Info:
Cornea Front
Rf: 7.68 mm K1: 44.0 D
Rs: 7.41 mm K2: 45.6 D
Rm: 7.54 mm Km: 44.8 D
QS: OK Axis (flat): 5.1° Astig: 1.6 D
Q-val. (8mm): -0.45 Rper: 7.91 mm Rmin: 7.34 mm
Cornea Back
Rf: 6.33 mm K1: -6.3 D
Rs: 5.88 mm K2: -6.8 D
Rm: 6.10 mm Km: -6.6 D
QS: OK Axis (flat): 3.0° Astig: 0.5 D
Q-val. (8mm): -0.53 Rper: 6.62 mm Rmin: 5.82 mm
Pachy x[mm] y[mm]
Pupil Center: + 492 µm +0.13 +0.12
Pachy Apex: 491 µm 0.00 0.00
Thinnest Locat.: ○ 488 µm +0.52 -0.46
K Max. (Front): 46.0 D 0.00 -0.13
Cornea Volume: 58.2 mm³ KPD: +1.3 D
Chamber Volume: 198 mm³ Angle: 37.2°
A. C. Depth (Int.): 3.41 mm Pupil Dia: 3.13 mm
Enter IOP IOP(Sum): +2.4 mmHg Lens Th.:
Elevation (Front) BFS=7.65 Float, Dia=8.00
Elevation (Back) BFS=6.20 Float, Dia=8.00
Sagittal Curvature (Front)
Corneal Thickness
OS
N T
2.5 µm Elevation Height
5.0 µm Elevation Height
0.50 D Curvature Fixed
10 µm Pachy. Rel
492
593
574
576

—Case 15—

Laser Vision Correction in Thin Corneas

When Does Thin Indicate Increased Risk?

A previous case in this book introduced the issues surrounding appropriate screening strategies to differentiate "normal" thin corneas from "suspicious" thin corneas. This case presents additional technologies that are available to differentiate "thin normal" corneas from "thin suspicious" corneas.

Case Analysis

- The estimated residual stromal bed (RSB) thickness is approximately 280 to 300 µm the right eye and 260 to 280 µm in the left eye.
- Case Figures show (A) normal topographic pattern in both eyes (symmetric bowtie). (B) Scheimpflug imaging (Pentacam; OCULUS Optikgerate GmbH) demonstrates a symmetric bowtie sagittal curvature pattern in both eyes, a mildly increased focal posterior elevation in both eyes, central corneal thickness of 473 µm in the right eye, and 492 µm in the left eye with a corneal thickness profile appears skewed inferotemporally in both eyes.

Pearl: *LASIK and surface ablation produce equivalent long-term outcomes; therefore, when corneal biomechanics are of some concern, choose surface ablation!*

Questions

1. Is this patient a candidate for refractive surgery? If so, what treatment options are available?

   Yes, this patient appears to be a candidate for refractive surgery. Based on his prescription, LASIK, surface ablation, and phakic IOL are possible options.

2. Considering all factors, what procedure would you recommend and why?

   Due to the corneal thickness with an estimated RSB thickness between 260 and 280 µm in both eyes with thin-flap LASIK, and some mildly suspicious findings on advanced testing, I would not offer LASIK but would offer surface ablation.

3. What additional information could be of particular utility in evaluating this patient for surgery?

   In this patient, additional biomechanical testing would be especially useful. These studies could include advanced Scheimpflug imaging, optical coherence tomography (OCT), and/or Ocular Response Analyzer (ORA; Reichert Technologies) analysis to further evaluate central and peripheral (relational) corneal thickness, as well as corneal hysteresis.

4. What are the most significant potential complications for each procedure available for this patient, based on his examination?

   The potential complications include the basic concerns regarding healing time and infection risk with surface ablation, and the potential increased risk of postoperative ectasia with surface ablation or LASIK, with greater ectasia risk with LASIK.

5. What special considerations are there for this patient regarding potential retreatment for postoperative ametropia?

   If this patient did undergo LASIK as primary surgery, he would not be a candidate for LASIK retreatment. Further, prior to retreatment a clear distinction would need to be made between residual ametropia or regression and early ectasia, where retreatment would be contraindicated. If the patient has surface ablation initially, then repeat surface ablation would be the best retreatment option, given the same caveats regarding early ectasia.

Laser Vision Correction in Thin, Mildly Suspicious Corneas

In this case, some initial findings are cause for concern and warrant a more detailed investigation in this patient, including a thin cornea centrally, the thinnest corneal point that is displaced from the center, and reduced relational corneal thickness when comparing inferior central values to superior central values. Figures Cases 15-1 to 15-3 display data generated from Scheimpflug, OCT, and ORA evaluations. In assessing these tests, there is a consistent pattern of displaced thinnest point on the cornea from center, as well as a less than normal thickening progression when moving from the center to the periphery in the inferotemporal quadrants of both eyes. This location is more worrisome than others because it is typically the weakest region of the cornea and is frequently the first location of focal thinning and steepening in keratoconus.

Taken together, these findings suggest that this patient's corneas may not be biomechanically normal, although no one specific test is definitive. Although the ORA Keratoconus Match Index provides an easy-to-read number, it has yet to be validated as definitive evidence of abnormality, and previous studies of ORA data have shown great overlap between normal and keratoconic populations. Therefore, this cornea can be accurately classified as "suspicious" rather than definitively normal or abnormal. Given that analysis, what is the best choice for surgery?

In this patient, the risk of ectasia after laser vision correction is unknown, but it is likely higher than the average patient for LASIK. Surface ablation carries a significantly lower (but undetermined) risk of ectasia than LASIK. However, ectasia can occur after surface ablation, and this patient should be counseled on the low, but possibly increased, risk of ectasia with any surgical procedure.

Patients with thin corneas and any suspicious findings on initial testing benefit from more advanced evaluation to obtain a better sense of their actual biomechanical status. Ideally, future testing will be able to directly address these issues and provide definitive answers on the level of risk in these suspicious individuals. For more information, see the section on Postoperative Corneal Ectasia in Chapter 5.

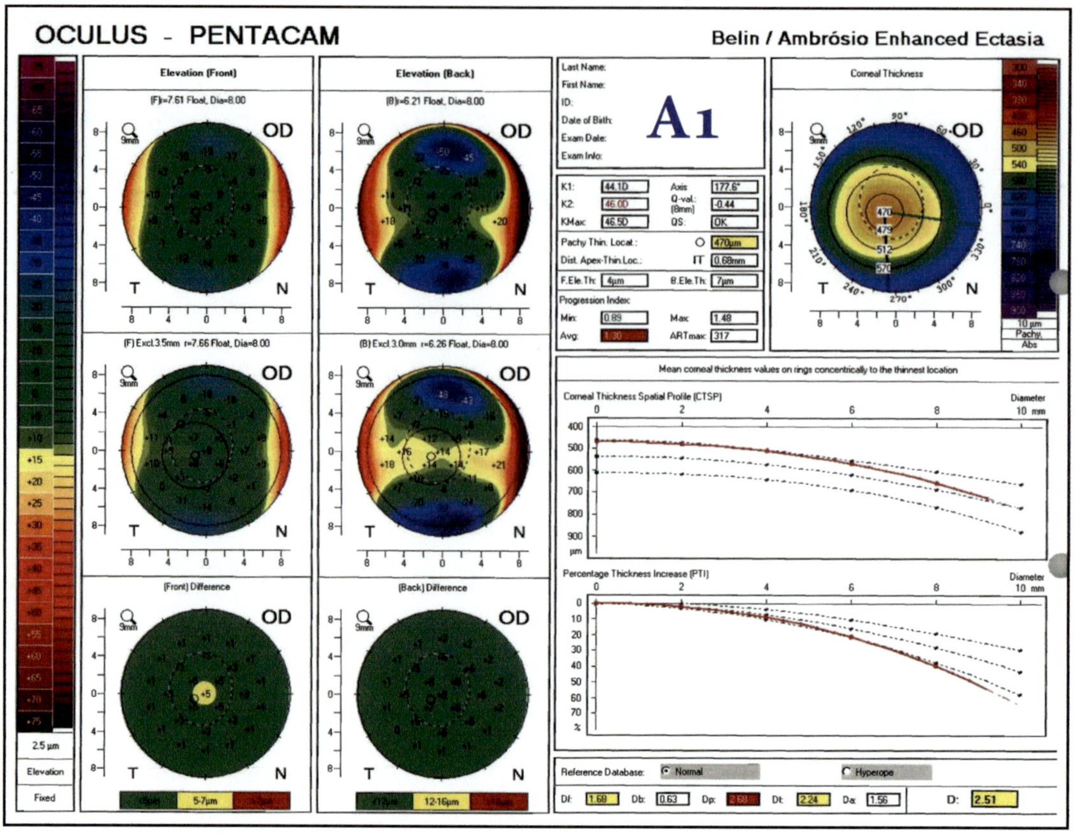

Case Figure 15-1. Scheimpflug imaging in the right and left eyes (expanded from Case Figure B, OD and OS) demonstrates (A1,A2) suspicious, but not definitive, findings on the Belin/Ambrosio enhanced display. Specifically, there is no major focal anterior or posterior elevation, but ARTMax is low in both eyes, and the "D" score is suspicious at 2.51 OD and 2.45 OS. Corneal thickness profile appears suspicious in both eyes. *(continued)*

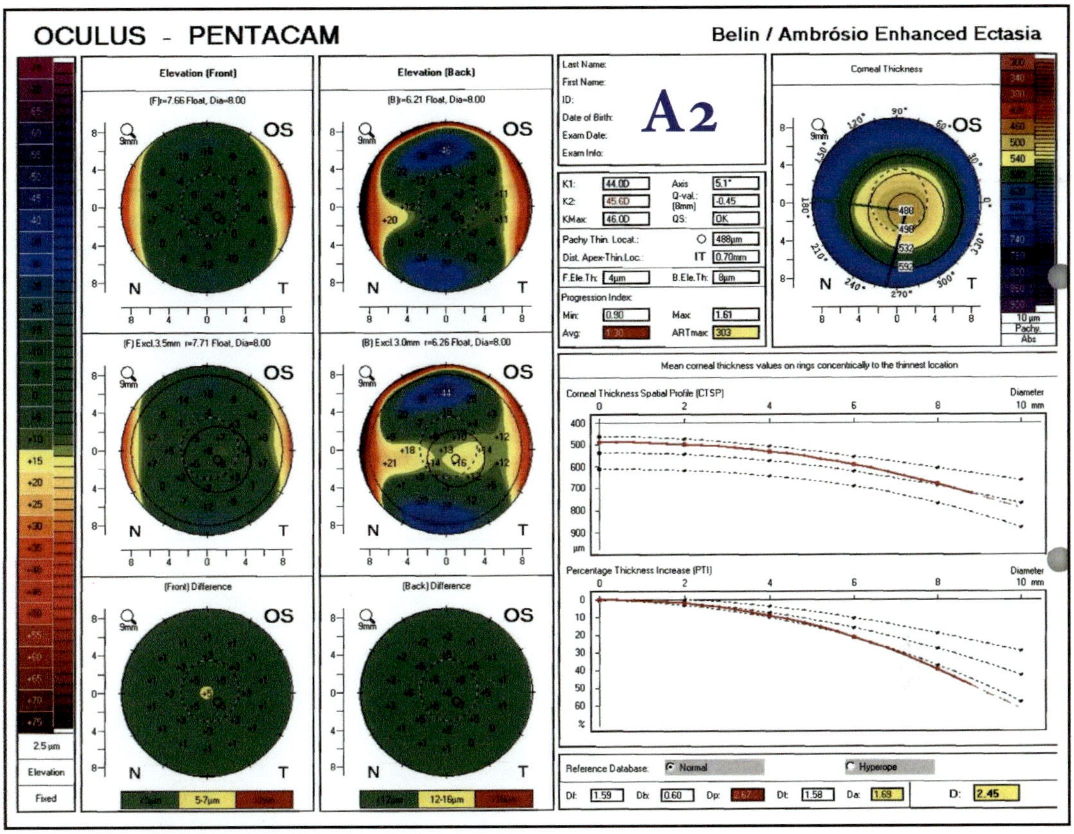

Case Figure 15-1 (continued).

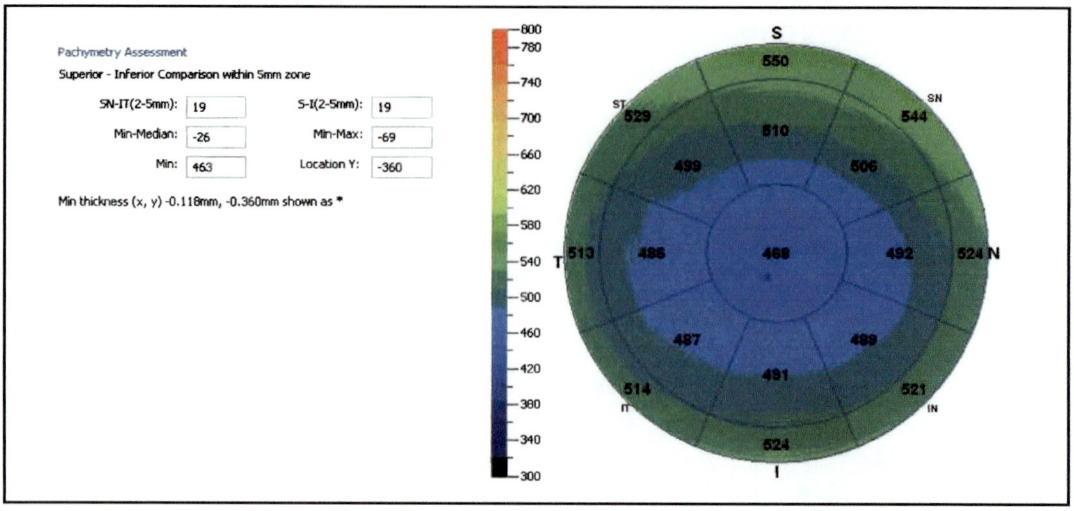

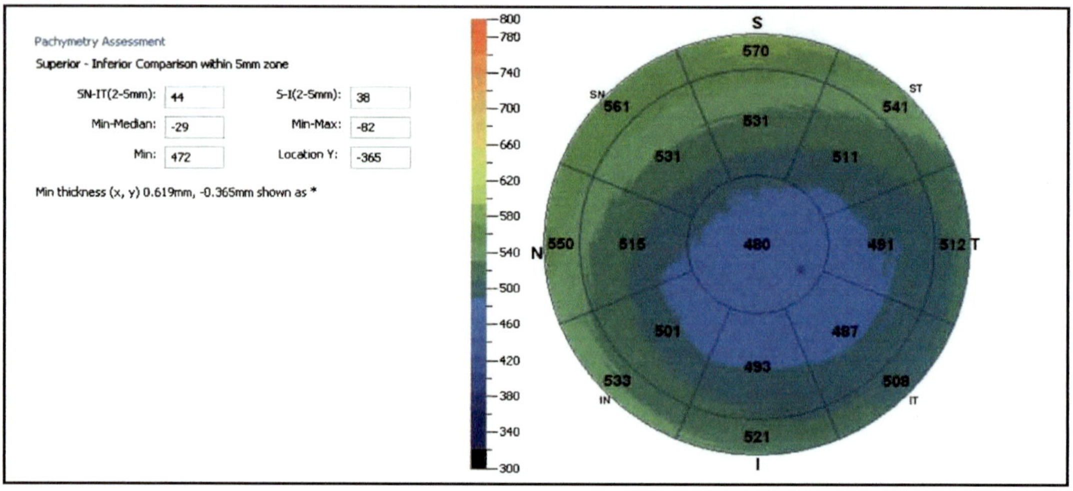

Case Figure 15-2. OCT images of the right and left eyes, with corneal thickness profiles that correlate well with the Pentacam maps, also exhibiting a suspicious corneal thickness profile in the inferotemporal direction, especially in the left eye.

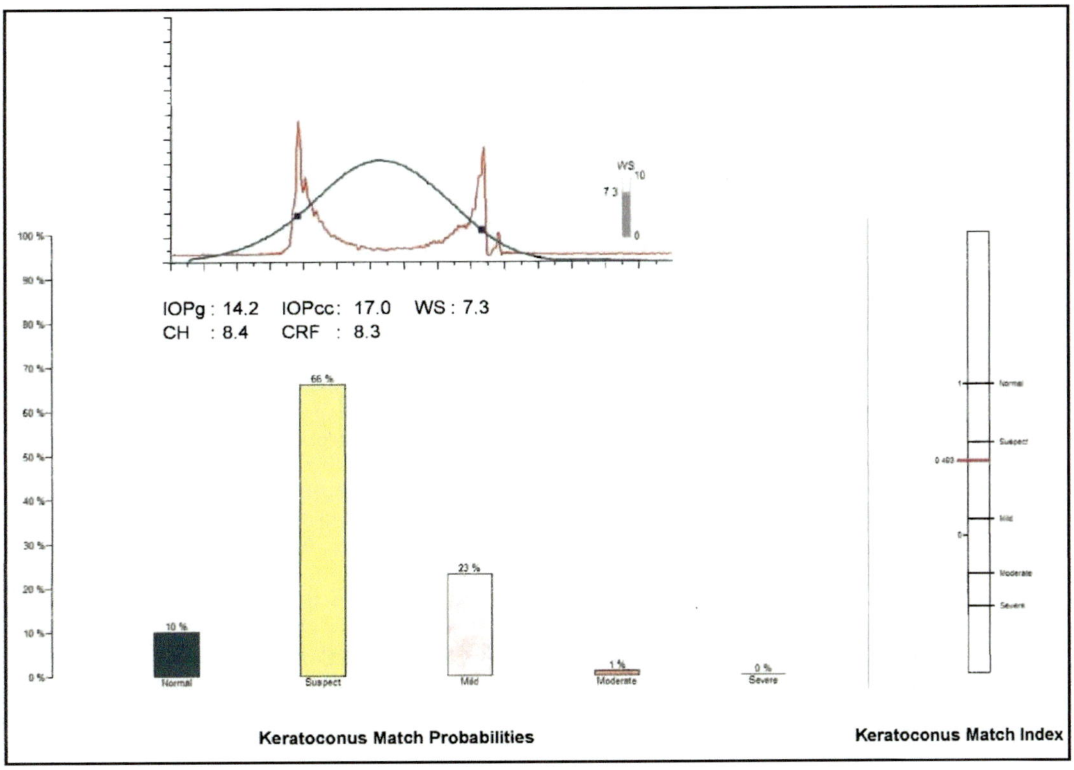

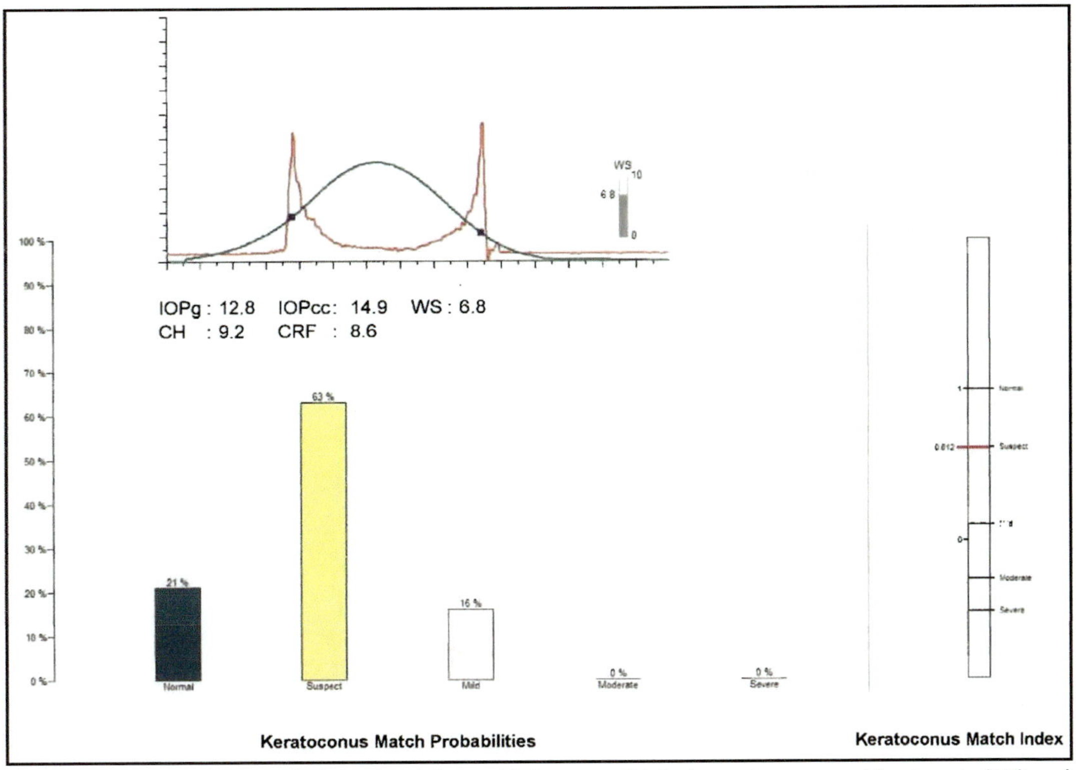

Case Figure 15-3. ORA analysis in the right and left eyes, which shows low corneal hysteresis (CH) and corneal resistance factor (CRF) values in both eyes and a Keratoconus Match Index in the suspicious to mild range in both eyes.

Bibliography

Ambrósio R Jr, Caiado AL, Guerra FP, et al. Novel pachymetric parameters based on corneal tomography for diagnosing keratoconus. *J Refract Surg.* 2011;27(10):753-758.

de Sanctis U, Missolungi A, Mutani B, Richiardi L, Grignolo FM. Reproducibility and repeatability of central corneal thickness measurement in keratoconus using the rotating Scheimpflug camera and ultrasound pachymetry. *Am J Ophthalmol.* 2007;144(5):712-718.

Fontes BM, Ambrósio R Jr, Jardim D, Velarde GC, Nosé W. Corneal biomechanical metrics and anterior segment parameters in mild keratoconus. *Ophthalmology.* 2010;117(4):673-679.

Fontes BM, Ambrósio R Jr, Velarde GC, Nosé W. Ocular response analyzer measurements in keratoconus with normal central corneal thickness compared with matched normal control eyes. *J Refract Surg.* 2011;27(3):209-215.

Kymionis GD, Tsiklis N, Karp CL, Kalyvianaki M, Pallikaris AI. Unilateral corneal ectasia after laser in situ keratomileusis in a patient with uncomplicated photorefractive keratectomy in the fellow eye. *J Cataract Refract Surg.* 2007;33(5):859-861.

Leccisotti A. Corneal ectasia after photorefractive keratectomy. *Graefes Arch Clin Exp Ophthalmol.* 2007;245(6):869-875.

Malecaze F, Coullet J, Calvas P, Fournié P, Arné JL, Brodaty C. Corneal ectasia after photorefractive keratectomy for low myopia. *Ophthalmology.* 2006;113(7):742-746.

Nam SM, Im CY, Lee HK, Kim EK, Kim TI, Seo KY. Accuracy of RTVue optical coherence tomography, Pentacam, and ultrasonic pachymetry for the measurement of central corneal thickness. Ophthalmology. 2010;117(11):2096-2103.

Navas A, Ariza E, Haber A, Fermón S, Velázquez R, Suárez R. Bilateral keratectasia after photorefractive keratectomy. *J Refract Surg.* 2007;23(9):941-943.

Randleman JB, Caster AI, Banning CS, Stulting RD. Corneal ectasia after photorefractive keratectomy. *J Cataract Refract Surg.* 2006;32(8):1395-1398.

Randleman JB, Woodward M, Lynn MJ, Stulting RD. Risk assessment for ectasia after corneal refractive surgery. *Ophthalmology.* 2008;115(1):37-50.

Reinstein DZ, Archer TJ, Gobbe M. Stability of LASIK in topographically suspect keratoconus confirmed non-keratoconic by Artemis VHF digital ultrasound epithelial thickness mapping: 1-year follow-up. *J Refract Surg.* 2009;25(7):569-577.

Sedaghat MR, Daneshvar R, Kargozar A, Derakhshan A, Daraei M. Comparison of central corneal thickness measurement using ultrasonic pachymetry, rotating Scheimpflug camera, and scanning-slit topography. *Am J Ophthalmol.* 2010;150(6):780-789.

Smadja D, Santhiago MR, Mello GR, Krueger RR, Colin J, Touboul D. Influence of the reference surface shape for discriminating between normal corneas, subclinical keratoconus, and keratoconus. *J Refract Surg.* 2013;29:274-81.

Smadja D, Touboul D, Cohen A, Doveh E, Santhiago MR, Mello GR, Krueger RR, Colin J. Detection of subclinical keratoconus using an automated decision tree classification. *Am J Ophthalmol.* 2013;156:237-246.

Smolek MK, McCarey BE. Interlamellar adhesive strength in human eyebank corneas. *Invest Ophthalmol Vis Sci.* 1990;31(6):1087-1095.

—Case 16—

A 37-year-old female desires refractive surgical correction. She has no significant family, past medical, or ocular history.

CASE HISTORY		
	Right Eye	**Left Eye**
Present correction method	CTL	CTL
Manifest refraction	-5.75 +1.75 x 145	-6.25 +1.50 x 082
CDVA (current)	20/20	20/20
Dominant eye	Right	
Ocular alignment	Orthophoric	Orthophoric
Keratometry		
Flat K	39.5 @ 160	40.2 @ 070
Steep K	40.5 @ 070	40.7 @ 160
Pupil size (bright)	4.2 mm	4.5 mm
Pupil size (dim)	6.4 mm	6.3 mm
Central corneal thickness	519 µm	527 µm
Physical examination	Normal	Normal
Estimated ablation depth	95 µm	95 µm

Questions

1. Is this patient a candidate for refractive surgery? If so, what treatment options are available?
2. Considering all factors, what procedure would you recommend and why?
3. What additional information could be of particular utility in evaluating this patient for surgery?
4. What special considerations are there for this patient regarding potential retreatment for postoperative ametropia?

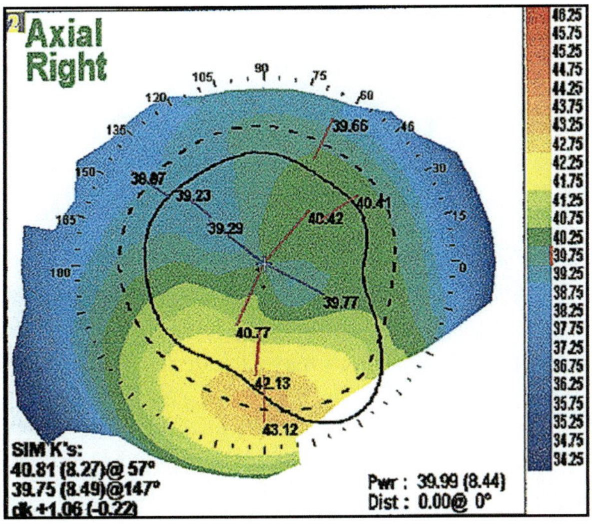
Axial
Right
SIM K's:
40.81 (8.27)@ 57°
39.75 (8.49)@147°
dk +1.06 (-0.22)
Pwr : 39.99 (8.44)
Dist : 0.00@ 0°

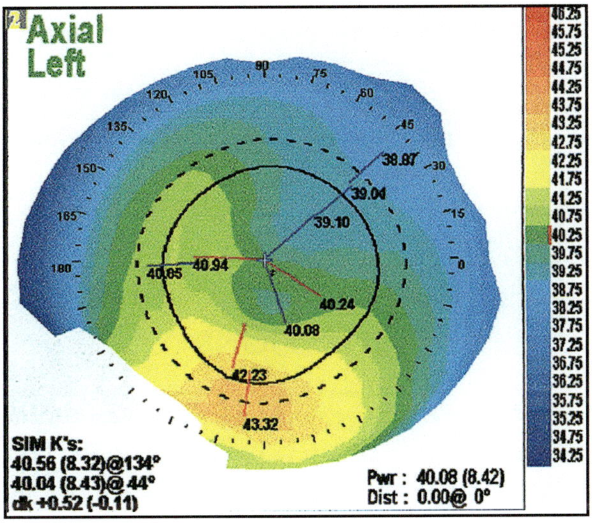
Axial
Left
SIM K's:
40.56 (8.32)@134°
40.04 (8.43)@ 44°
dk +0.52 (-0.11)
Pwr : 40.08 (8.42)
Dist : 0.00@ 0°

—CASE 16—

Screening for Ectasia Risk

Abnormal Preoperative Topography

Postoperative ectasia after corneal refractive surgery (ectasia), especially LASIK, remains a rare but potentially severe complication. Much of the time spent on patient screening protocols is used to identify "high-risk" individuals, which may exclude them from LASIK and potentially all corneal refractive surgery, depending on the degree of abnormality present. Screening techniques, technologies, and strategies have evolved over time, and although some elements of the process are well accepted, others are still in evolution and remain the topic of great debate.

Case Analysis

- The estimated residual stromal bed (RSB) thickness is approximately 305 to 325 μm in the right eye and 310 to 330 μm in the left eye.
- Case Figures show topographic images of the right and left eyes demonstrating significant inferior steepening >4.00 diopters (D) with skewed radial axes in both eyes.

Pearl: *Always view topographic patterns as stand-alone entities first, and do NOT normalize suspicious patterns with additional patient data!*

QUESTIONS

1. Is this patient a candidate for refractive surgery? If so, what treatment options are available?

   No, not at this time. This patient is not a good candidate for laser vision correction (LVC). Based on the topographic findings, this patient is at significant risk of developing postoperative ectasia after corneal refractive surgery. The patient is potentially a candidate for phakic intraocular lens (PIOL) implantation; however, astigmatism would be significant after a nontoric PIOL is implanted.

2. Considering all factors, what procedure would you recommend and why?

   I would not recommend any refractive surgery at this time. When toric PIOLs become available, the patient could then elect this option.

3. What additional information could be of particular utility in evaluating this patient for surgery?

   Although this case appears fairly straightforward regarding biomechanical evaluation, additional tomographic results may be of further value in borderline cases.

4. What special considerations are there for this patient regarding potential retreatment for postoperative ametropia?

   If the patient had PIOL implants, she would not be a suitable candidate for fine-tuning with excimer laser correction. Therefore, the patient would be unlikely to obtain full correction due to the amount of astigmatism present.

Screening for Ectasia Risk

Ectasia is a known complication after corneal refractive surgery that can occur in the absence of any known risk factors, but most frequently occurs in patients with abnormal preoperative topography in isolation or combined with other recognized risk factors (discussed more fully in Chapters 3 and 5). The incidence of ectasia after LASIK is not firmly established, but rough estimates are approximately 1/2500 cases overall, with a much lower incidence in patients without risk factors. Therefore, all patients should be informed about the low, but possible risk, of ectasia after uneventful and initially successful surgery. The risk of ectasia after surface ablation is also not firmly established; however, available evidence supports an even lower ectasia risk with surface ablation procedures.

A variety of modalities are used for ectasia screening, all of which are fully discussed in Chapter 3. The most common screening modalities include Placido-based topography (Case Figure), scanning slit-beam technology (Orbscan II, Bausch & Lomb) (Case Figure 16-1), and Scheimpflug tomography (Case Figure 16-2). In this case presentation, Placido imaging clearly demonstrates a significant anterior curvature abnormality, with inferior steepening >4.00 D and skewed radial axes in both eyes. These findings meet the topographic criteria for abnormal topography as forme fruste keratoconus. These Placido-based findings have been evaluated in detail and have been confirmed as risk factors for ectasia after LASIK in multiple case-control studies.

The need for additional testing is minimal in this patient with clearly abnormal topographic mapping. Case Figures 16-1 and 16-2 (also from this patient) demonstrate notable abnormalities in every map, including the corneal thickness profile and anterior (front) and posterior (back) elevation maps.

The primary shortcoming of stand-alone Placido topography is the lack of regional corneal thickness data, as only central thicknesses are otherwise routinely measured. For that reason, most practitioners utilize some form of regional corneal thickness measurements, either those included in scanning slit-beam and Scheimpflug devices or in newer anterior segment OCT imaging devices. In less clear cases, advanced testing, including advanced corneal thickness spatial profiles, with OCT and ORA may be of benefit in discriminating the low-risk patient from the moderate-risk patient.

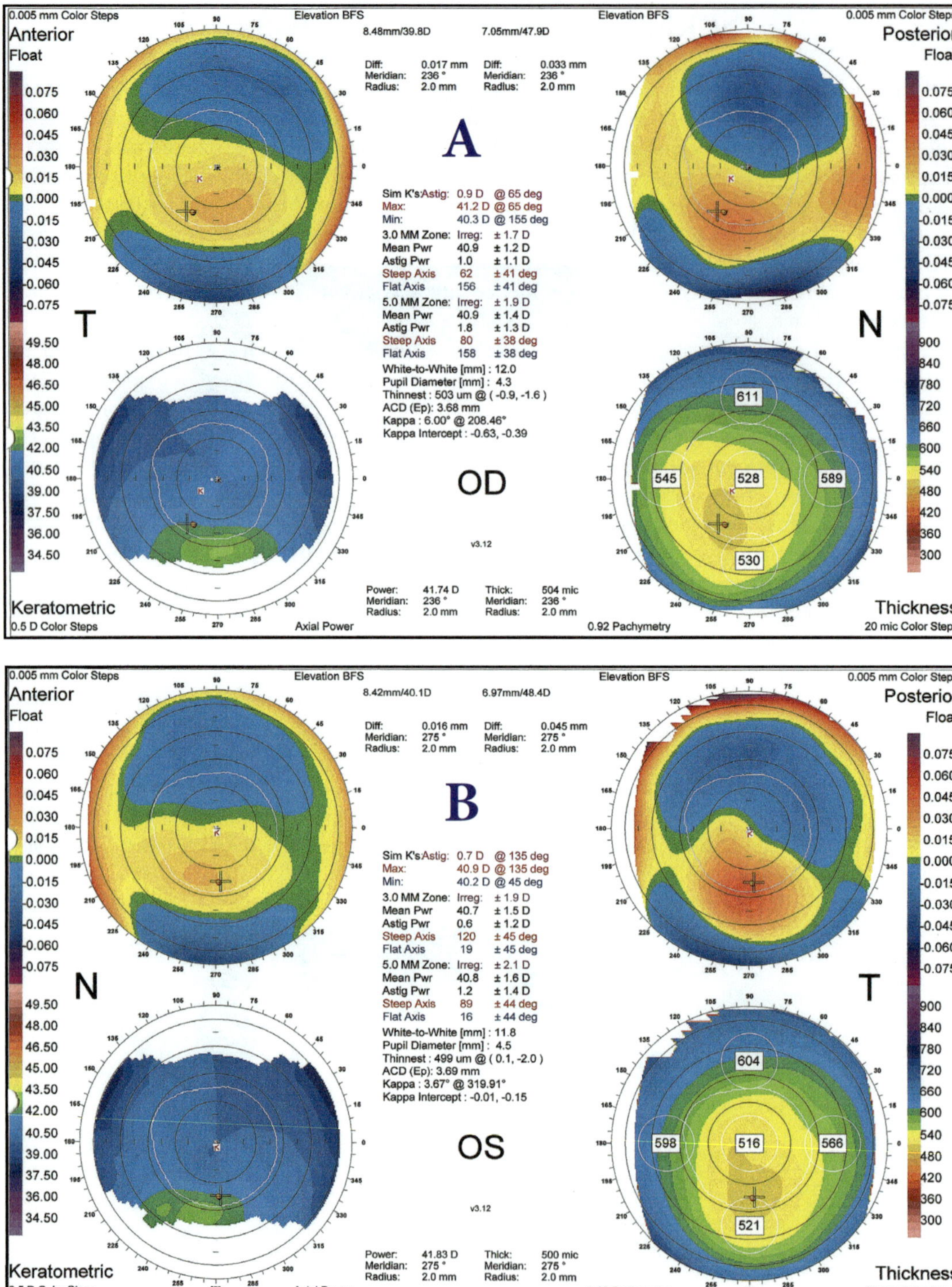

Case Figure 16-1. Placido and scanning slit-beam imaging (Orbscan II) of the (A) right and (B) left eyes demonstrate similar findings on the keratometric map (lower left), with 2.00 D of focal inferior steepening with inferior data loss, inferiorly displaced thinnest corneal pachymetry on the thickness map (lower right), and inferiorly displaced focal steepening on the anterior (upper left) and posterior (upper right) float maps.

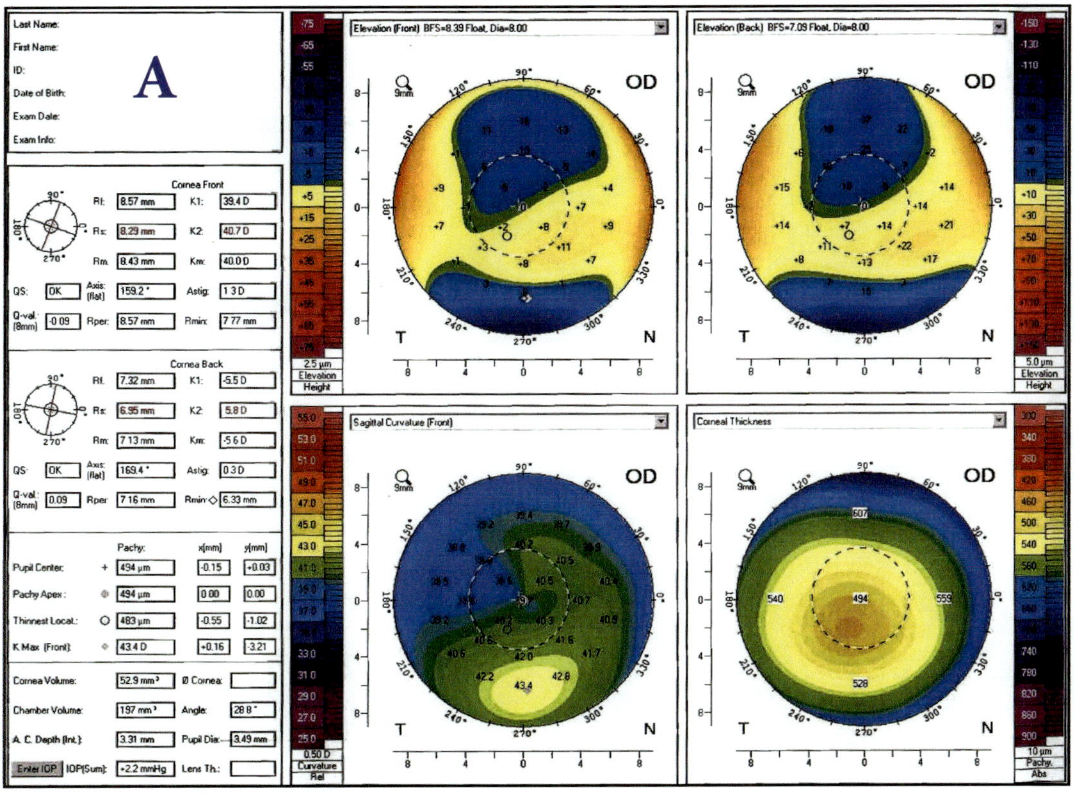

Case Figure 16-2. (A) Scheimpflug tomography (Pentacam) of the (A) right and (B) left eyes demonstrate analogous findings on the sagittal curvature map (lower left), inferiorly displaced thinnest corneal point on the corneal thickness map (lower right), and moderate focal steepening on the front (upper left) and back (upper right) elevation maps. *(continued)*

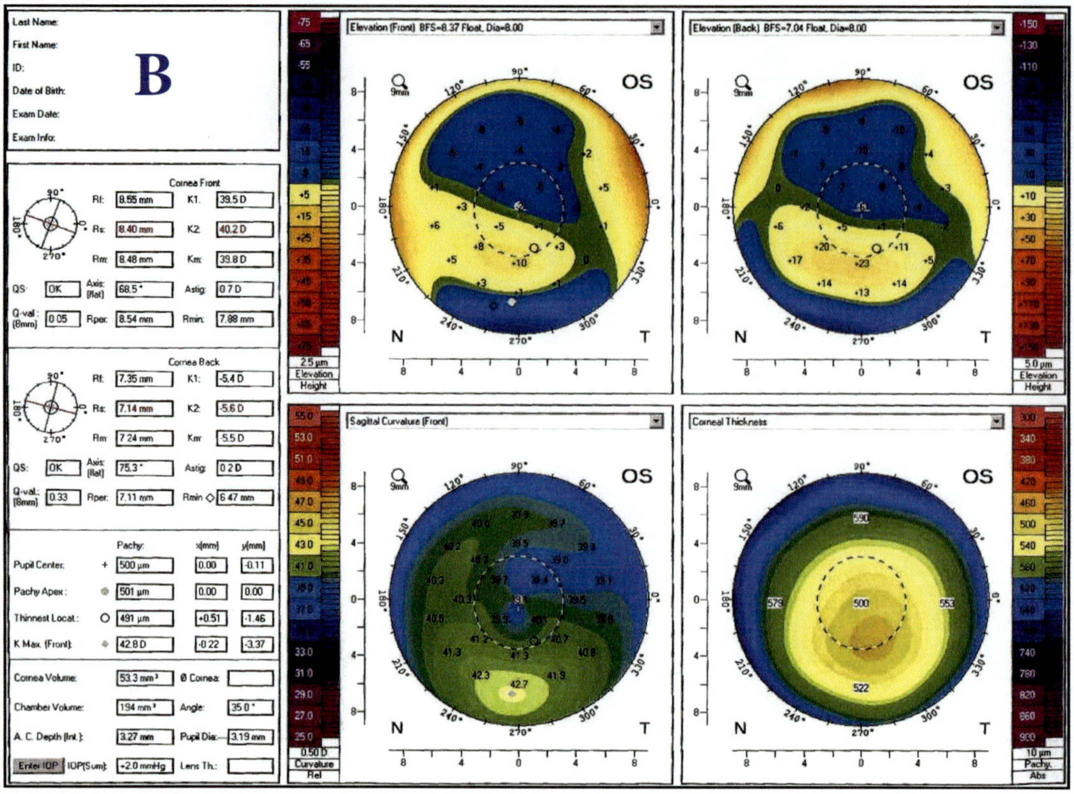

Case Figure 16-2 (continued). (B)

BIBLIOGRAPHY

Ambrósio R Jr, Nogueira LP, Caldas DL, Fontes BM, Luz A, Cazal JO, Alves MR, Belin MW. Evaluation of corneal shape and biomechanics before LASIK. *Int Ophthalmol Clin.* 2011;51(2):11-38.

Binder PS, Lindstrom RL, Stulting RD, et al. Keratoconus and corneal ectasia after LASIK. *J Refract Surg.* 2005;21(6):749-752.

Rabinowitz YS. Videokeratographic indices to aid in screening for keratoconus. J Refract Surg. 1995;11(5):371-379.

Rabinowitz YS, McDonnell PJ. Computer-assisted corneal topography in keratoconus. *Refract Corneal Surg.* 1989;5(6):400-408.

Rabinowitz YS, Yang H, Brickman Y, et al. Videokeratography database of normal human corneas. *Br J Ophthalmol* 1996;80(7):610-616.

Randleman JB, Russell B, Ward MA, Thompson KP, Stulting RD. Risk factors and prognosis for corneal ectasia after LASIK. *Ophthalmology* 2003;110(2):267-275.

Randleman JB, Trattler WB, Stulting RD. Validation of the Ectasia Risk Assessment Score System for preoperative laser in situ keratomileusis screening. *Am J Ophthalmol.* 2008;145(5):813-818.

Randleman JB, Woodward M, Lynn MJ, Stulting RD. Risk assessment for ectasia after corneal refractive surgery. *Ophthalmology.* 2008;115(1):37-50.

—Case 17—

A 28-year-old female desires refractive surgical correction. She has no significant family, past medical, or ocular history.

CASE HISTORY		
	Right Eye	**Left Eye**
Present correction method	CTL	CTL
Manifest refraction	-6.50 +0.50 x 050	-6.75 +0.50 x 075
CDVA (current)	20/15	20/15
Dominant eye	Right	
Ocular alignment	Orthophoric	Orthophoric
Keratometry		
Flat K	44.5 @ 174	44.4 @ 009
Steep K	45.4 @ 084	45.75 @ 099
Pupil size (bright)	4.3 mm	4.2 mm
Pupil size (dim)	6.5 mm	6.4 mm
Central corneal thickness	516 µm	518 µm
Physical examination	Normal	Normal
Estimated ablation depth	100 µm	105 µm

Questions

1. Is this patient a candidate for refractive surgery? If so, what treatment options are available?
2. What, if any, additional testing would you perform on this patient, assuming all testing modalities were available?
3. Considering all factors, what procedure would you recommend and why?
4. What special considerations are there for this patient regarding potential retreatment for postoperative ametropia?

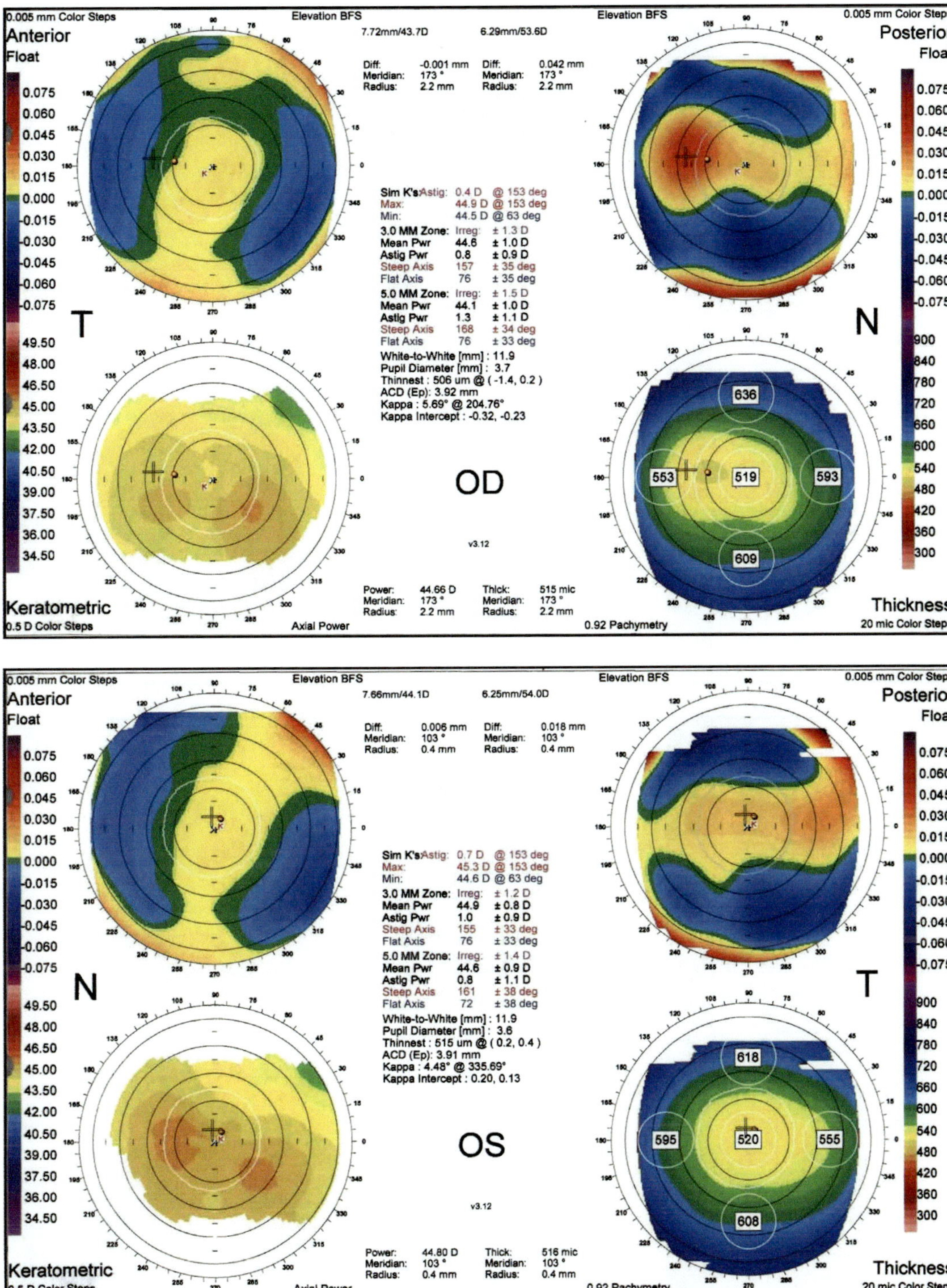
0.005 mm Color Steps
Anterior
Float
Elevation BFS
7.72mm/43.7D
6.29mm/53.6D
Diff: -0.001 mm
Meridian: 173 °
Radius: 2.2 mm
Diff: 0.042 mm
Meridian: 173 °
Radius: 2.2 mm
Elevation BFS
0.005 mm Color Steps
Posterior
Float
T
N
Sim K's Astig: 0.4 D @ 153 deg
Max: 44.9 D @ 153 deg
Min: 44.5 D @ 63 deg
3.0 MM Zone: Irreg: ± 1.3 D
Mean Pwr 44.6 ± 1.0 D
Astig Pwr 0.8 ± 0.9 D
Steep Axis 157 ± 35 deg
Flat Axis 76 ± 35 deg
5.0 MM Zone: Irreg: ± 1.5 D
Mean Pwr 44.1 ± 1.0 D
Astig Pwr 1.3 ± 1.1 D
Steep Axis 168 ± 34 deg
Flat Axis 76 ± 33 deg
White-to-White [mm] : 11.9
Pupil Diameter [mm] : 3.7
Thinnest : 506 um @ (-1.4, 0.2)
ACD (Ep): 3.92 mm
Kappa : 5.69° @ 204.76°
Kappa Intercept : -0.32, -0.23
OD
v3.12
636
553
519
593
609
Power: 44.66 D
Meridian: 173 °
Radius: 2.2 mm
Thick: 515 mic
Meridian: 173 °
Radius: 2.2 mm
Keratometric
0.5 D Color Steps
Axial Power
0.92 Pachymetry
Thickness
20 mic Color Steps
0.005 mm Color Steps
Anterior
Float
Elevation BFS
7.66mm/44.1D
6.25mm/54.0D
Diff: 0.006 mm
Meridian: 103 °
Radius: 0.4 mm
Diff: 0.018 mm
Meridian: 103 °
Radius: 0.4 mm
Elevation BFS
0.005 mm Color Steps
Posterior
Float
N
T
Sim K's Astig: 0.7 D @ 153 deg
Max: 45.3 D @ 153 deg
Min: 44.6 D @ 63 deg
3.0 MM Zone: Irreg: ± 1.2 D
Mean Pwr 44.9 ± 0.8 D
Astig Pwr 1.0 ± 0.9 D
Steep Axis 155 ± 33 deg
Flat Axis 76 ± 33 deg
5.0 MM Zone: Irreg: ± 1.4 D
Mean Pwr 44.6 ± 0.9 D
Astig Pwr 0.8 ± 1.1 D
Steep Axis 161 ± 38 deg
Flat Axis 72 ± 38 deg
White-to-White [mm] : 11.9
Pupil Diameter [mm] : 3.6
Thinnest : 515 um @ (0.2, 0.4)
ACD (Ep): 3.91 mm
Kappa : 4.48° @ 335.69°
Kappa Intercept : 0.20, 0.13
OS
v3.12
618
595
520
555
608
Power: 44.80 D
Meridian: 103 °
Radius: 0.4 mm
Thick: 516 mic
Meridian: 103 °
Radius: 0.4 mm
Keratometric
0.5 D Color Steps
Axial Power
0.92 Pachymetry
Thickness
20 mic Color Steps

A

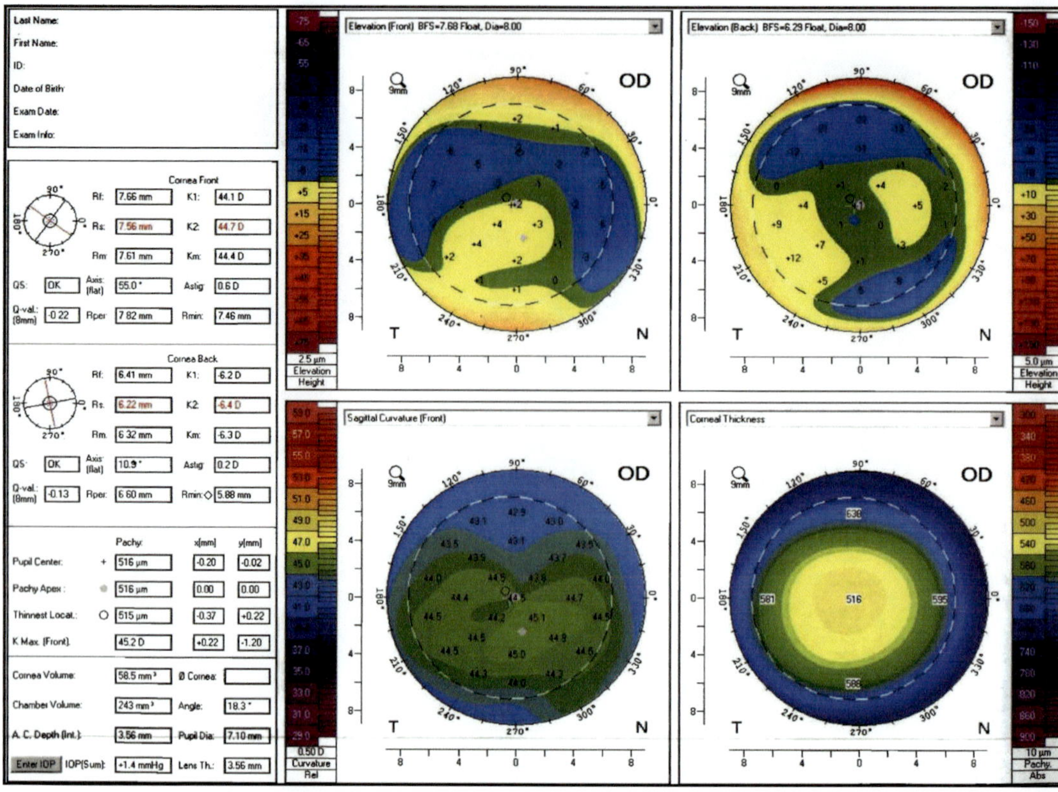
Last Name:
First Name:
ID:
Date of Birth:
Exam Date:
Exam Info:
Cornea Front
Rf: 7.66 mm K1: 44.1 D
Rs: 7.56 mm K2: 44.7 D
Rm: 7.61 mm Km: 44.4 D
QS: OK Axis (flat): 55.0° Astig: 0.6 D
Q-val. (8mm): -0.22 Rper: 7.82 mm Rmin: 7.46 mm
Cornea Back
Rf: 6.41 mm K1: -6.2 D
Rs: 6.22 mm K2: -6.4 D
Rm: 6.32 mm Km: -6.3 D
QS: OK Axis (flat): 10.9° Astig: 0.2 D
Q-val. (8mm): -0.13 Rper: 6.60 mm Rmin: 5.88 mm
Pachy: x[mm] y[mm]
Pupil Center: + 516 µm -0.20 -0.02
Pachy Apex: 516 µm 0.00 0.00
Thinnest Locat.: 515 µm -0.37 +0.22
K Max. (Front): 45.2 D +0.22 -1.20
Cornea Volume: 58.5 mm³ Ø Cornea:
Chamber Volume: 243 mm³ Angle: 18.3°
A. C. Depth (Int.): 3.56 mm Pupil Dia: 7.10 mm
Enter IOP IOP(Sum): +1.4 mmHg Lens Th.: 3.56 mm
Elevation (Front) BFS=7.68 Float, Dia=8.00
Elevation (Back) BFS=6.29 Float, Dia=8.00
Sagittal Curvature (Front)
Corneal Thickness
OD
T
N
2.5 µm Elevation Height
5.0 µm Elevation Height
0.50 D Curvature Rel
10 µm Pachy. Abs

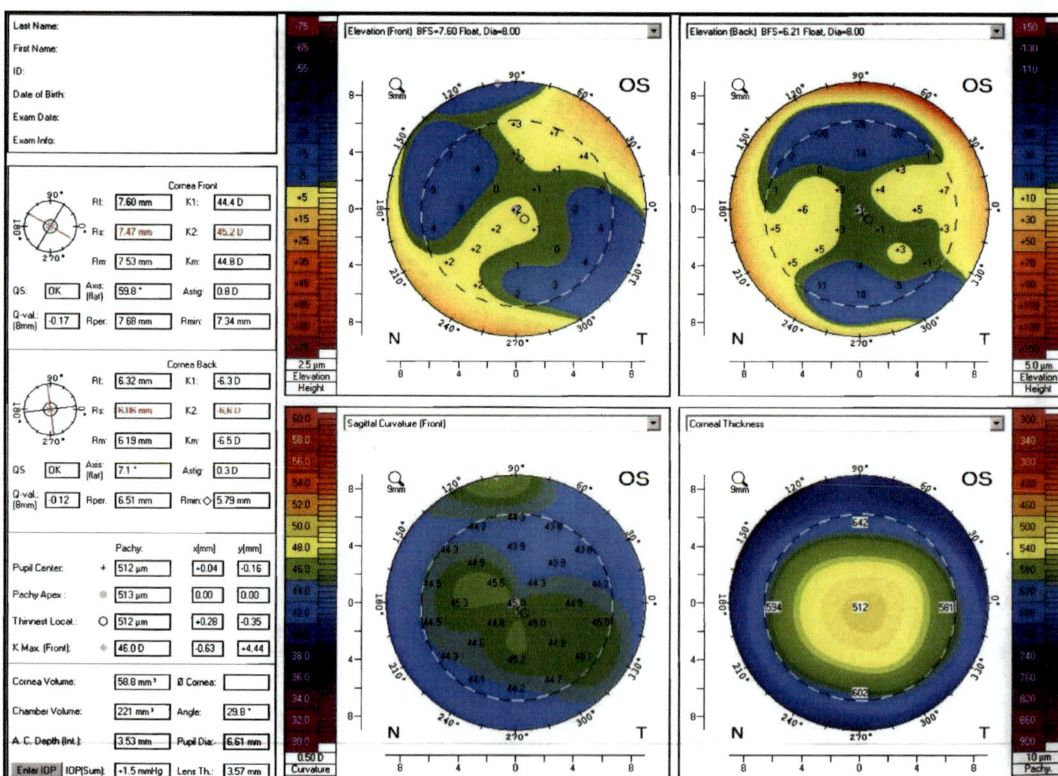
Last Name:
First Name:
ID:
Date of Birth:
Exam Date:
Exam Info:
Cornea Front
Rf: 7.60 mm K1: 44.4 D
Rs: 7.47 mm K2: 45.2 D
Rm: 7.53 mm Km: 44.8 D
QS: OK Axis (flat): 59.8° Astig: 0.8 D
Q-val. (8mm): -0.17 Rper: 7.68 mm Rmin: 7.34 mm
Cornea Back
Rf: 6.32 mm K1: -6.3 D
Rm: 6.19 mm Km: -6.5 D
QS: OK Axis (flat): 7.1° Astig: 0.3 D
Q-val. (8mm): -0.12 Rper: 6.51 mm Rmin: 5.79 mm
Pachy: x[mm] y[mm]
Pupil Center: + 512 µm +0.04 -0.16
Pachy Apex: 513 µm 0.00 0.00
Thinnest Locat.: 512 µm +0.28 -0.35
K Max. (Front): 46.0 D -0.63 +4.44
Cornea Volume: 58.8 mm³ Ø Cornea:
Chamber Volume: 221 mm³ Angle: 29.8°
A. C. Depth (Int.): 3.53 mm Pupil Dia: 6.61 mm
Enter IOP IOP(Sum): +1.5 mmHg Lens Th.: 3.57 mm
Elevation (Front) BFS=7.60 Float, Dia=8.00
Elevation (Back) BFS=6.21 Float, Dia=8.00
Sagittal Curvature (Front)
Corneal Thickness
OS
N
T
2.5 µm Elevation Height
5.0 µm Elevation Height
0.50 D Curvature Rel
10 µm Pachy. Abs

B

—CASE 17—

Screening for Ectasia Risk

Advanced Biomechanical Evaluation in Suspicious Cases

Many patients have suspicious topographic patterns. In these less definitive cases, increased awareness of additional screening parameters is necessary, and additional screening technologies may improve distinguishing between higher risk patients and those with normal risk.

Case Analysis

- The estimated residual stromal bed (RSB) thickness is approximately 290 to 310 µm in both eyes.
- Case Figure A shows Placido and scanning slit-beam imaging (Orbscan II; Bausch & Lomb) of the right eye demonstrating inferior steepening of up to 1.00 D with an inferiorly displaced, skewed radial axis on the keratometric map (lower left); temporally displaced thinnest corneal pachymetry on the thickness map (lower right), with abnormal central/peripheral thickening temporally; a normal anterior (upper left) float map; and a temporally displaced focal steepening on the posterior (upper right) float map. The left eye demonstrates similar, but more subtle, variations of the same findings displayed in the right eye.
- Case Figure B shows Scheimpflug-based imaging (Pentacam; OCULUS Optikgerate GmbH) of the right and left eyes demonstrating analogous findings on the sagittal curvature maps (lower left), with approximately 1.00 D of inferior steepening and skewed axes in both eyes; mild inferotemporal displacement of the thickness map profile, but with centered thinnest points (lower right); and unremarkable front (upper left) and back (upper right) elevation maps.

Pearl: *When in doubt, utilize additional screening technologies to gain a more complete determination of corneal biomechanics before surgery!*

QUESTIONS

1. Is this patient a candidate for refractive surgery? If so, what treatment options are available for this patient?

    This patient is a suspicious candidate based on topography alone, without definitive abnormality but with subtle suspicious patterns in both eyes. The corneal thickness profile is of concern in the scanning slit images but not in the Scheimpflug images. Although this patient is technically a candidate for surface ablation, LASIK, or phakic intraocular lens (PIOL) implantation based on refractive error, she would benefit from additional diagnostic testing prior to proceeding with any surgery.

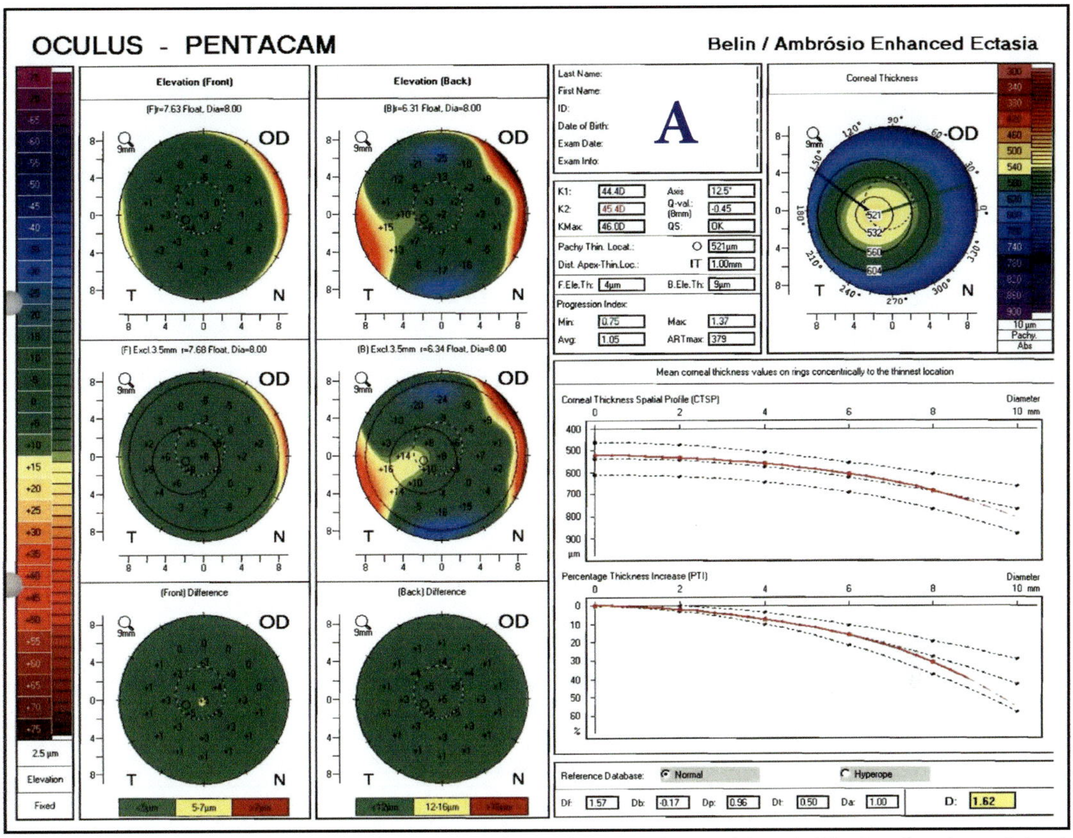

Case Figure 17-1. (A) Scheimpflug (Pentacam) Belin/Ambrosio Enhanced Ectasia Display showing minimal focal anterior or posterior elevations, a lower ARTMax (relational thickness) score, and a suspicious "D" value. *(continued)*

2. What, if any, additional testing would you perform on this patient, assuming all testing modalities were available?

   In this individual I would look at additional parameters on Scheimpflug imaging, including relational corneal thickness and posterior elevation evaluation (Case Figure 17-1) and corneal thickness spatial profile (Case Figure 17-2). In addition, anterior segment optical coherence tomography (OCT) would be of benefit (see Case Figure 17-2), and the Ocular Response Analyzer (ORA; OCULUS Optikgerate GmbH) could be of use (Case Figure 17-3).

3. Considering all factors, what procedure would you recommend and why?

   Based on suspicious topographic patterns, coupled with suspicious testing with each technology (corneal thickness profiles as demonstrated by scanning slit, Scheimpflug, and OCT imaging, and ORA analysis), and patient age, I would not offer this patient laser vision correction. The patient is potentially a candidate for a PIOL implantation, pending appropriate endothelial cell counts.

4. What special considerations are there for this patient regarding potential retreatment for postoperative ametropia?

   Although the risk of a small surface ablation is not definitive, the patient is unlikely to be a reasonable candidate for any retreatment with the excimer laser.

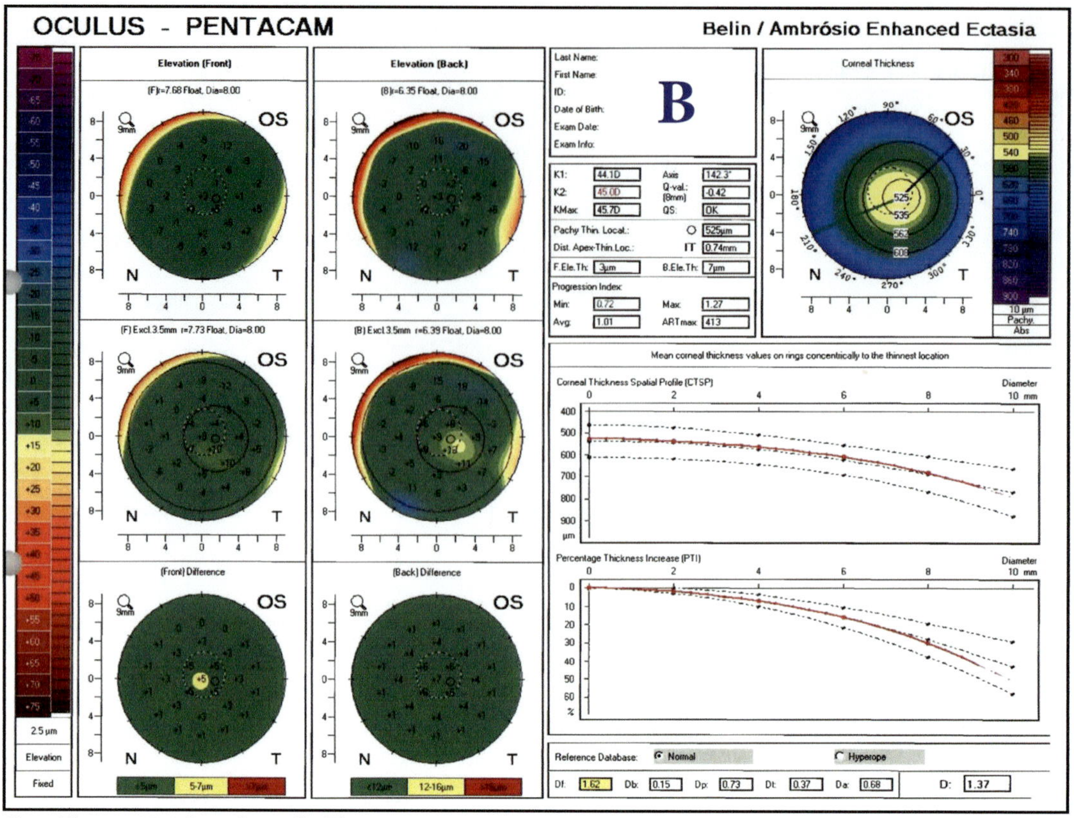

Case Figure 17-1 (continued). (B)

Advanced Corneal Biomechanical Evaluation

In cases without definitively recognized Placido-based topographic abnormalities, data are lacking about actual risk estimates, and great debate exists as to the best screening strategies for these individuals (discussed in Chapter 3). The "best" additional testing remains to be determined, and for most practices, it is cost prohibitive to acquire all of the of imaging devices that are available on the market.

In this case, a mildly suspicious topographic abnormality in a younger patient raises red flags for ectasia risk. The risk score calculated by the Ectasia Risk Score System (ERSS) is 3, with 1 point added each for age (28 years), asymmetric topography, and estimated RSB (approximately 290 µm) using a conservative flap thickness estimate, or 5 using the same scoring parameters but scoring the topographic image "3" based on skewed axis and inferior steepening. There remains variation in how even experienced examiners are scoring images such as these. Thus, the risk score is either "moderate" or "high" depending on this critical metric.

Based on the best information available currently, corneal thickness profiles appear to be the next best data to evaluate. A variety of parameters for scanning slit-beam technology have been reported, but these remain to be validated. Scanning slit-beam imaging is particularly sensitive to corneal clarity and appears to generate the greatest artifact and thus the overall risk when used in isolation. Scheimpflug imaging appears to be less influenced by other factors, but it is not immune to generating artifact. In this case, both Scheimpflug corneal thickness spatial relationships and OCT demonstrate suspicious regional thickness profiles. In Case Figure 17-2, the "drooping" red line, viewed from right to left, signifies that central corneal thickness is thinner than would be anticipated, based on peripheral thickness. In Case Figure 17-2, the OCT regional profiles

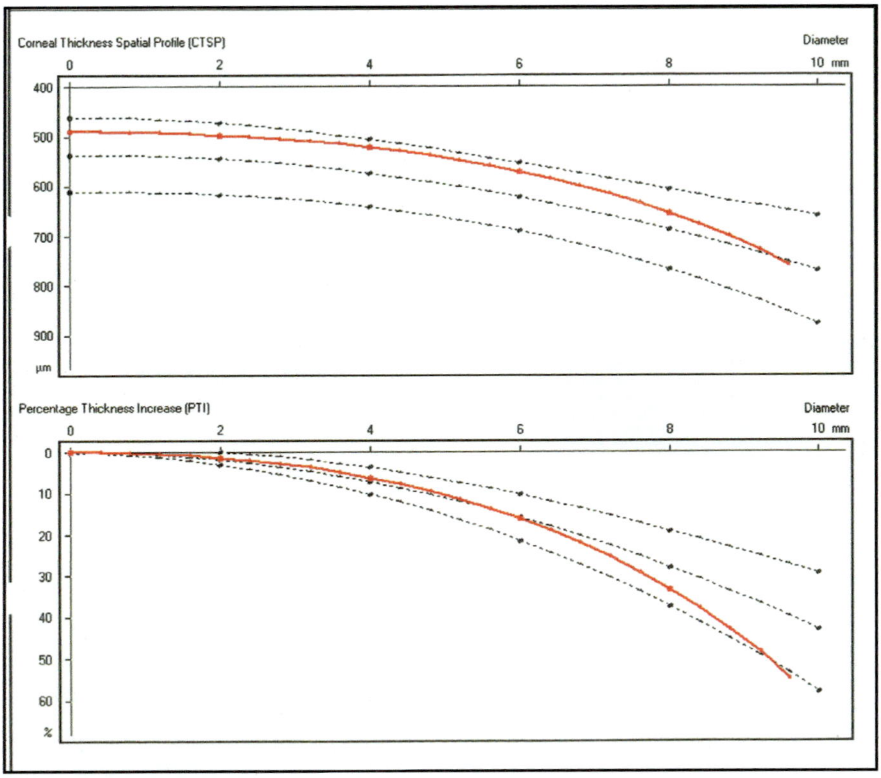

Case Figure 17-2. Scheimpflug (Pentacam) corneal thickness spatial profile maps from a similar patient demonstrate an abnormal center-to-peripheral thickness ratio, demonstrated by the abnormal "drooping" of the red thickness line as it extends from left to right.

minimally increase in thickness when moving from the center to the inferotemporal quadrant, especially when compared with the corresponding superior area thickening. Suspicious corneal thickness profiles have been associated with keratoconus-suspect eyes.

The role of "direct" biomechanical measurement with the ORA remains less well defined (Case Figure 17-4). Although in population studies, the ORA can distinguish keratoconic corneas from normal, the significant overlap limits the utility for individual eyes. Advanced device parameters, including the Keratoconus Match Indices (KMI) and Keratoconus Match Probabilities (KMP) may improve screening sensitivity, but they also remain to be validated.

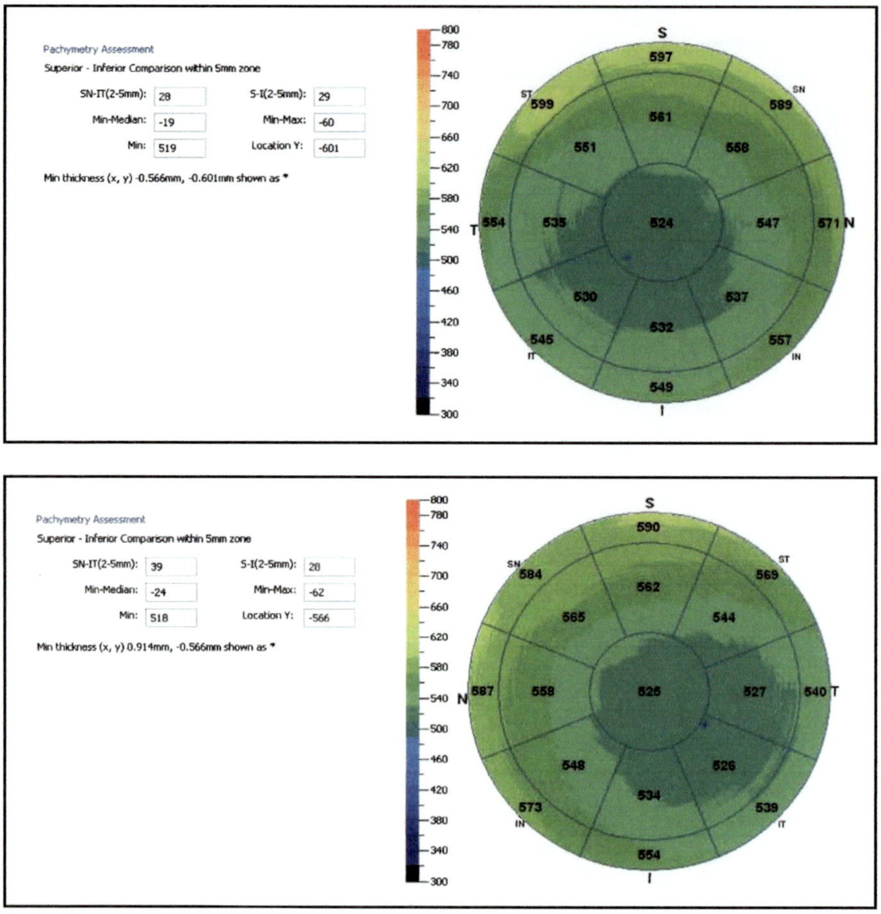

Case Figure 17-3. Anterior segment OCT demonstrating suspicious thickness progression from the center to periphery in the inferotemporal direction in both eyes (left more so than right), compared with corresponding regions superiorly.

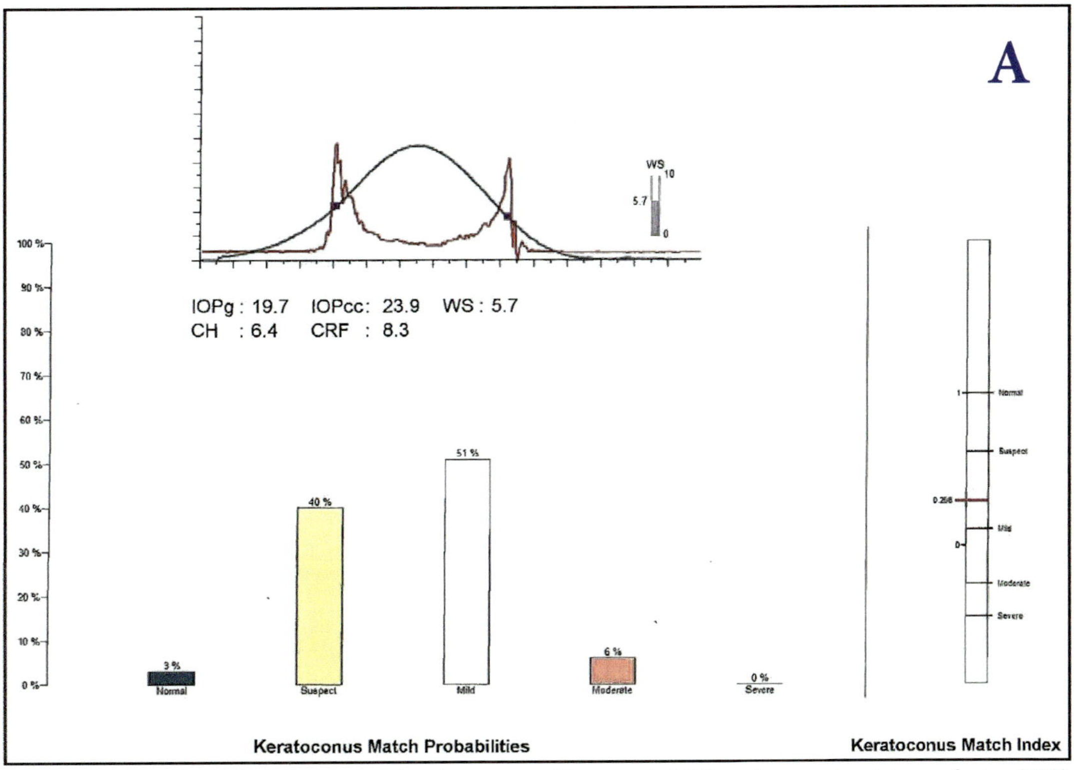

Case Figure 17-4. (A) ORA demonstrating low corneal hysteresis (CH) and corneal resistance factor (CRF) in both eyes and abnormal KMI and KMP readings. *(continued)*

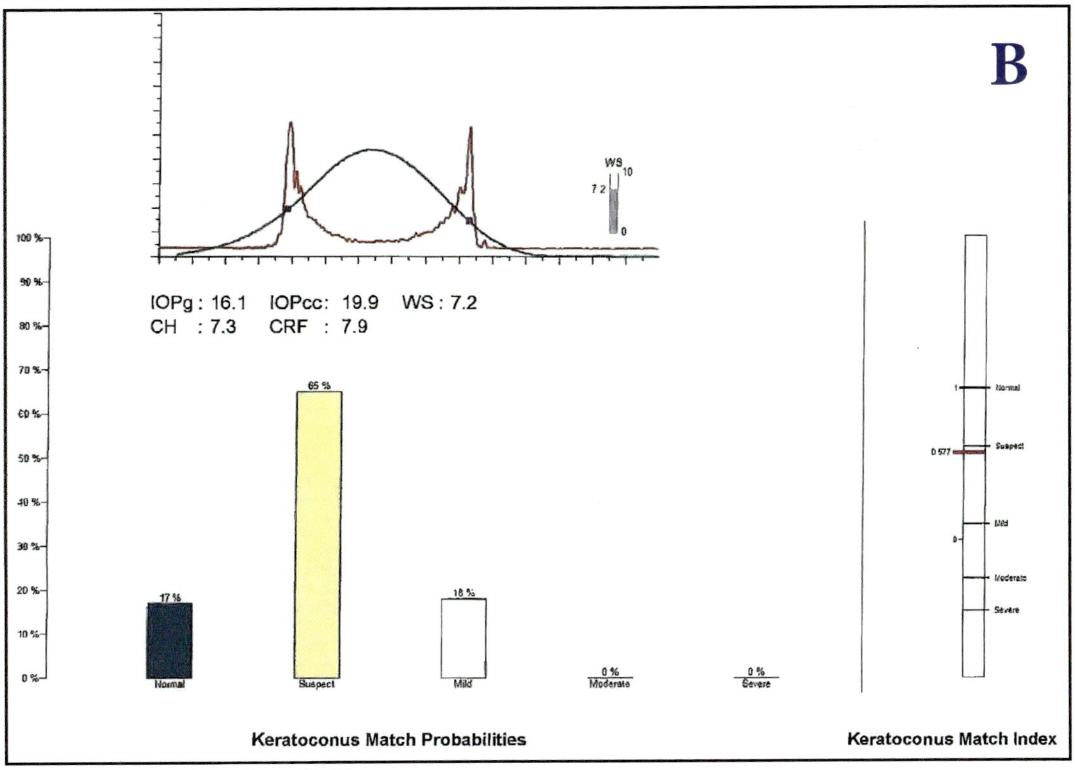

Case Figure 17-4 (continued). (B)

Bibliography

Ambrósio R Jr, Alonso RS, Luz A, Coca Velarde LG. Corneal-thickness spatial profile and corneal-volume distribution: Tomographic indices to detect keratoconus. *J Cataract Refract Surg.* 2006;32(11):1851-1859.

Ambrósio R Jr, Caiado AL, Guerra FP, et al. Novel pachymetric parameters based on corneal tomography for diagnosing keratoconus. *J Refract Surg.* 2011;27(1):753-758.

Ambrósio R Jr, Klyce SD, Wilson SE. Corneal topographic and pachymetric screening of keratorefractive patients. *J Refract Surg.* 2003;19(1):24-29.

Ambrósio, RA Jr, Randleman JB. Screening for ectasia risk: what are we screening for and how should we screen for it? *J Refract Surg.* 2013;29(4):230-232.

Hardten DR, Gosavi VV. Photorefractive keratectomy in eyes with atypical topography. *J Cataract Refract Surg.* 2009;35(8):1437-1444.

Li Y, Meisler DM, Tang M, et al. Keratoconus diagnosis with optical coherence tomography pachymetry mapping. *Ophthalmology.* 2008;115(12):2159-2166.

Liu Z, Huang AJ, Pflugfelder SC. Evaluation of corneal thickness and topography in normal eyes using the Orbscan corneal topography system. *Br J Ophthalmol.* 1999;83(7):774-778.

Ramos IC, Correa R, Guerra FP, et al. Variability of subjective classifications of corneal topography maps from LASIK candidates. *J Refract Surg.* 2013 Aug 30:1-7.

Saad A, Gatinel D. Topographic and tomographic properties of forme fruste keratoconus corneas. *Invest Ophthalmol Vis Sci.* 2010;51(11):5546-5553.

Saad A, Lteif Y, Azan E, Gatinel D. Biomechanical properties of keratoconus suspect eyes. *Invest Ophthalmol Vis Sci.* 2010;51(6):2912-2916.

Sonmez B, Doan MP, Hamilton DR. Identification of scanning slit-beam topographic parameters important in distinguishing normal from keratoconic corneal morphologic features. *Am J Ophthalmol.* 2007;143(3):401-408.

—Case 18—

A 29-year-old male desires refractive surgical correction. He admits to poor contact lens hygiene and wearing patterns, and he frequently sleeps in his lenses. He has no significant family or past medical history. The patient was at another facility and brought with him the results of the testing that was performed, which is included with the testing done today.

CASE HISTORY		
	Right Eye	**Left Eye**
Present correction method	CTL	CTL
Manifest refraction	-5.25 +0.50 x 080	-5.25 +1.00 x 085
CDVA (current)	20/20	20/20
Dominant eye		Left
Ocular alignment	Orthophoric	Orthophoric
Keratometry		
Flat K	42.5 @ 005	42.0 @ 180
Steep K	43.0 @ 095	43.0 @ 090
Pupil size (bright)	3.9 mm	3.7 mm
Pupil size (dim)	5.3 mm	5.0 mm
Central corneal thickness	521 µm	516 µm
Physical examination	Normal	Normal
Estimated ablation depth	80 µm	80 µm

Questions

1. Is this patient a candidate for refractive surgery? If so, what treatment options are available?
2. Considering all factors, what procedure would you recommend and why?
3. What are the most significant potential complications for each procedure available for this patient, based on the examination?

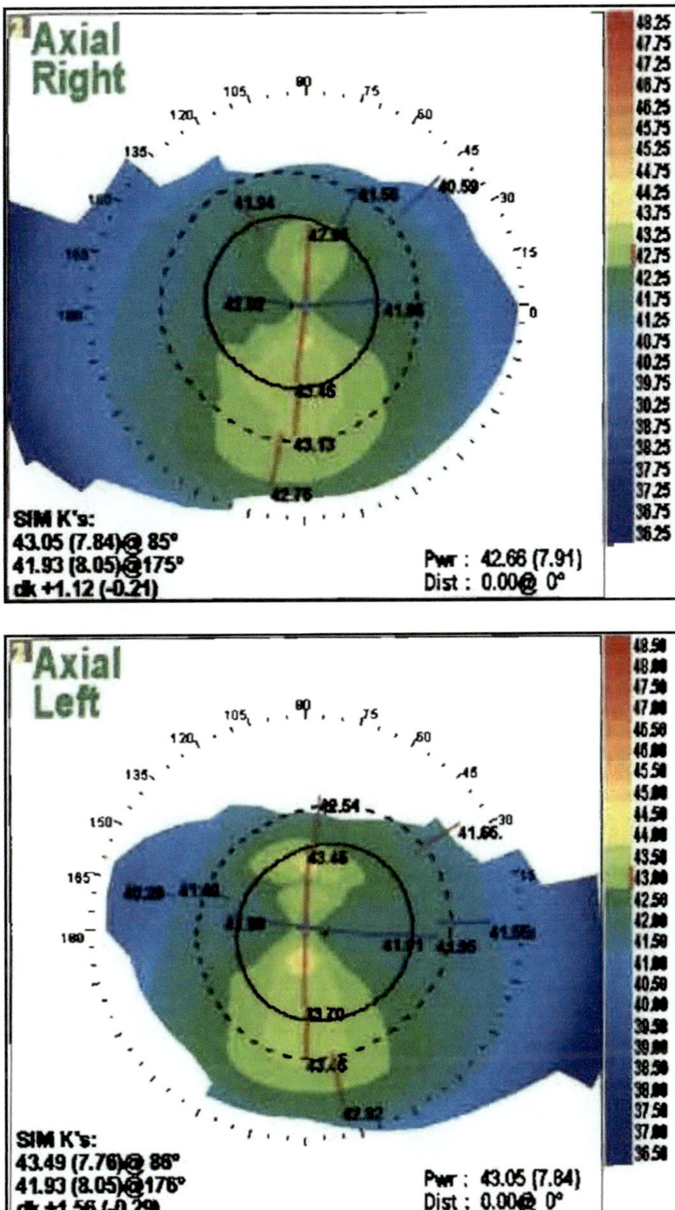
Axial Right
SIM K's:
43.05 (7.84)@ 85°
41.93 (8.05)@175°
dk +1.12 (-0.21)
Pwr : 42.66 (7.91)
Dist : 0.00@ 0°
Axial Left
SIM K's:
43.49 (7.76)@ 86°
41.93 (8.05)@176°
dk +1.56 (-0.29)
Pwr : 43.05 (7.84)
Dist : 0.00@ 0°

A

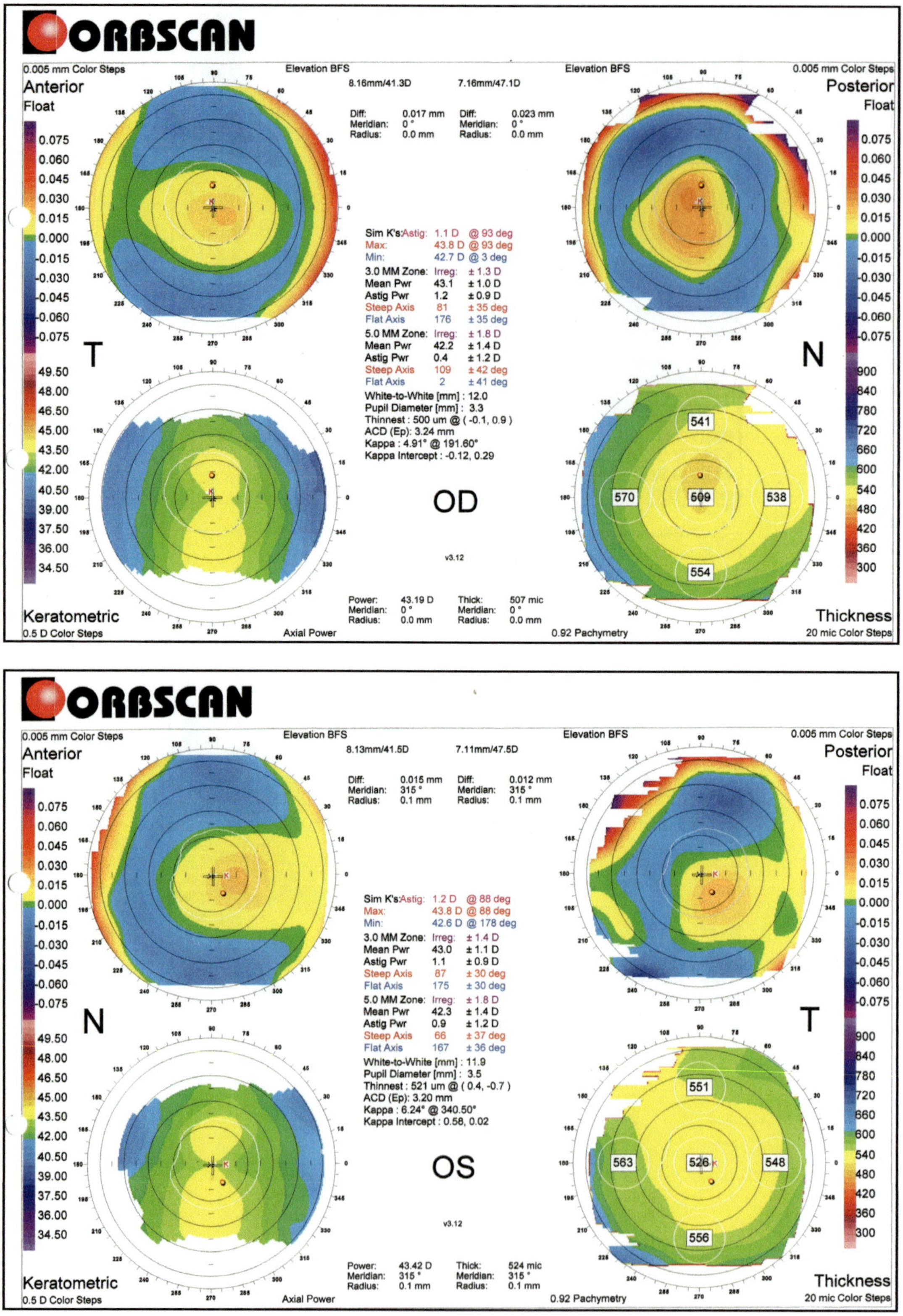
ORBSCAN
0.005 mm Color Steps
Anterior
Float
Elevation BFS
8.16mm/41.3D
7.16mm/47.1D
Elevation BFS
0.005 mm Color Steps
Posterior
Float
Diff: 0.017 mm
Meridian: 0 °
Radius: 0.0 mm
Diff: 0.023 mm
Meridian: 0 °
Radius: 0.0 mm
Sim K's:Astig: 1.1 D @ 93 deg
Max: 43.8 D @ 93 deg
Min: 42.7 D @ 3 deg
3.0 MM Zone: Irreg: ± 1.3 D
Mean Pwr 43.1 ± 1.0 D
Astig Pwr 1.2 ± 0.9 D
Steep Axis 81 ± 35 deg
Flat Axis 176 ± 35 deg
5.0 MM Zone: Irreg: ± 1.8 D
Mean Pwr 42.2 ± 1.4 D
Astig Pwr 0.4 ± 1.2 D
Steep Axis 109 ± 42 deg
Flat Axis 2 ± 41 deg
White-to-White [mm] : 12.0
Pupil Diameter [mm] : 3.3
Thinnest : 500 um @ (-0.1, 0.9)
ACD (Ep): 3.24 mm
Kappa : 4.91° @ 191.60°
Kappa Intercept : -0.12, 0.29
T
N
OD
v3.12
541
570
509
538
554
Power: 43.19 D
Meridian: 0 °
Radius: 0.0 mm
Thick: 507 mic
Meridian: 0 °
Radius: 0.0 mm
Keratometric
0.5 D Color Steps
Axial Power
0.92 Pachymetry
Thickness
20 mic Color Steps
ORBSCAN
0.005 mm Color Steps
Anterior
Float
Elevation BFS
8.13mm/41.5D
7.11mm/47.5D
Elevation BFS
0.005 mm Color Steps
Posterior
Float
Diff: 0.015 mm
Meridian: 315 °
Radius: 0.1 mm
Diff: 0.012 mm
Meridian: 315 °
Radius: 0.1 mm
Sim K's:Astig: 1.2 D @ 88 deg
Max: 43.8 D @ 88 deg
Min: 42.6 D @ 178 deg
3.0 MM Zone: Irreg: ± 1.4 D
Mean Pwr 43.0 ± 1.1 D
Astig Pwr 1.1 ± 0.9 D
Steep Axis 87 ± 30 deg
Flat Axis 175 ± 30 deg
5.0 MM Zone: Irreg: ± 1.8 D
Mean Pwr 42.3 ± 1.4 D
Astig Pwr 0.9 ± 1.2 D
Steep Axis 66 ± 37 deg
Flat Axis 167 ± 36 deg
White-to-White [mm] : 11.9
Pupil Diameter [mm] : 3.5
Thinnest : 521 um @ (0.4, -0.7)
ACD (Ep): 3.20 mm
Kappa : 6.24° @ 340.50°
Kappa Intercept : 0.58, 0.02
N
T
OS
v3.12
551
563
526
548
556
Power: 43.42 D
Meridian: 315 °
Radius: 0.1 mm
Thick: 524 mic
Meridian: 315 °
Radius: 0.1 mm
Keratometric
0.5 D Color Steps
Axial Power
0.92 Pachymetry
Thickness
20 mic Color Steps

B

C

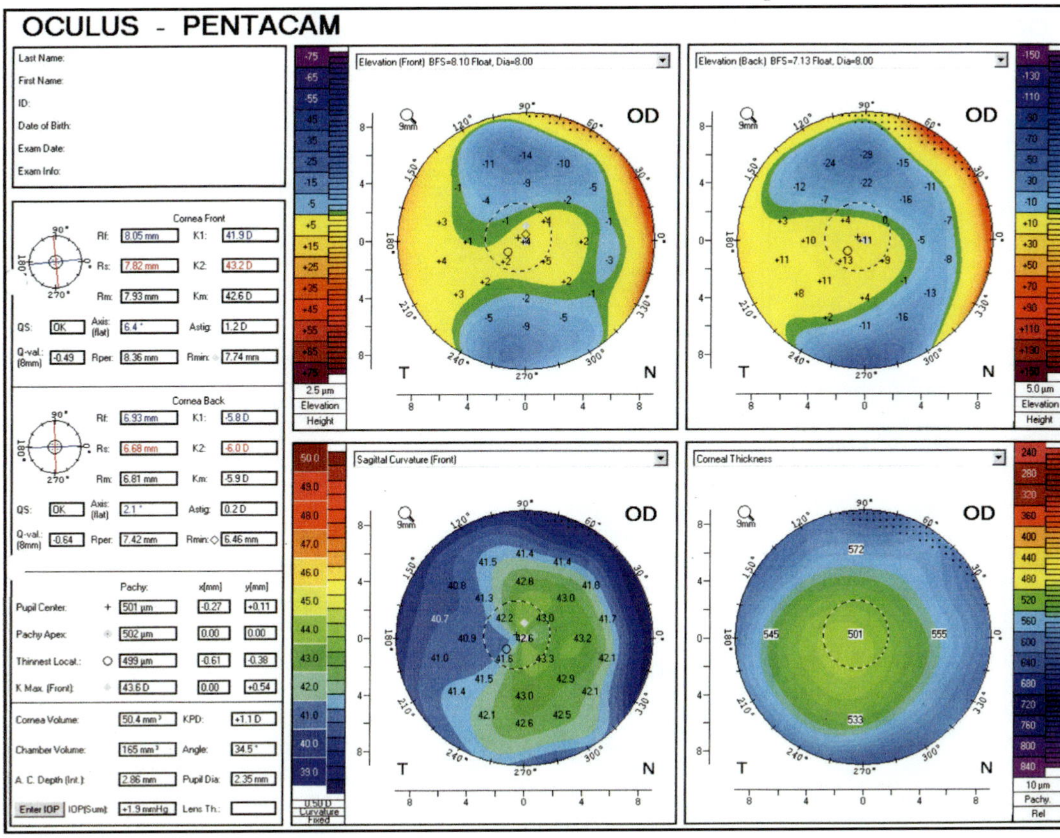
OCULUS - PENTACAM
Last Name:
First Name:
ID:
Date of Birth:
Exam Date:
Exam Info:
Cornea Front
Rf: 8.05 mm K1: 41.9 D
Rs: 7.82 mm K2: 43.2 D
Rm: 7.93 mm Km: 42.6 D
QS: OK Axis (flat): 6.4° Astig: 1.2 D
Q-val. (8mm): -0.49 Rper: 8.36 mm Rmin: 7.74 mm
Cornea Back
Rf: 6.93 mm K1: -5.8 D
Rs: 6.68 mm K2: -6.0 D
Rm: 6.81 mm Km: -5.9 D
QS: OK Axis (flat): 2.1° Astig: 0.2 D
Q-val. (8mm): -0.64 Rper: 7.42 mm Rmin: 6.46 mm
Pachy: x[mm] y[mm]
Pupil Center: 501 µm -0.27 +0.11
Pachy Apex: 502 µm 0.00 0.00
Thinnest Locat.: 499 µm -0.61 -0.38
K Max. (Front): 43.6 D 0.00 +0.54
Cornea Volume: 50.4 mm³ KPD: +1.1 D
Chamber Volume: 165 mm³ Angle: 34.5°
A. C. Depth (Int.): 2.86 mm Pupil Dia: 2.35 mm
Enter IOP IOP(Sum): +1.9 mmHg Lens Th.:
Elevation (Front) BFS=8.10 Float, Dia=8.00
Elevation (Back) BFS=7.13 Float, Dia=8.00
Sagittal Curvature (Front)
Corneal Thickness
OD
T
N
2.5 µm Elevation Height
5.0 µm Elevation Height
0.50 D Curvature Fixed
10 µm Pachy. Rel

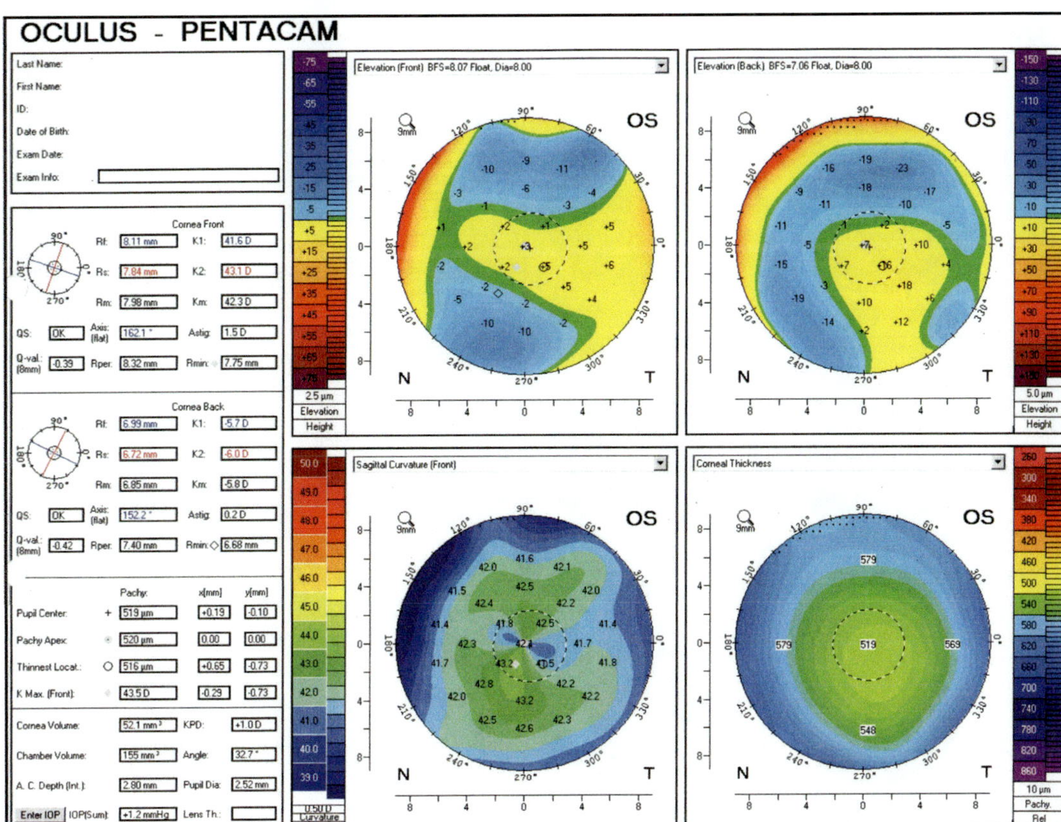
OCULUS - PENTACAM
Last Name:
First Name:
ID:
Date of Birth:
Exam Date:
Exam Info:
Cornea Front
Rf: 8.11 mm K1: 41.6 D
Rs: 7.84 mm K2: 43.1 D
Rm: 7.98 mm Km: 42.3 D
QS: OK Axis (flat): 162.1° Astig: 1.5 D
Q-val. (8mm): -0.39 Rper: 8.32 mm Rmin: 7.75 mm
Cornea Back
Rf: 6.99 mm K1: -5.7 D
Rs: 6.72 mm K2: -6.0 D
Rm: 6.85 mm Km: -5.8 D
QS: OK Axis (flat): 152.2° Astig: 0.2 D
Q-val. (8mm): -0.42 Rper: 7.40 mm Rmin: 6.68 mm
Pachy: x[mm] y[mm]
Pupil Center: 519 µm +0.19 -0.10
Pachy Apex: 520 µm 0.00 0.00
Thinnest Locat.: 516 µm +0.65 -0.73
K Max. (Front): 43.5 D -0.29 -0.73
Cornea Volume: 52.1 mm³ KPD: +1.0 D
Chamber Volume: 155 mm³ Angle: 32.7°
A. C. Depth (Int.): 2.80 mm Pupil Dia: 2.52 mm
Enter IOP IOP(Sum): +1.2 mmHg Lens Th.:
Elevation (Front) BFS=8.07 Float, Dia=8.00
Elevation (Back) BFS=7.06 Float, Dia=8.00
Sagittal Curvature (Front)
Corneal Thickness
OS
N
T
2.5 µm Elevation Height
5.0 µm Elevation Height
0.50 D Curvature Fixed
10 µm Pachy. Rel

D

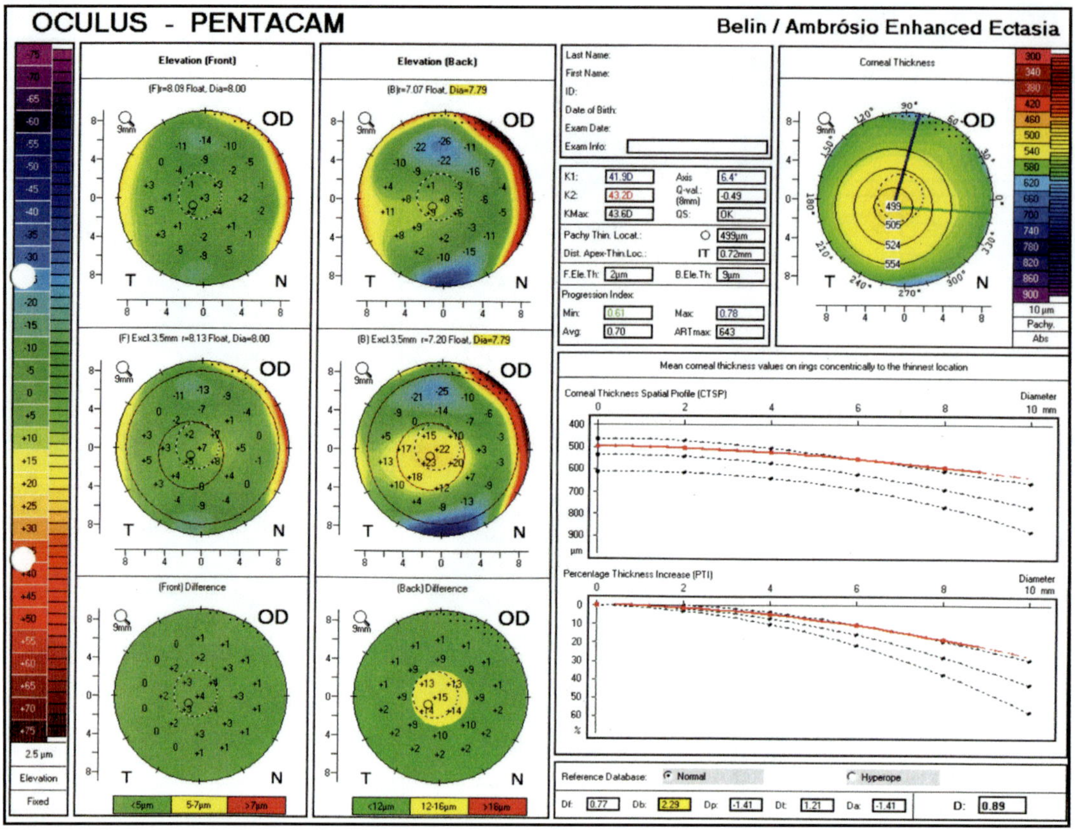
OCULUS - PENTACAM
Belin / Ambrósio Enhanced Ectasia
Elevation (Front)
Elevation (Back)
Corneal Thickness
OD
(F)r=8.09 Float, Dia=8.00
(B)r=7.07 Float, Dia=7.79
(F) Excl.3.5mm r=8.13 Float, Dia=8.00
(B) Excl.3.5mm r=7.20 Float, Dia=7.79
(Front) Difference
(Back) Difference
Last Name:
First Name:
ID:
Date of Birth:
Exam Date:
Exam Info:
K1: 41.9D
K2: 43.2D
KMax: 43.6D
Axis: 6.4°
Q-val.: (8mm) -0.49
QS: OK
Pachy Thin. Locat.: 499µm
Dist. Apex-Thin.Loc.: 0.72mm
F.Ele.Th: 2µm
B.Ele.Th: 9µm
Progression Index
Min: 0.61
Max: 0.78
Avg: 0.70
ARTmax: 643
Mean corneal thickness values on rings concentrically to the thinnest location
Corneal Thickness Spatial Profile (CTSP)
Percentage Thickness Increase (PTI)
Diameter 10 mm
Reference Database: Normal
Hyperope
Df: 0.77
Db: 2.29
Dp: -1.41
Dt: 1.21
Da: -1.41
D: 0.89
<5µm
5-7µm
>7µm
<12µm
12-16µm
>16µm
2.5 µm
Elevation
Fixed
10 µm
Pachy.
Abs

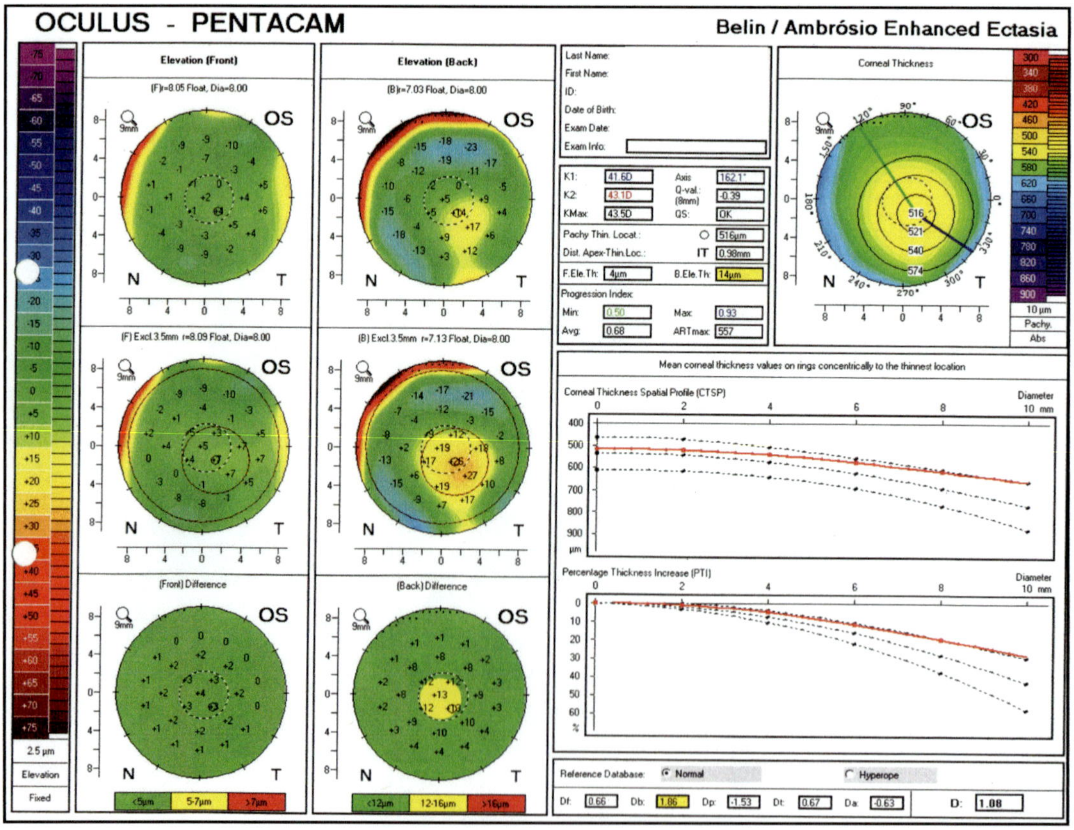
OCULUS - PENTACAM
Belin / Ambrósio Enhanced Ectasia
Elevation (Front)
Elevation (Back)
Corneal Thickness
OS
(F)r=8.05 Float, Dia=8.00
(B)r=7.03 Float, Dia=8.00
(F) Excl.3.5mm r=8.09 Float, Dia=8.00
(B) Excl.3.5mm r=7.13 Float, Dia=8.00
(Front) Difference
(Back) Difference
Last Name:
First Name:
ID:
Date of Birth:
Exam Date:
Exam Info:
K1: 41.6D
K2: 43.1D
KMax: 43.5D
Axis: 162.1°
Q-val.: (8mm) -0.39
QS: OK
Pachy Thin. Locat.: 516µm
Dist. Apex-Thin.Loc.: 0.98mm
F.Ele.Th: 4µm
B.Ele.Th: 14µm
Progression Index
Min: 0.50
Max: 0.93
Avg: 0.68
ARTmax: 557
Mean corneal thickness values on rings concentrically to the thinnest location
Corneal Thickness Spatial Profile (CTSP)
Percentage Thickness Increase (PTI)
Diameter 10 mm
Reference Database: Normal
Hyperope
Df: 0.66
Db: 1.86
Dp: -1.53
Dt: 0.67
Da: -0.63
D: 1.08
<5µm
5-7µm
>7µm
<12µm
12-16µm
>16µm
2.5 µm
Elevation
Fixed
10 µm
Pachy.
Abs

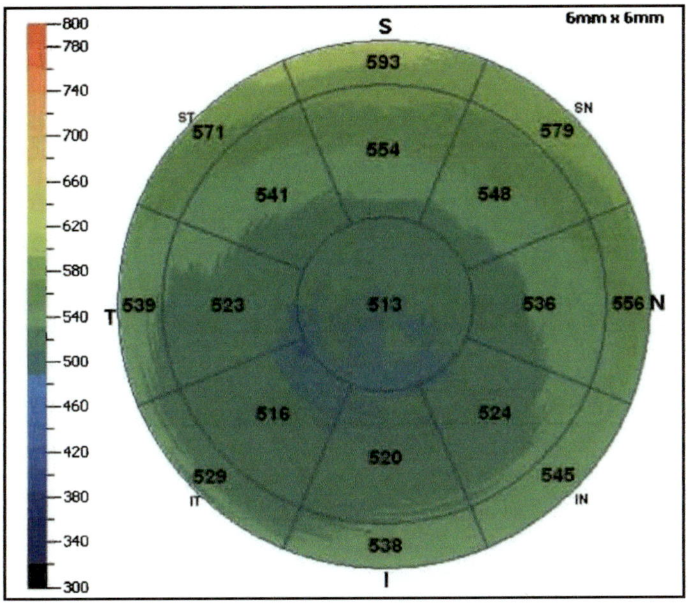
6mm x 6mm
S
593
571
554
579
541
548
T 539
523
513
536
556 N
516
524
520
529
545
538
I
800
780
740
700
660
620
580
540
500
460
420
380
340
300

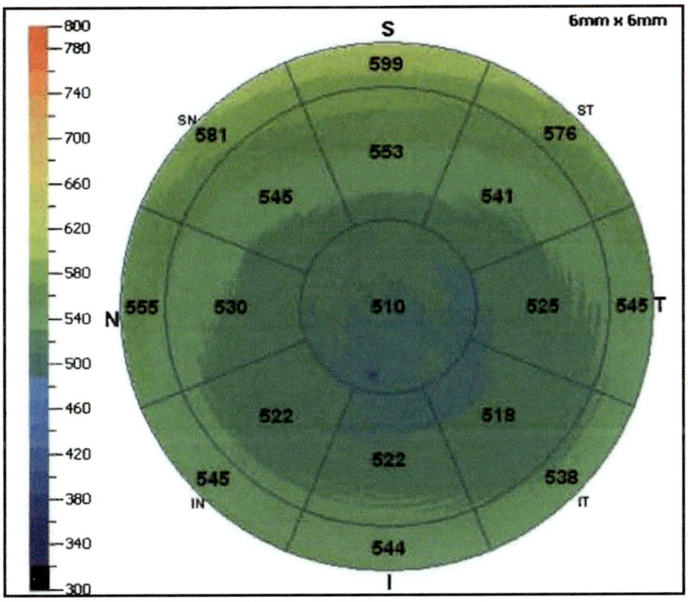
6mm x 6mm
S
599
581
553
576
545
541
N 555
530
510
525
545 T
522
518
522
545
538
544
I
800
780
740
700
660
620
580
540
500
460
420
380
340
300

E

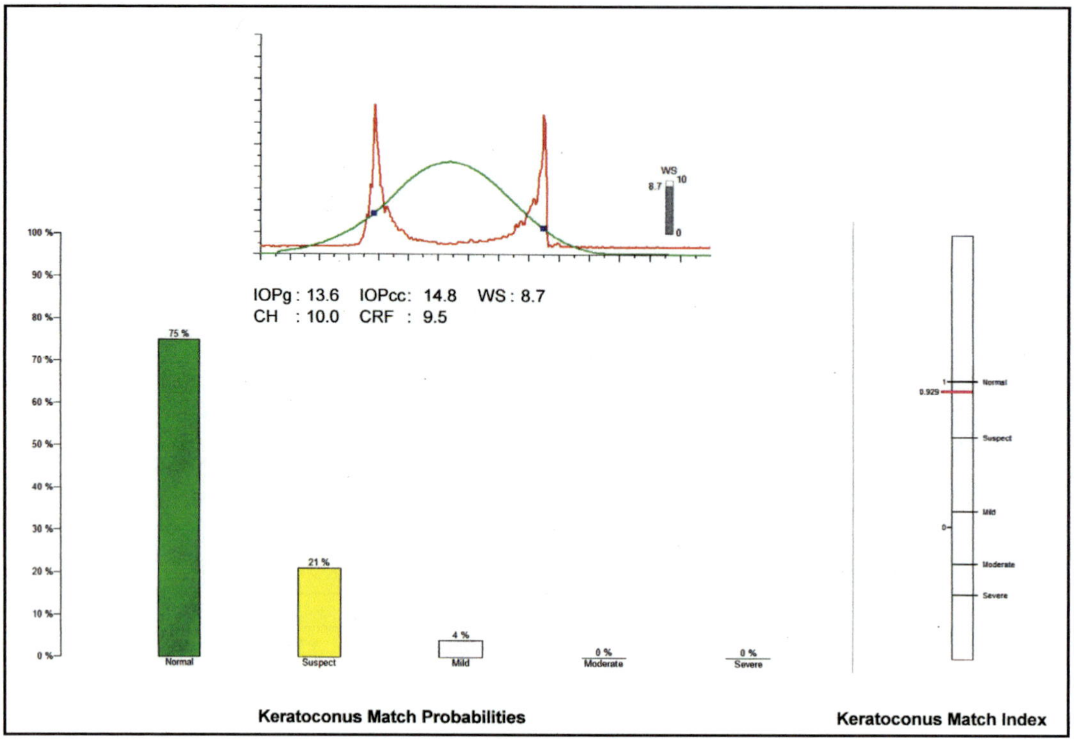
WS
8.7
10
0
IOPg : 13.6 IOPcc: 14.8 WS : 8.7
CH : 10.0 CRF : 9.5
100 %
90 %
80 %
70 %
60 %
50 %
40 %
30 %
20 %
10 %
0 %
75 %
21 %
4 %
0 %
0 %
Normal
Suspect
Mild
Moderate
Severe
Keratoconus Match Probabilities
1
0.929
0
Normal
Suspect
Mild
Moderate
Severe
Keratoconus Match Index

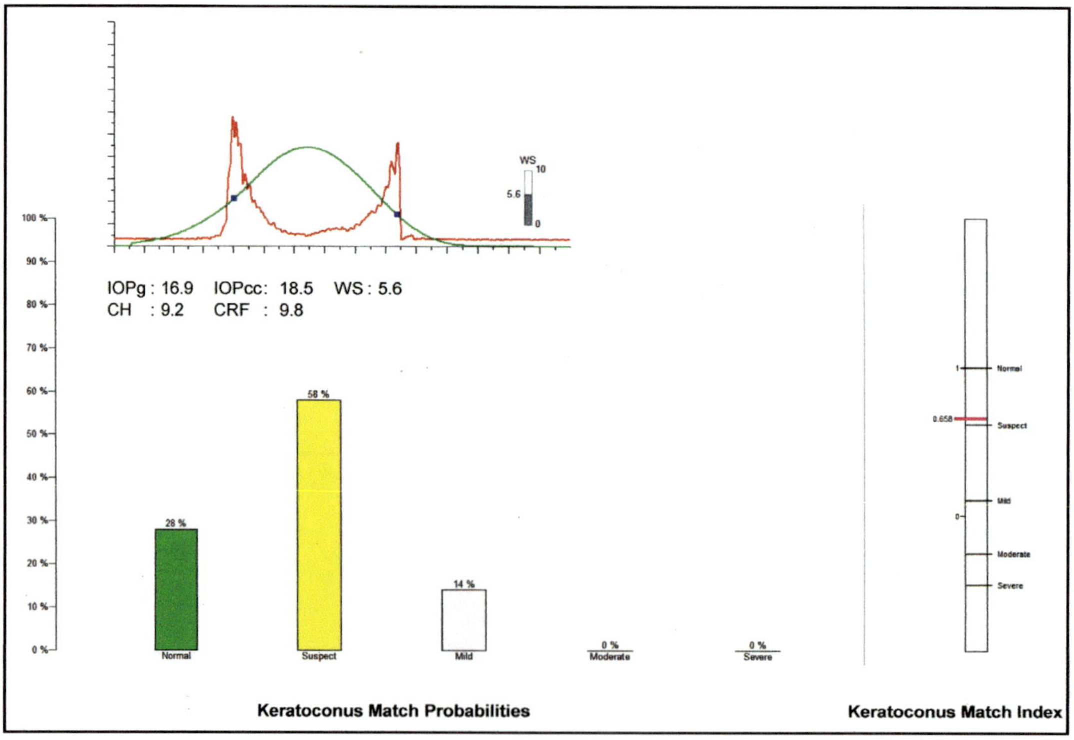
WS
5.6
10
0
IOPg : 16.9 IOPcc: 18.5 WS : 5.6
CH : 9.2 CRF : 9.8
100 %
90 %
80 %
70 %
60 %
50 %
40 %
30 %
20 %
10 %
0 %
28 %
58 %
14 %
0 %
0 %
Normal
Suspect
Mild
Moderate
Severe
Keratoconus Match Probabilities
1
0.658
0
Normal
Suspect
Mild
Moderate
Severe
Keratoconus Match Index

F

—Case 18—

Screening for Ectasia Risk

When Is Too Much Evaluation Too Much?

With the advent of multiple screening technologies available, it can become overwhelming to determine the difference between clinically significant asymmetry and normal variation. Although in many cases additional screening can prove useful, in others it can simply confuse the situation and override basic patient screening strategies that have been validated and proven useful over time.

Case Analysis

- The estimated residual stromal bed (RSB) thickness is approximately 315 to 335 µm in both eyes.
- Case Figure A shows Placido imaging of the right and left eyes demonstrating symmetric bowtie with-the-rule patterns in both eyes.
- Case Figure B shows scanning slit-beam images from the Orbscan II (Bausch & Lomb) demonstrating similar symmetric bowtie with-the-rule keratometric patterns in both eyes. Central corneal thickness is less than measured with ultrasound pachymetry, and there are some findings of borderline significance on thickness progression and posterior float in both eyes.
- Case Figure C shows Scheimpflug based imaging (Pentacam) of the right and left eyes demonstrating analogous findings on the sagittal curvature maps (lower left), compared with previous images. Corneal thickness is unremarkable in both eyes. There is a slight increase in posterior elevation (+13 µm in the right eye and +18 µm in the left eye).
- Case Figure D shows Belin/Ambrosio enhanced ectasia display of the right and left eyes. There is an increased posterior elevation difference (15 µm in the right eye and 13 µm in the left eye), but the ARTmax and D indices (discussed next) are unremarkable for either eye.
- Case Figure E shows OCT images demonstrating mildly suspicious thickness progression from the center to the periphery in both eyes, with relative symmetry between eyes.
- Case Figure F shows ORA images of the (A) right and (B) left eyes demonstrating moderately low corneal hysteresis (CH) and corneal resistance factor (CRF) in the 9 to 10 range for both eyes, with suspicious Keratoconus Match Index and Keratoconus Match Probabilities measures in both eyes.

Pearl: *Screening for ectasia risk is an important part, but just one part, of the overall screening process—keep it and the overall surgical risk in appropriate perspective!*

Questions

1. Is this patient a candidate for refractive surgery? If so, what treatment options are available for this patient?

    Yes, this patient is a candidate for refractive surgery. Corneal biomechanical testing appears minimally concerning when taken in aggregate. All other patient screening parameters appear normal. This patient is a candidate for surface ablation, LASIK, or phakic intraocular lens (PIOL) implantation, based on refractive error.

2. Considering all factors, what procedure would you recommend and why?

    This patient is probably suitable for any of the above-mentioned procedures. The risks and benefits of each procedure should therefore be explored with the patient.

3. What are the most significant potential complications for each procedure available for this patient, based on the examination?

    Surface ablation carries a higher risk of infection and visually significant haze, although this is unlikely to occur. LASIK carries a higher risk of ectasia, but there is no clear evidence that this patient's risk would be elevated more than average. Phakic IOL implantation carries additional intraocular risks and is overall the highest-risk procedure for this patient.

Keeping Ectasia Risk Screening in Perspective

Ectasia has received significant attention over the past 10 years, and in some instances it appears that it is the primary, almost exclusive, consideration for some refractive surgeons and patients. Although this cautious approach is warranted to some extent, in some instances, the relative risk of ectasia may be overstated, especially when considering other risks from having or not having surgery.

In this patient, the risk score, calculated with the Ectasia Risk Score System (ERSS), is 1 (low risk) based on age (29 years), normal topographic pattern, normal corneal and RSB thickness, and moderate myopic refraction. Placido imaging is normal, symmetrical, and reproducible between measuring systems. The advanced biomechanical testing obtained is not definitive or particularly additive to the screening process.

Corneal thickness and regional profiles by all devices appear relatively normal, although there is some variability between devices. The Belin/Ambrosio Enhanced Ectasia Display has been introduced as an advanced measurement system to elaborate on regional corneal thickness and posterior elevation findings. This display provides 2 primary metrics, "D" and "ARTMax," which are automatically generated and flagged as normal (white), suspicious (yellow), or abnormal (red), based on their values. Although an attractive metric, the values remain to be validated as a screening device for ectasia risk, and even in cases with clear topographic abnormalities by all other testing, these values may not identify patients as abnormal.

The ORA assessment in this case by CH and CRF values is borderline suspicious and is suspicious by KMI and KMP, but without firm data to support these ORA findings, it is difficult to rely on this test when others are normal. Various other diagnostic modalities have been identified, including epithelial thickness profiles and higher-order aberrations. The degree to which these become a part of routine clinical practice remains to be determined.

In this patient, an admitted contact lens abuser, the risk of surgery should be weighed against the risk of not performing surgery and relegating him to continued contact lens wear. The relative safety of contact lens wear and LASIK remains a topic of debate; however, literature exists that demonstrates that LASIK is as safe as routine contact lens wear for most patients and safer than improper contact lens wear. The risk of infection is approximately 10 times greater after surface ablation than after LASIK, and, in normal cases, healing time and visual recovery are significantly prolonged. The relative risks for all of this patient's options suggest that LASIK is as safe as other alternatives for vision correction, except for full-time spectacle wear.

Bibliography

Ambrósio R Jr, Caiado AL, Guerra FP, et al. Novel pachymetric parameters based on corneal tomography for diagnosing keratoconus. *J Refract Surg.* 2011;27(1):753-758.

Fontes BM, Ambrósio R Jr, Jardim D, Velarde GC, Nosé W. Corneal biomechanical metrics and anterior segment parameters in mild keratoconus. *Ophthalmology.* 2010;117(4):673-679.

Fontes BM, Ambrósio R Jr, Velarde GC, Nosé W. Ocular response analyzer measurements in keratoconus with normal central corneal thickness compared with matched normal control eyes. *J Refract Surg.* 2011;27(3):209-215.

Guilbert E, Saad A, Grise-Dulac A, Gatinel D. Corneal thickness, curvature, and elevation readings in normal corneas: combined Placido-Scheimpflug system versus combined Placido-scanning-slit system. *J Cataract Refract Surg.* 2012;38(7):1198-1206.

Mathers WD, Fraunfelder FW, Rich LF. Risk of LASIK surgery vs contact lenses. *Arch Ophthalmol.* 2006;124(10):1510-1511.

McGee HT, Mathers WD. Laser in situ keratomileusis versus long-term contact lens wear: decision analysis. *J Cataract Refract Surg.* 2009;35(11):1860-1867.

Reinstein DZ, Archer TJ, Gobbe M. Corneal epithelial thickness profile in the diagnosis of keratoconus. *J Refract Surg.* 2009;25(7):604-610.

Reinstein DZ, Archer TJ, Gobbe M, Silverman RH, Coleman DJ. Epithelial thickness in the normal cornea: three-dimensional display with Artemis very high-frequency digital ultrasound. *J Refract Surg.* 2008;24(6):571-581.

Reinstein DZ, Couch DG, Archer T. Direct residual stromal thickness measurement for assessing suitability for LASIK enhancement by Artemis 3D very high-frequency digital ultrasound arc scanning. *J Cataract Refract Surg.* 2006;32(11):1884-1888.

Reinstein DZ, Gobbe M, Archer TJ, Silverman RH, Coleman DJ. Epithelial, stromal, and total corneal thickness in keratoconus: three-dimensional display with artemis very-high frequency digital ultrasound. *J Refract Surg.* 2010;26(4):259-271.

Rocha KM, Perez-Straziota CE, Stulting RD, Randleman JB. SD-OCT analysis of regional epithelial thickness profiles in keratoconus, postoperative corneal ectasia, and normal eyes. *J Refract Surg.* 2013;29(3):173-179.

Saad A, Gatinel D. Evaluation of total and corneal wavefront high order aberrations for the detection of forme fruste keratoconus. *Invest Ophthalmol Vis Sci.* 2012 17;53(6):2978-2992.

Part 2
Postoperative Evaluations

—Case 19—

A 31-year-old male desires refractive surgical correction. He had LASIK approximately 3 to 4 years ago, with an original prescription of approximately -6.00 diopters (D) in both eyes. He reported good visual acuity initially, but he has experienced a gradual decrease in vision, especially at night, for the past year.

Case History		
	Right Eye	**Left Eye**
UDVA	20/40	20/40
Manifest refraction	-1.50 +0.75 x 095	-1.50 sphere
CDVA	20/20	20/20
CNVA	20/20	20/20
Cycloplegic refraction	-1.00 +0.75 x 095	-1.00 sphere
Cycloplegic CDVA	20/15	20/20
Keratometry		
Flat K	42.25 @ 150	42.5 @ 040
Steep K	43.00 @ 060	43.0 @ 130
Central corneal thickness	460 µm	465 µm
Physical examination	LASIK scar barely visible inferiorly	LASIK scar barely visible inferiorly
Estimated ablation depth	20 µm	15 µm

Questions

1. Is this patient a candidate for refractive surgery retreatment? If so, what treatment options are available?
2. What additional testing may be useful to help determine your course of action?
3. Considering all factors, what procedure would you recommend and why?
4. What are the most likely causes for this refractive error at this time point after LASIK?
5. How would your management change if this patient were 5 to 7 years out after surgery? 10 to 12 years?

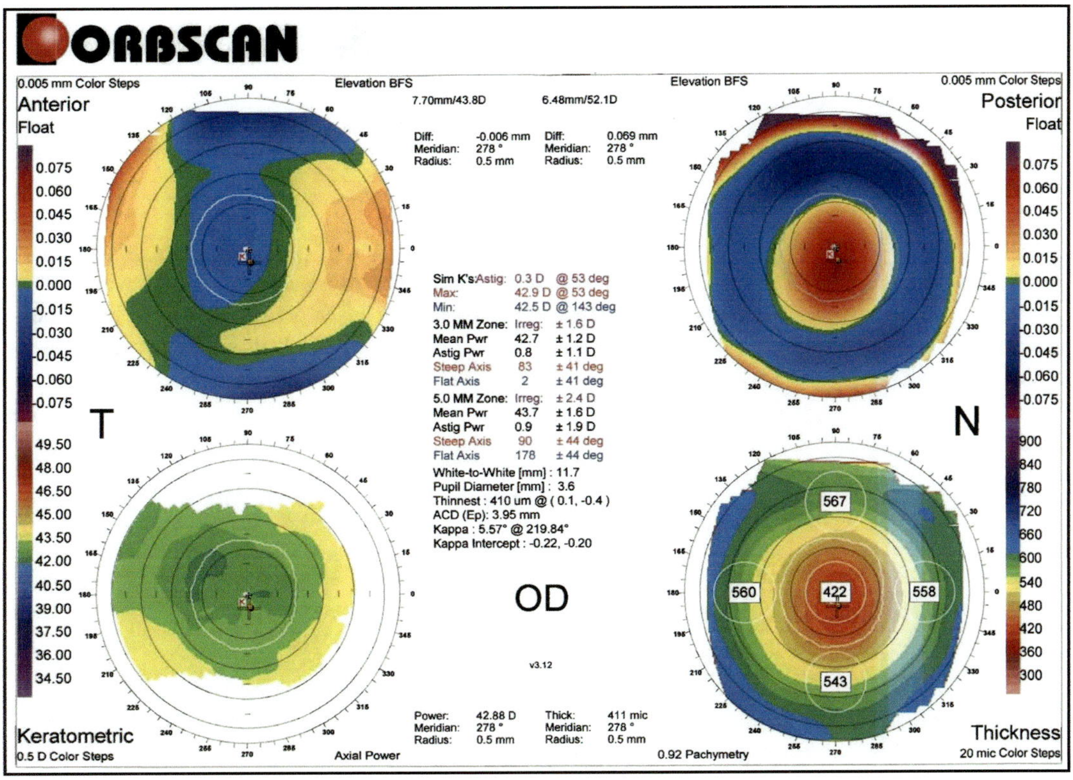
ORBSCAN
0.005 mm Color Steps
Anterior
Float
Elevation BFS
7.70mm/43.8D
6.48mm/52.1D
Diff: -0.006 mm
Meridian: 278 °
Radius: 0.5 mm
Diff: 0.069 mm
Meridian: 278 °
Radius: 0.5 mm
Elevation BFS
0.005 mm Color Steps
Posterior
Float
Sim K's Astig: 0.3 D @ 53 deg
Max: 42.9 D @ 53 deg
Min: 42.5 D @ 143 deg
3.0 MM Zone: Irreg: ± 1.6 D
Mean Pwr 42.7 ± 1.2 D
Astig Pwr 0.8 ± 1.1 D
Steep Axis 83 ± 41 deg
Flat Axis 2 ± 41 deg
5.0 MM Zone: Irreg: ± 2.4 D
Mean Pwr 43.7 ± 1.6 D
Astig Pwr 0.9 ± 1.9 D
Steep Axis 90 ± 44 deg
Flat Axis 178 ± 44 deg
White-to-White [mm] : 11.7
Pupil Diameter [mm] : 3.6
Thinnest : 410 um @ (0.1, -0.4)
ACD (Ep): 3.95 mm
Kappa : 5.57° @ 219.84°
Kappa Intercept : -0.22, -0.20
T
N
OD
v3.12
567
560
422
558
543
Power: 42.88 D
Meridian: 278 °
Radius: 0.5 mm
Thick: 411 mic
Meridian: 278 °
Radius: 0.5 mm
Keratometric
0.5 D Color Steps
Axial Power
0.92 Pachymetry
Thickness
20 mic Color Steps

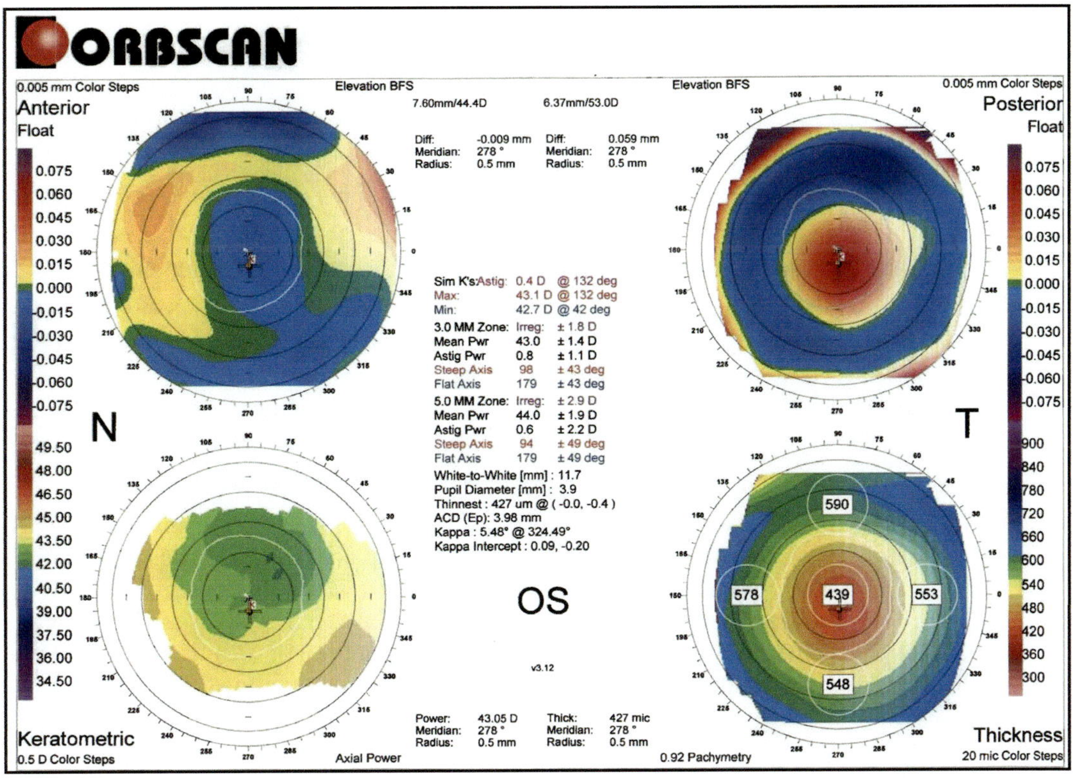
ORBSCAN
0.005 mm Color Steps
Anterior
Float
Elevation BFS
7.60mm/44.4D
6.37mm/53.0D
Diff: -0.009 mm
Meridian: 278 °
Radius: 0.5 mm
Diff: 0.059 mm
Meridian: 278 °
Radius: 0.5 mm
Elevation BFS
0.005 mm Color Steps
Posterior
Float
Sim K's Astig: 0.4 D @ 132 deg
Max: 43.1 D @ 132 deg
Min: 42.7 D @ 42 deg
3.0 MM Zone: Irreg: ± 1.8 D
Mean Pwr 43.0 ± 1.4 D
Astig Pwr 0.8 ± 1.1 D
Steep Axis 98 ± 43 deg
Flat Axis 179 ± 43 deg
5.0 MM Zone: Irreg: ± 2.9 D
Mean Pwr 44.0 ± 1.9 D
Astig Pwr 0.6 ± 2.2 D
Steep Axis 94 ± 49 deg
Flat Axis 179 ± 49 deg
White-to-White [mm] : 11.7
Pupil Diameter [mm] : 3.9
Thinnest : 427 um @ (-0.0, -0.4)
ACD (Ep): 3.98 mm
Kappa : 5.48° @ 324.49°
Kappa Intercept : 0.09, -0.20
N
T
OS
v3.12
590
578
439
553
548
Power: 43.05 D
Meridian: 278 °
Radius: 0.5 mm
Thick: 427 mic
Meridian: 278 °
Radius: 0.5 mm
Keratometric
0.5 D Color Steps
Axial Power
0.92 Pachymetry
Thickness
20 mic Color Steps

—Case 19—
Retreatment After LASIK

Residual ametropia after initial laser refractive surgery is the most common issue warranting intervention. Retreatment (or enhancement) rates after excimer laser procedures vary by indication and patient expectations, but generally are less than 5% for all procedures. This rate appears stable over time.

Case Analysis

- The current estimated residual stromal bed (RSB) thickness is approximately 310 μm in both eyes.
- After retreatment with LASIK, the RSB thickness is approximately 290 to 300 μm in both eyes.
- Case Figures show normal topographic patterns after myopic LASIK, with well-centered central flattening and thinning.

Pearl: *Confirm flap thickness and actual RSB prior to considering LASIK retreatment, and do not lift flaps that have been in place for many years!*

Questions

1. Is this patient a candidate for refractive surgery retreatment? If so, what treatment options are available for this patient?

   Yes; based on refraction, pachymetry, and topography, this patient is a reasonable candidate for laser vision correction retreatment.

2. What additional testing may be useful to help determine your course of action?

   If one were considering retreatment with flap lift, it would be useful to obtain data to confirm the flap thickness and RSB thickness at the time of initial LASIK. This can be achieved by obtaining old records, if flap thickness was directly measured, or by current direct flap measurement, using anterior segment optical coherence tomography (OCT), very high-frequency ultrasound, or confocal microscopy.

3. Considering all factors, what procedure would you recommend and why?

   Assuming RSB is adequate, 3 to 4 years after LASIK either retreatment with flap lift or photorefractive keratectomy (PRK) over the flap are options. Performing LASIK again by creating a new flap is NOT an option, as stromal tissue between flaps may be lost, resulting in significant irregular astigmatism. An informed discussion with the patient, focusing on the increased rate of epithelial ingrowth with flap lift and infection and residual ametropia with PRK, is necessary to determine the best course.

4. What are the most likely causes for this refractive error at this time point after LASIK?

   The most likely causes are residual myopic astigmatism or regression. All patients presenting with myopia and astigmatism after LASIK must be screened to preclude early ectasia before retreatment. Cataract development can also cause myopic shifts after LASIK, although it is not commonly seen in younger patients.

5. How would your management change if this patient were 5 to 7 years out after surgery? 10 to 12 years?

   At some time point after LASIK, it is no longer reasonable to relift the original flap; in these cases, surface ablation over the flap is the best treatment option. The exact timing for this is still under debate. Most surgeons no longer advocate flap lift at 5 or more years after primary LASIK, and very few advocate flap lift at 10 years after LASIK due to increased risk of epithelial ingrowth and irregular astigmatism from flap healing issues.

Retreatment (Enhancement) After LASIK and Photorefractive Keratectomy

The incidence of retreatment after LASIK or PRK has decreased steadily over the years, and recent studies quote retreatment rates as less than 5% overall, with equivalent rates for LASIK and PRK. Patients with hyperopia or high astigmatism have a higher likelihood of requiring retreatment than patients with myopia.

Reported enhancement rates among publications and refractive surgery centers differ, based on specific criteria for retreatment. Discrepancy also exists in the literature regarding enhancement rates for patients selecting monovision, but these individuals may be more sensitive to smaller degrees of ametropia in their distance eye and therefore have a higher retreatment rate. Long-term follow-up studies have demonstrated good stability over time, without increasing late retreatment rates.

Treatment options depend on the timing of retreatment, corneal anatomy, and risk profiles. Flap lift is commonly performed early in the postoperative course, but it is not advisable after many years. In between, there are differing opinions as to when it is still safe to relift a flap. Some surgeons recommend no flap relift after 1 year, whereas others regard flap relift as an option up to 5 years. Recent reports have found that the risk of epithelial ingrowth increases significantly (but remains low) at 3 years after LASIK.

Residual stromal bed thickness must be adequate and should be determined prior to flap lift. This can be accomplished through direct measurements with OCT or confocal microscopy or from old records (if the flap was directly measured at the time of initial surgery). It is not appropriate to rely on corneal thickness measurements obtained at the time of retreatment only, as epithelial hypertrophy may unduly affect these measurements and result in an artificially thick estimated RSB.

Photorefractive keratectomy on top of the flap is a reasonable approach at any time point. However, patients with previous LASIK should be counseled about the prolonged healing process, which may be longer and more variable than for primary PRK treatments. Early data suggest that PRK after LASIK may not be as accurate as after primary PRK. Further, the risk of infection is significantly higher for PRK than LASIK retreatment. Postoperative haze was once considered a contraindication to PRK after LASIK, but this appears to be minimal due to modern laser platforms and the adjuvant use of mitomycin C for appropriate cases.

Microkeratome flap recut is not a viable retreatment option, as significant irregular astigmatism or scarring may result in the interface between the 2 flaps with an intermediary sliver of stromal tissue, which may be lost during retreatment. Currently, new flap creation with a femtosecond laser is not encouraged; however, with more advances in corneal measurements and flap creation precision, this may become an option in the future. Some surgeons have advocated making a new femtosecond laser side cut only and lifting the original flap with a new edge; however, these results are mixed, and this technique requires a sufficiently large initial flap to contain the entire second treatment under the new, smaller flap edge.

For all patients undergoing retreatment, early ectasia or other reasons for ametropia must be ruled out, including cataract development. Careful evaluation of corneal topography is necessary, as "normal" postoperative topographic patterns are different from preoperative patterns, with central flattening and concomitant thinning after myopic LASIK and central steepening without concomitant thinning in hyperopic LASIK. Patterns exhibiting steepening with corresponding thinning are of concern, and comparison with preoperative topographies is essential to determine actual focal corneal shape changes in these eyes.

Bibliography

Avila M, Li Y, Song JC, Huang D. High-speed optical coherence tomography for management after laser in situ keratomileusis. *J Cataract Refract Surg.* 2006;32(11):1836-1842.

Braun EH, Lee J, Steinert RF. Monovision in LASIK. *Ophthalmology.* 2008;115(7):1196-1202.

Davis EA, Hardten DR, Lindstrom M, Samuelson TW, Lindstrom RL. Lasik enhancements: a comparison of lifting to recutting the flap. *Ophthalmology.* 2002;109(12):2308-2313.

Hersh PS, Fry KL, Bishop DS. Incidence and associations of retreatment after LASIK. *Ophthalmology.* 2003;110(4):748-754.

Jin GJ, Merkley KH. Retreatment after wavefront-guided and standard myopic LASIK. *Ophthalmology.* 2006;113(9):1623-1628.

Randleman JB, Hewitt SM, Lynn MJ, Thompson KP, Stulting RD. A comparison of 2 methods for estimating residual stromal bed thickness before repeat LASIK. *Ophthalmology.* 2005;112(1):98-103.

Randleman JB, White AJ, Jr., Lynn MJ, Hu MH, Stulting RD. Incidence, outcomes, and risk factors for retreatment after wavefront-optimized ablations with PRK and LASIK. *J Refract Surg.* 2009;25(3):273-276.

Rubinfeld RS, Hardten DR, Donnenfeld ED, et al. To lift or recut: changing trends in LASIK enhancement. *J Cataract Refract Surg.* 2003;29(12):2306-2317.

Santhiago MR, Smadja D, Zaleski K, Espana EM, Armstrong BK, Wilson SE. Flap relift for retreatment after femtosecond laser-assisted LASIK. *J Refract Surg.* 2012;28(7):482-487.

Steinert RF, Fynn-Thompson N. Relationship between preoperative aberrations and postoperative refractive error in enhancement of previous laser in situ keratomileusis with the LADARVision system. *J Cataract Refract Surg.* 2008;34(8):1267-1272.

—CASE 20—

A 48-year-old female complains of blurred vision bilaterally at 6 months after photorefractive keratectomy (PRK). At the time of initial surgery, manifest and cycloplegic refractions were equal at -10.50 diopters (D) in the right eye and -9.50 +0.50 x 165 in the left eye. The laser was set to treat -9.50 D sphere in the right eye and -8.50 +0.50 x 165 in the left eye, for a target of plano for both eyes. The patient desires further refractive surgical correction, if possible.

CASE HISTORY		
	Right Eye	**Left Eye**
UDVA	20/60	20/50
Manifest refraction	+2.00 +0.50 x 080	+1.25 sphere
CDVA (current)	20/20	20/20
Cycloplegic refraction	+2.00 +0.50 x 080	+1.25 sphere
Cycloplegic CDVA	20/20	20/20
Keratometry		
Flat K	38.00 @ 180	39.00 @ 180
Steep K	38.25 @ 90	39.50 @ 90
Central corneal thickness	450 µm	455 µm
Physical examination	Normal	Normal
Estimated ablation depth	30 µm	30 µm

QUESTIONS

1. Is this patient a candidate for refractive surgery retreatment? If so, what treatment options are available?
2. Considering all factors, what procedure would you recommend and why?
3. What would you program the laser to treat, assuming the patient still desires full distance correction bilaterally?
4. What changes could you make to prevent this outcome after initial treatment?

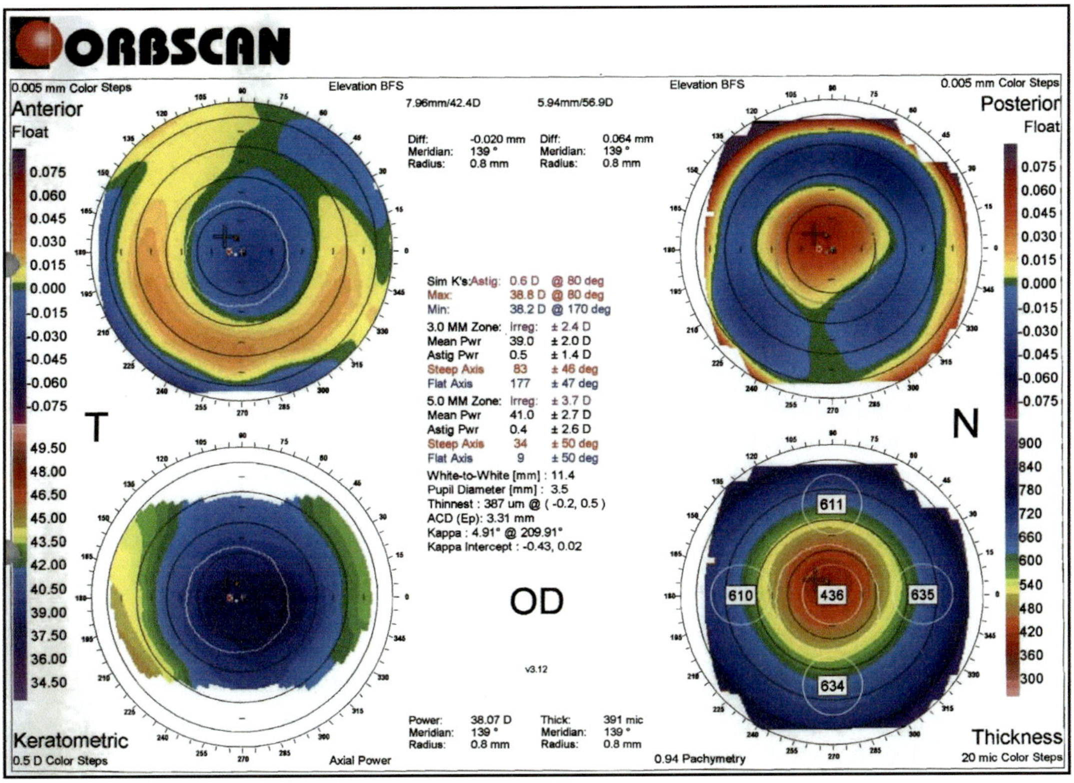
ORBSCAN
0.005 mm Color Steps
Anterior
Float
Elevation BFS
7.96mm/42.4D
5.94mm/56.9D
Elevation BFS
0.005 mm Color Steps
Posterior
Float
Diff: -0.020 mm
Meridian: 139 °
Radius: 0.8 mm
Diff: 0.064 mm
Meridian: 139 °
Radius: 0.8 mm
Sim K's:Astig: 0.6 D @ 80 deg
Max: 38.8 D @ 80 deg
Min: 38.2 D @ 170 deg
3.0 MM Zone: Irreg: ± 2.4 D
Mean Pwr 39.0 ± 2.0 D
Astig Pwr 0.5 ± 1.4 D
Steep Axis 83 ± 46 deg
Flat Axis 177 ± 47 deg
5.0 MM Zone: Irreg: ± 3.7 D
Mean Pwr 41.0 ± 2.7 D
Astig Pwr 0.4 ± 2.6 D
Steep Axis 34 ± 50 deg
Flat Axis 9 ± 50 deg
White-to-White [mm] : 11.4
Pupil Diameter [mm] : 3.5
Thinnest : 387 um @ (-0.2, 0.5)
ACD (Ep): 3.31 mm
Kappa : 4.91° @ 209.91°
Kappa Intercept : -0.43, 0.02
T
N
OD
v3.12
611
610
436
635
634
Power: 38.07 D
Meridian: 139 °
Radius: 0.8 mm
Thick: 391 mic
Meridian: 139 °
Radius: 0.8 mm
Keratometric
0.5 D Color Steps
Axial Power
0.94 Pachymetry
Thickness
20 mic Color Steps

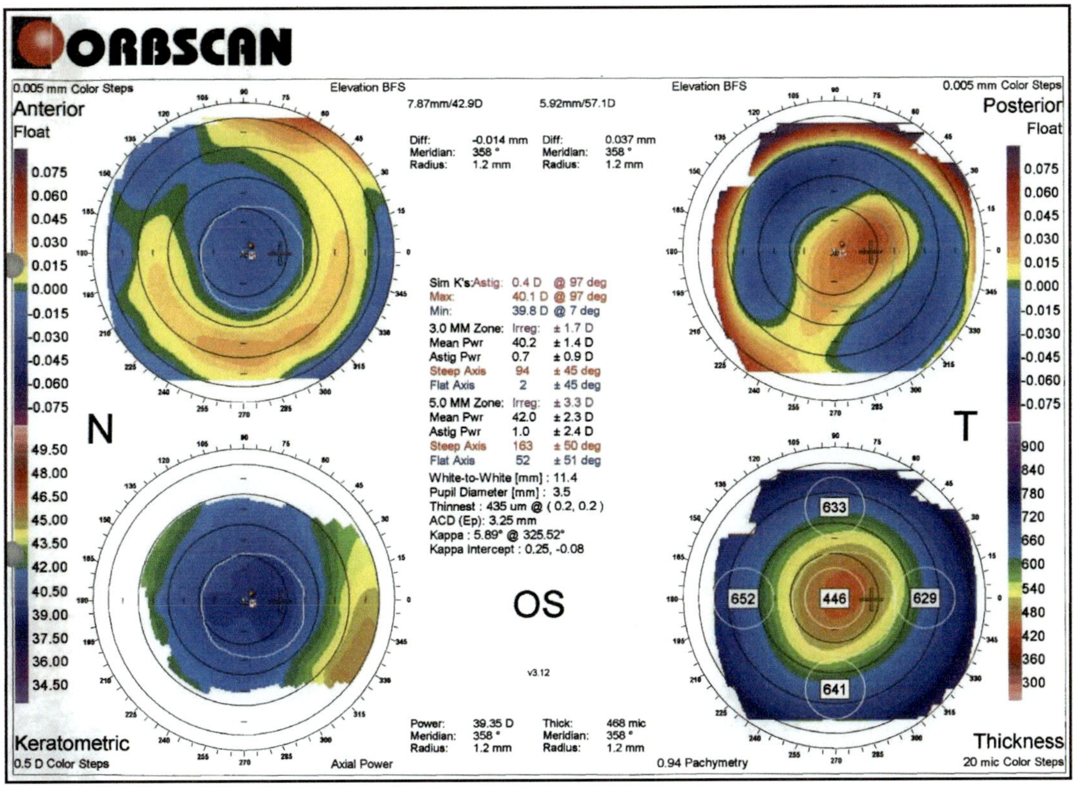
ORBSCAN
0.005 mm Color Steps
Anterior
Float
Elevation BFS
7.87mm/42.9D
5.92mm/57.1D
Elevation BFS
0.005 mm Color Steps
Posterior
Float
Diff: -0.014 mm
Meridian: 358 °
Radius: 1.2 mm
Diff: 0.037 mm
Meridian: 358 °
Radius: 1.2 mm
Sim K's:Astig: 0.4 D @ 97 deg
Max: 40.1 D @ 97 deg
Min: 39.8 D @ 7 deg
3.0 MM Zone: Irreg: ± 1.7 D
Mean Pwr 40.2 ± 1.4 D
Astig Pwr 0.7 ± 0.9 D
Steep Axis 94 ± 45 deg
Flat Axis 2 ± 45 deg
5.0 MM Zone: Irreg: ± 3.3 D
Mean Pwr 42.0 ± 2.3 D
Astig Pwr 1.0 ± 2.4 D
Steep Axis 163 ± 50 deg
Flat Axis 52 ± 51 deg
White-to-White [mm] : 11.4
Pupil Diameter [mm] : 3.5
Thinnest : 435 um @ (0.2, 0.2)
ACD (Ep): 3.25 mm
Kappa : 5.89° @ 325.52°
Kappa Intercept : 0.25, -0.08
N
T
OS
v3.12
633
652
446
629
641
Power: 39.35 D
Meridian: 358 °
Radius: 1.2 mm
Thick: 468 mic
Meridian: 358 °
Radius: 1.2 mm
Keratometric
0.5 D Color Steps
Axial Power
0.94 Pachymetry
Thickness
20 mic Color Steps

—Case 20—

Overcorrection After Laser Vision Correction

Undercorrection, resulting in residual refractive error (eg, myopia after initial myopic treatment), or overcorrection, resulting in induced or consecutive refractive error (eg, hyperopia after initial myopic treatment), is possible after LASIK and surface ablation procedures. These variations from target usually result from variation in patient response to laser ablation. Retreatment is possible after both LASIK and surface ablation procedures, but the type of refractive error (residual or induced) should be recognized, and other patient factors, such as age and refractive target, should be taken into account when planning retreatment, especially for overcorrections.

Case Analysis

- The current estimated residual stromal bed (RSB) thickness is >400 μm in both eyes.
- Post-retreatment RSB thickness (PRK) is >400 μm in both eyes.
- Post-retreatment RSB thickness (LASIK) is approximately 330 μm in both eyes.
- Case Figures show normal topographic patterns after myopic laser vision correction, with central flattening and thinning.

Pearl: *When retreating an overcorrected patient, consider reducing the planned ablation by 10% to prevent repeat overcorrection!*

Questions

1. Is this patient a candidate for refractive surgery retreatment? If so, what treatment options are available?

   Yes, this patient is a candidate for retreatment when she has a stable refraction. She is theoretically a candidate for PRK or LASIK retreatment.

2. Considering all factors, what procedure would you recommend and why?

   Because the patient had PRK initially, she is a candidate for PRK retreatment, and that would be my first choice. LASIK is an option, and RSB thickness would be well above 300 μm (indicating she had thick corneas before the initial treatment). However, before considering LASIK, it would be imperative to review her preoperative topographies to determine what, if any, screening issues led the initial surgeon to choose PRK as the primary treatment.

3. What would you program the laser to treat, assuming the patient still desires full distance correction bilaterally?

   This patient was overcorrected, so one can assume that she is an "over responder" to laser ablation. Therefore, the laser should be programmed to reduce the chance for another overcorrection. Many surgeons reduce the planned ablation by 10% when treating overcorrections. However, because this patient is 48 years old, she will most likely tolerate a small amount of myopia rather than hyperopia, so minimal adjustments to the treatment refraction are best.

4. What changes could you make to prevent this type of issue after initial treatment?

   This patient was a high myope who had PRK treatment. Each surgeon should evaluate his or her own outcomes and determine whether nomogram adjustments are needed to maximize outcomes, especially for higher treatments.

Retreatment for Overcorrection After Laser Vision Correction

Although the overall process of retreatment does not differ significantly between residual and consecutive refractive errors, there are additional factors to consider for overcorrections. First, a different ablation pattern will be applied to the cornea, either hyperopic (peripheral) ablation after initial (central) myopic ablation or vice versa. This is usually only of major concern for initial high hyperopic ablations because significant irregular astigmatism can result if the optical zone is displaced or irregular. Second, a variety of factors can result in overcorrection, including the variability of patient response to the excimer laser (most common), laser calibration issues, variable stromal bed dehydration due to varying surgical time from case to case, or the need for nomogram adjustments by the surgeon. Each of these factors must be evaluated to determine the mechanism of initial overcorrection and to plan appropriately for retreatment.

Many surgeons reduce the planned retreatment ablation by 10% for patients with an initial overcorrection; however, patient factors, such as age and refractive target goals, should be considered. In young patients, small levels of hyperopia are well tolerated, whereas in patients over 40 years old, small amounts of myopia are better tolerated in one or both eyes. If the patient desires monovision, he or she is likely to be more tolerant of myopia in the near eye, less tolerant of myopia in the distance eye, and less tolerant of significant anisometropia.

The use of mitomycin C (MMC) has minimized variability in refractive outcomes after PRK; however, higher surface ablations are still more prone to overcorrection than with LASIK. Repeat PRK is more prone to corneal haze, and MMC should be considered for retreatment, even if it was not used initially.

Finally, overcorrections do occur, and this should not stimulate panic in surgeons. However, closely monitoring one's refractive outcomes and making necessary nomogram adjustments, as well as standardizing one's surgical technique and time, will minimize these occurrences.

Bibliography

Alió JL, Muftuoglu O, Ortiz D, et al. Ten-year follow-up of photorefractive keratectomy for myopia of more than -6 diopters. *Am J Ophthalmol.* 2008;145(1):37-45.

Alió JL, Muftuoglu O, Ortiz D, et al. Ten-year follow-up of laser in situ keratomileusis for myopia of up to -10 diopters. *Am J Ophthalmol.* 2008;145(1):46-54.

Biebesheimer JB, Kang TS, Huang CY, Yu F, Hamilton DR. Development of an advanced nomogram for myopic astigmatic wavefront-guided laser in situ keratomileusis (LASIK). Ophthalmic Surg Lasers Imaging. 2011;42(3):241-247.

Chang JS, Lau SY. Conductive keratoplasty to treat hyperopic overcorrection after LASIK for myopia. *J Refract Surg.* 2011;27(1):49-55.

Ditzen K, Handzel A, Pieger S. Laser in situ keratomileusis nomogram development. *J Refract Surg.* 1999;15(2 Suppl):S197-S201.

Jabbur NS, Sakatani K, O'Brien TP. Survey of complications and recommendations for management in dissatisfied patients seeking a consultation after refractive surgery. *J Cataract Refract Surg.* 2004;30(9):1867-1874.

Lapid-Gortzak R, van der Linden JW, van der Meulen IJ, Nieuwendaal CP. Advanced personalized nomogram for myopic laser surgery: first 100 eyes. *J Cataract Refract Surg.* 2008;34(11):1881-1885.

Leccisotti A. Mitomycin C in photorefractive keratectomy: effect on epithelialization and predictability. *Cornea.* 2008;27(3):288-291.

Netto MV, Mohan RR, Ambrósio R Jr, Hutcheon AE, Zieske JD, Wilson SE. Wound healing in the cornea: a review of refractive surgery complications and new prospects for therapy. *Cornea.* 2005;24(5):509-522.

Rojas MC, Haw WW, Manche EE. Laser in situ keratomileusis enhancement for consecutive hyperopia after myopic overcorrection. *J Cataract Refract Surg.* 2002;28(1):37-43.

Taneri S, Zieske JD, Azar DT. Evolution, techniques, clinical outcomes, and pathophysiology of LASEK: review of the literature. *Surv Ophthalmol.* 2004;49(6):576-602.

—Case 21—

A 30-year-old male presents with complaints of blurred vision after LASIK 9 weeks earlier. At the time of the initial surgery, manifest and cycloplegic refractions were equal at -3.25 +1.00 x 060 in the right eye and -3.00 +0.50 x 115 in the left eye. The laser was set to treat -3.25 +1.00 x 060 in the right eye and -3.00 +0.50 x 115 in the left eye, for a target of plano for both eyes.

Case History		
	Right Eye	**Left Eye**
UDVA	20/50	20/40
UNVA	20/20	20/20
Manifest refraction	-1.00 sphere	-0.75 sphere
Manifest CDVA	20/20	20/20
Cycloplegic refraction	Plano	Plano
Cycloplegic CDVA	20/15	20/20
Central corneal thickness	466 µm	469 µm
Physical examination	Normal	Normal
Estimated ablation depth	15 µm	15 µm

Questions

1. Is this patient a candidate for refractive surgery retreatment? If so, what treatment options are available?
2. What additional testing may be useful to help determine your course of action?
3. Considering all factors, what procedure would you recommend and why?
4. What are the most likely causes for this refractive error at this time point after LASIK?
5. What would you program the laser to treat, assuming the patient still desires full distance correction bilaterally?

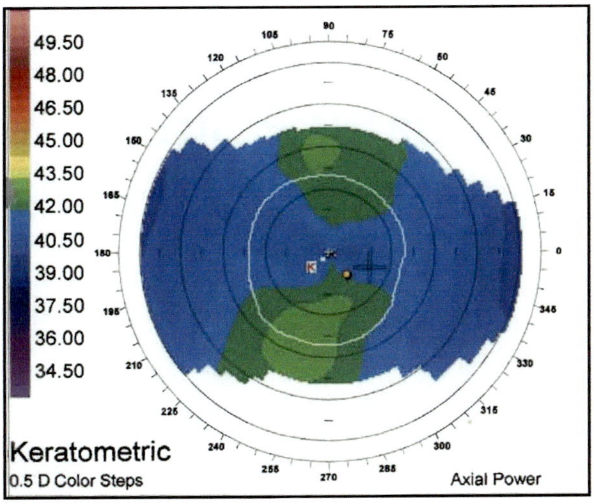
49.50
48.00
46.50
45.00
43.50
42.00
40.50
39.00
37.50
36.00
34.50
Keratometric
0.5 D Color Steps
Axial Power

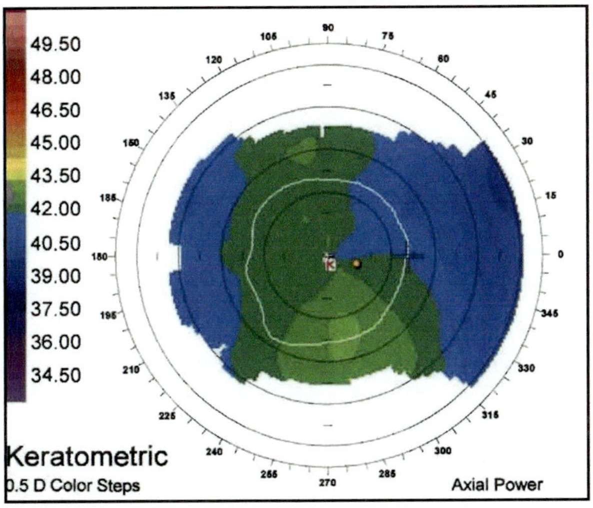
49.50
48.00
46.50
45.00
43.50
42.00
40.50
39.00
37.50
36.00
34.50
Keratometric
0.5 D Color Steps
Axial Power

—Case 21—
Accommodative Spasm After Laser Vision Correction

Accommodative spasm is an infrequent occurrence after laser vision correction, but it most commonly presents as apparent residual myopia, usually in younger patients, after an otherwise successful surgery.

Case Analysis

- Case Figures show normal topographic patterns after myopic LASIK, with central flattening and thinning.

Pearl: *Accommodative spasm occurs infrequently but is more common than reported—cycloplegics may be needed therapeutically and ALL patients need a cycloplegic refraction prior to considering retreatment!*

Questions

1. Is this patient a candidate for refractive surgery retreatment? If so, what treatment options are available?

   No, this patient is not a candidate for retreatment. Based on the cycloplegic refraction, this patient has accommodative spasm, not residual refractive error. Laser retreatment would not be beneficial and would ultimately lead to overcorrection when the spasm resolves.

2. What additional testing may be useful to help determine your course of action?

   The diagnosis is made by cycloplegic refraction. However, a prolonged trial of topical cycloplegic drops can help in less definitive cases.

3. Considering all factors, what procedure would you recommend and why?

   I would recommend that the patient perform distance-viewing exercises, such as looking out the window or taking breaks from reading or from viewing a computer screen, on a scheduled basis throughout the day. For persistent cases, topical cycloplegic drops taken for a short course will be effective.

4. What would you program the laser to treat, assuming the patient still desires full distance correction bilaterally?

   None! Do not retreat at the current time!

Accommodative Spasm After Laser Vision Correction

A rare, or at least an uncommonly reported phenomenon, accommodative spasm can present as residual or consecutive myopia after refractive surgery. The mechanism for this is unclear. Most reports of accommodative spasm in the literature occur in the setting of head trauma, systemic diseases, or as a side effect from certain medication use. However, none of these are frequent mechanisms for accommodative spasm after laser vision correction. Patients occasionally report headaches, in addition to blurred distance vision. The condition is generally benign and reverses over time, but it must be ruled out prior to performing surgical retreatment. Cycloplegic refraction is necessary for all primary procedures and retreatments.

In many cases, the situation will resolve spontaneously or with simple eye exercises to force distance viewing and to take breaks from near tasks. In some instances, a course of topical cycloplegic drops are necessary to reverse the spasm. Cyclopentolate is usually preferred due to its shorter duration of action. When used, these drops should be tapered so as not to induce spasm when discontinued.

Bibliography

Airiani S, Braunstein RE. Accommodative spasm after laser-assisted in situ keratomileusis (LASIK). *Am J Ophthalmol.* 2006;141(6):1163-1164.

Kanda H, Kobayashi M, Mihashi T, Morimoto T, Nishida K, Fujikado T. Serial measurements of accommodation by open-field Hartmann-Shack wavefront aberrometer in eyes with accommodative spasm. *Jpn J Ophthalmol.* 2012;56(6):617-263.

Ninomiya S, Fujikado T, Kuroda T, et al. Wavefront analysis in eyes with accommodative spasm. *Am J Ophthalmol.* 2003;136(6):1161-1163.

Prakash G, Sharma N, Sharma P, Choudhary V, Titiyal JS. Accommodative spasm after laser-assisted in situ keratomileusis (LASIK). *Am J Ophthalmol.* 2007;143(3):540; author reply 540-541.

Rutstein RP, Daum KM, Amos JF. Accommodative spasm: a study of 17 cases. *J Am Optom Assoc.* 1988;59(7):527-538.

—Case 22—

A 41-year-old female complains of extreme glare and poor night vision 4 months after bilateral photorefractive keratectomy (PRK). Her preoperative prescription was approximately -8.75 diopters (D) in both eyes. Surgery was performed using the VISX Star S3 laser (Abbott Medical Optics), with a conventional ablation profile and application of mitomycin C for 12 seconds. She states that her night vision has improved somewhat since surgery, but she is still highly symptomatic and is seeking options for treatment.

CASE HISTORY		
	Right Eye	**Left Eye**
UDVA	20/40	20/25
Manifest refraction	-0.50 +1.00 x 082	-0.25 +0.75 x 074
CDVA (current)	20/20	20/20
CNVA (current)	20/20	20/20
Dominant eye	Right	
Keratometry		
Flat K	37.50 @ 030	37.00 @ 070
Steep K	37.75 @ 120	37.5 @ 160
Pupil size (bright)	4.8 mm	4.5 mm
Pupil size (dim)	7.0 mm	7.1 mm
Central corneal thickness	390 μm	379 μm
Physical examination	Normal	Normal
Estimated ablation depth	15 μm	10 μm

Questions

1. What factors likely contribute to this patient's complaints?
2. What further testing may help to identify primary causes for these complaints?
3. What treatment options are available for this patient?
4. Is this patient a candidate for refractive surgery retreatment to ameliorate her symptoms?
5. Considering all factors, what would you recommend and why?

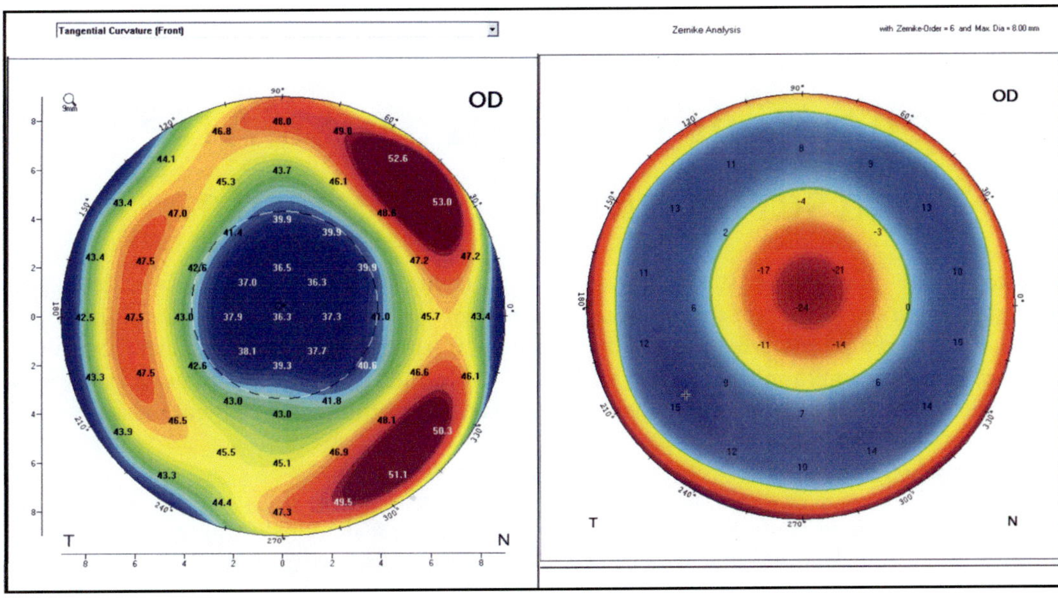
Tangential Curvature (Front)
Zernike Analysis
with Zernike-Order = 6 and Max. Dia = 8.00 mm
OD
T
N
OD
T
N

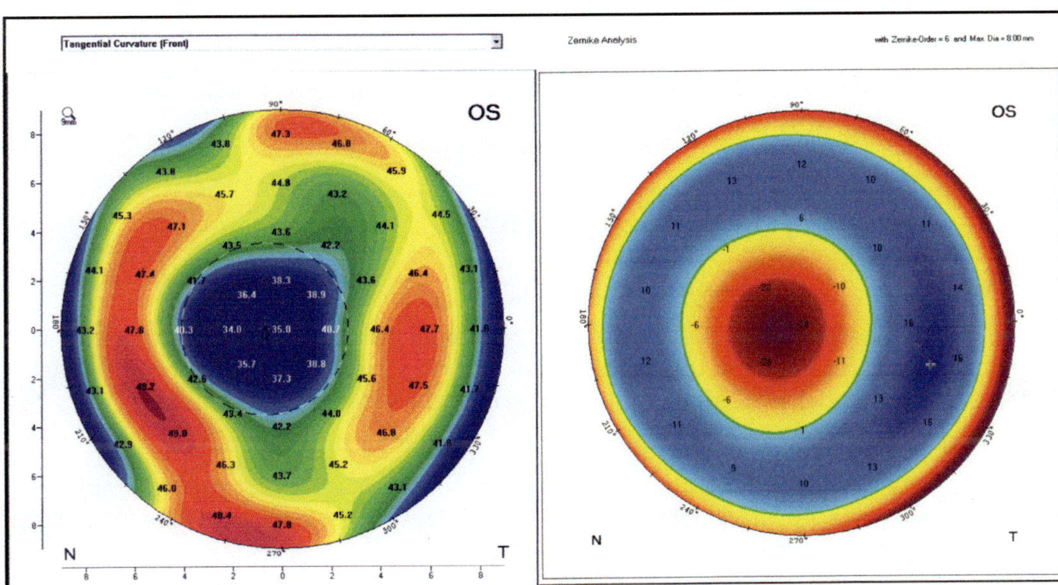
Tangential Curvature (Front)
Zernike Analysis
with Zernike-Order = 6 and Max. Dia = 8.00 mm
OS
N
T
OS
N
T

—Case 22—

Night Vision Complaints After Laser Vision Correction

Postoperative glare, halos, starbursts, and night driving problems, generically called *night vision complaints* (NVC), affect a small number of patients and are likely multifactorial in origin. Although these symptoms are occasionally caused by intrinsic issues from excimer laser ablation, they are more commonly associated with identifiable and treatable conditions. A systematic approach to evaluation will direct management and maximally optimize the patient's visual acuity.

Case Analysis

- Case Figures show postoperative topography (left images) demonstrating a focal ablation with an abrupt drop-off that is common for a conventional ablation with no blend zone. Significantly positive postoperative higher-order aberrations (HOAs; right images) are seen in both eyes outside the treatment zone.

Pearl: *Night vision complaints have not been correlated with pupil size; however, small optical zones without peripheral ablations increase the risk of NVC!*

Questions

1. What factors likely contribute to this patient's complaints?

   The reasons for NVC 4 months after PRK could include residual refractive error, dry eye, corneal haze, or induced NVC from excimer laser treatment of high myopia with a conventional ablation profile, a small optical zone, and no blend zone.

2. What further testing may help identify primary causes for these complaints?

   Dry eye testing, including Schirmer's test, tear break-up time, corneal staining with vital dyes, cycloplegic refraction, and careful evaluation for corneal haze may help to identify the causes for the patient's complaints.

3. What treatment options are available for this patient?

   The treatment options include medical treatment for ocular surface disease (if present or suspected), prescribing a temporary trial of spectacles use, eventual treatment of corneal haze (if present), and/or topical brimonidine drops to use at dusk.

4. Is this patient a candidate for refractive surgery retreatment to ameliorate her symptoms?

   At 3 months after high myopic PRK treatment, it is too early to consider retreatment. When the patient is stable, if residual refractive error is the most bothersome symptom, further wavefront-optimized or wavefront-guided ablation therapy may be warranted. If it is warranted, the patient's optical zone could potentially be enlarged with topography-guided ablation (as an off label treatment in the United States).

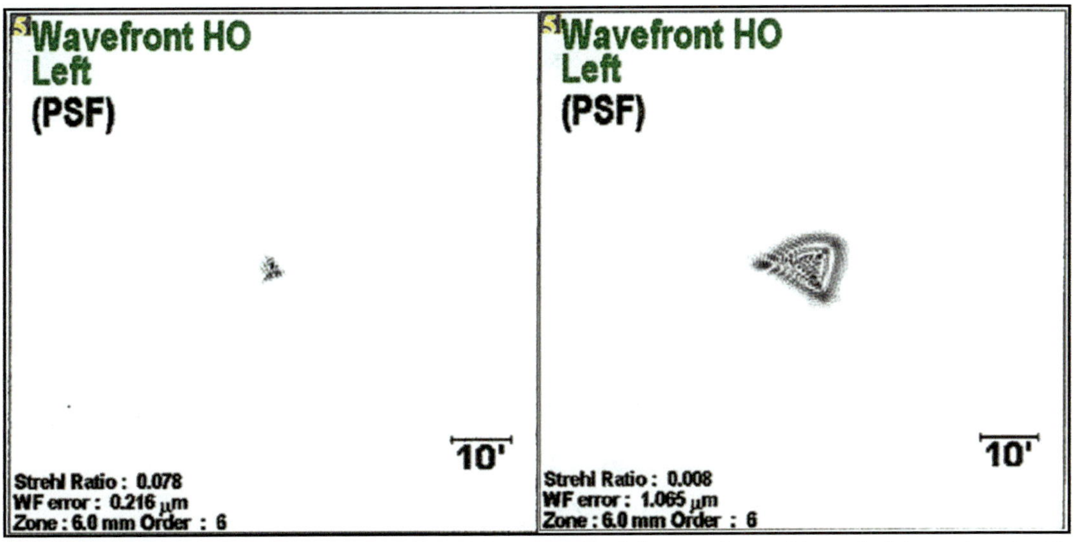

Case Figure 22-1. Postoperative point spread function (PSF) for a patient without (left image) and with (right image) NVC. The PSF approximates how an individual might perceive light emanating from a single point source; the larger the PSF, the greater the potential NVC.

5. Considering all factors, what procedure would you recommend and why?

   Assuming there is no significant ocular surface disease, I would prescribe trial spectacles for both diagnostic and therapeutic reasons, and include a trial of brimonidine if symptoms persist with use of spectacles. Most NVC symptoms improve over time, either due to actual improvement or neural adaptation. The symptoms may not resolve, but they should not worsen over time. As discussed, eventual retreatment is possible of residual ametropia is impacting NVC

Night Vision Complaints After Laser Vision Correction

As discussed in Case 8, NVC are rare, but potentially highly symptomatic, even after an otherwise uneventful laser vision correction (LVC). The cause may be multifactorial and may include residual ametropia, ocular surface dysfunction, corneal haze, irregular ablations (small optical zones, decentered ablations, central islands), or intrinsic issues related to excimer laser ablation. Case Figure 22-1 shows the postoperative point spread function (PSF), which approximates how an individual might perceive light emanating from a point source, in a patient with and without NVC.

Prevention of Night Vision Complaints

Patients should be counseled about the possibility of NVC prior to all LVC; however, patients at higher risk, including those with larger myopic refractive errors and patients with preoperative night vision symptoms, warrant additional discussion and planning.

Conventional ablations induce more HOAs than wavefront-guided or wavefront-optimized treatments and increase the likelihood of NVC. Conventional ablation should be avoided when possible, especially in patients with higher refractive errors. If insufficient corneal tissue is

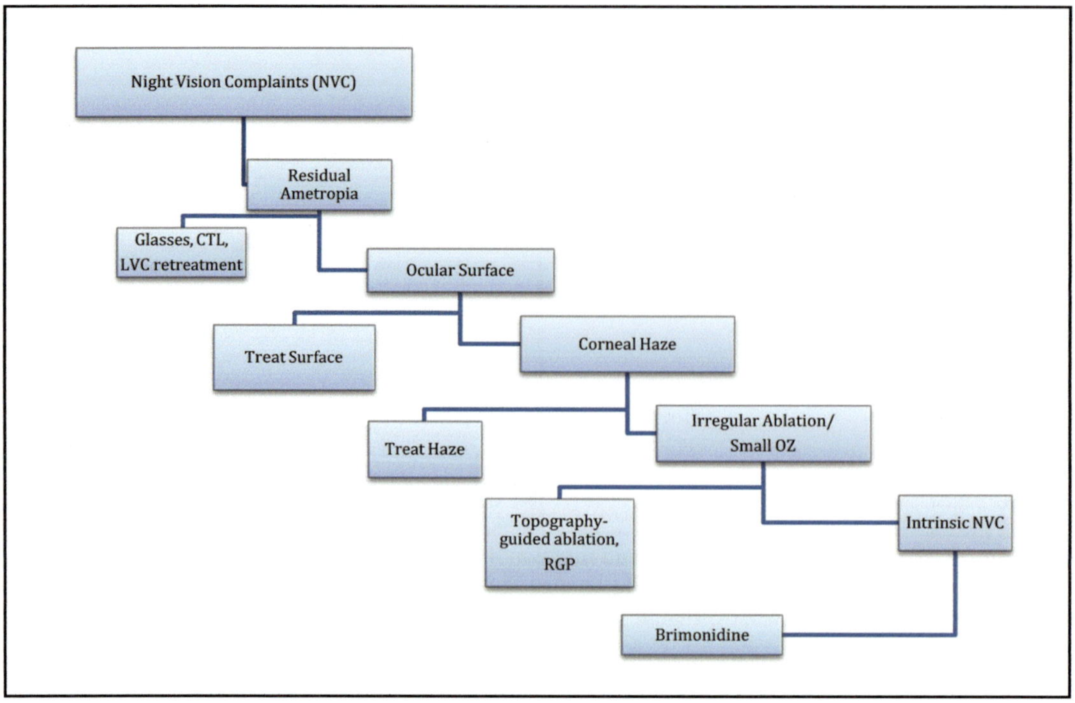

Case Figure 22-2. Decision tree for NVC diagnosis and management after LVC.

available to safely perform LVC, phakic intraocular lens implantation should be considered. Small optical zones increase the risk of NVC in all eyes and should be avoided as well.

Management of Night Vision Complaints

Case Figure 22-2 demonstrates a step-wise approach to NVC diagnosis and management. Straightforward issues should be addressed first, including residual refractive error and ocular surface dysfunction, as these are the most likely findings and causes for patient dissatisfaction after LVC. Topography-guided ablations have shown promise in enlarging smaller optical zones and improving centration for decentered ablations. Although large pupils have not been directly correlated with NVC, reducing scotopic pupil size through constriction (with miotics, such as pilocarpine) or preventing dilation (with alpha agonists, such as brimonidine) can be effective in minimizing symptoms. For intractable cases, rigid gas permeable contact lens wear may improve symptoms.

Bibliography

Chen X, Stojanovic A, Zhou W, Utheim TP, Stojanovic F, Wang Q. Transepithelial, topography-guided ablation in the treatment of visual disturbances in LASIK flap or interface complications. *J Refract Surg.* 2012;28(2):120-126.

Edwards JD, Burka JM, Bower KS, Stutzman RD, Sediq DA, Rabin JC. Effect of brimonidine tartrate 0.15% on night-vision difficulty and contrast testing after refractive surgery. *J Cataract Refract Surg.* 2008;34(9):1538-1541.

Jabbur NS, Sakatani K, O'Brien TP. Survey of complications and recommendations for management in dissatisfied patients seeking a consultation after refractive surgery. *J Cataract Refract Surg.* 2004;30(9):1867-1874.

Lee JH, You YS, Choe CM, Lee ES. Efficacy of brimonidine tartrate 0.2% ophthalmic solution in reducing halos after laser in situ keratomileusis. *J Cataract Refract Surg.* 2008;34(6):963-967.

Levinson BA, Rapuano CJ, Cohen EJ, Hammersmith KM, Ayres BD, Laibson PR. Referrals to the Wills Eye Institute Cornea Service after laser in situ keratomileusis: reasons for patient dissatisfaction. *J Cataract Refract Surg.* 2008;34(1):32-39.

Pasquali T, Krueger R. Topography-guided laser refractive surgery. *Curr Opin Ophthalmol.* 2012;23(4):264-268.

Perez-Straziota CE, Randleman JB, Stulting RD. Visual acuity and higher-order aberrations with wavefront-guided and wavefront-optimized laser in situ keratomileusis. *J Cataract and Refract Surg.* 2010;36(3):437-441.

Randleman JB, Hu MH, Loft ES, Perez-Straziota CE, White AJ, Stulting RD. High order aberrations after wavefront-optimized advanced surface ablation and laser in situ keratomileusis. *J Cataract Refract Surg.* 2009;35(2):260-264.

Tan G, Chen X, Xie RZ, et al. Reverse geometry rigid gas permeable contact lens wear reduces high-order aberrations and the associated symptoms in post-LASIK patients. *Curr Eye Res.* 2010;35(1):9-16.

Tan J, Simon D, Mrochen M, Por YM. Clinical results of topography-based customized ablations for myopia and myopic astigmatism. *J Refract Surg.* 2012;28(11):S829-S836.

—Case 23—

A 34-year-old female presents on day 1 after bilateral myopic LASIK for manifest refraction of -7.50 +1.50 x 090 in the right eye and -8.75 +1.00 x 090 in the left eye. She is generally happy with her vision but notes some fogginess and blur in the left eye more than the right. She also has mild foreign body sensation in both eyes.

Current medications: Topical antibiotic and topical steroid four times daily in both eyes, frequent artificial tear use.

Case History		
	Right Eye	**Left Eye**
UDVA	20/30	20/40
Manifest refraction	Plano	Plano
CDVA	20/30	20/40
Physical examination	Normal	See Figure

Questions

1. Given the patient's presentation and clinical appearance, what is the most likely diagnosis?
2. What elements of the case (findings, symptoms, etc) are most important in helping you to differentiate between the possible etiologies of this patient's symptoms?
3. What is the best course of action at this juncture for this patient?
4. What is the next intervention if your initial treatment plan is not successful?
5. What is the primary concern for this patient if she is not treated appropriately?

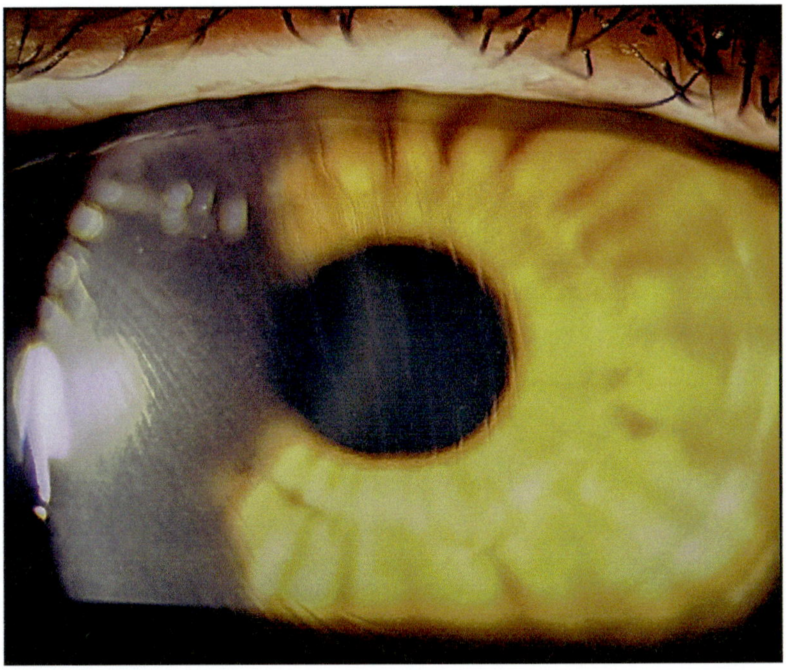

—CASE 23—
Flap Stria

Flap stria is the most common abnormal finding on the first postoperative day, which requires flap repositioning (refloat) in up to 1% of cases. Striae can be microstriae, which do not require intervention, or macrostriae from partial flap slippage, which do require repositioning to maximize visual outcomes. The timing of intervention may dictate success with simple repositioning versus more invasive techniques to eradicate striae.

Case Analysis

- Case Figure shows a slit-lamp image of the left eye depicting flap striae. The striae are oriented vertically and appear to emanate from the nasal region of the cornea, which corresponds to the hinge location.

Pearl: *Flap striae will NOT appear resolved immediately after flap lift; in fact, they will likely appear worse!*

QUESTIONS

1. Given the patient's presentation and clinical appearance, what is the most likely diagnosis?

   Flap striae.

2. What elements of the case (findings, symptoms, etc) are most important in helping you to differentiate between the possible etiologies of this patient's symptoms?

   The patient's symptoms and visual acuity are the most important elements to consider when evaluating striae. Mild blurred vision is expected on postoperative day 1. Significant striae will distort visual acuity and usually cause some degree of foreign body sensation or discomfort as a result of the flap not being in the correct position, with resultant exposed stromal bed.

3. What is the best course of action at this juncture for this patient?

   Given the patient's different acuity between eyes, mild symptoms, and flap appearance, it is best to reposition the left flap. This could be performed at the slit lamp, but positioning in the laser suite under the operating microscope is generally preferable when possible.

4. What is the next intervention if your initial treatment plan is not successful?

   If flap lift and repositioning is not successful in eradicating the flap striae, the patient may require flap suturing to place the striae under tension and ultimately smooth the flap.

5. What is the primary concern for this patient if she is not treated appropriately?

   Persistent macrostriae will reduce visual acuity and visual quality. Displaced flaps increase the risk of epithelial ingrowth if not repositioned. Further, if suboptimally treated, the striae will become increasingly difficult to eradicate and may require modified phototherapeutic keratectomy or concomitant epithelial removal with flap suturing at a later time to improve visual acuity.

Flap Striae: Observation Versus Intervention

The reported incidence is approximately 1%. Striae occur more often in older patients and patients with preoperative hyperopia and may be more common after flap creation with a mechanical microkeratome. Flap dislocations have also been associated with preoperative or intraoperative use of brimonidine, which is administered by some surgeons to decrease the incidence of subconjunctival hemorrhage from suction during LASIK flap creation.

Flap microstriae rarely impact visual acuity and can simply be observed. Flap macrostriae outside of the visual axis, without a demonstrable gutter between the flap edge and the flap bed, can also be observed without intervention. However, when flap striae appear visually significant or when a gutter exists, the flap should be repositioned to avoid long-term visual sequelae. Flaps may be repositioned with or without therapeutic bandage contact lens placement. Many surgeons use bandage contact lenses to facilitate flap stability for the first day after flap reposition, although this may increase the risk for epithelial ingrowth or infection.

When to Lift the Flap (Indications for Flap Lift/Reposition)

1. Visually significant macrostriae.
2. Striae that are accompanied with significant foreign body sensation.
3. Striae that are accompanied by a visible gutter at edge of flap.

When Not to Lift the Flap

Lifting the flap increases the likelihood of epithelial ingrowth, infection, and potential flap adherence problems and should not be done without a definitive indication. Flaps should not be lifted in the following situations:

1. There are no subjective complaints (vision or discomfort) and objective visual acuity is good.
2. Uncertainty exists as to the relationship between the flap appearance and visual complaints.
3. No visible gutter at the flap edge.

Patients with striae of undetermined significance should be closely monitored over the first postoperative week; if no resolution occurs, they should have flap lift with reposition.

Bibliography

Albelda-Vallés JC, Martin-Reyes C, Ramos F, Beltran J, Llovet F, Baviera J. Effect of preoperative keratometric power on intraoperative complications in LASIK in 34,099 eyes. *J Refract Surg.* 2007;23(6):592-597.

Clare G, Moore TC, Grills C, Leccisotti A, Moore JE, Schallhorn S. Early flap displacement after LASIK. *Ophthalmology.* 2011;118(9):1760-1765.

Davies JB, Randleman JB. Successful delayed surgical revision of a dislocated LASIK flap. *Ophthalmic Surg Lasers Imaging.* 2008;39(3):221-224.

Lin RT, Maloney RK. Flap complications associated with lamellar refractive surgery. *Am J Ophthalmol.* 1999;127(2):129-136.

Moshirfar M, Gardiner JP, Schliesser JA, et al. Laser in situ keratomileusis flap complications using mechanical microkeratome versus femtosecond laser: retrospective comparison. *J Cataract Refract Surg.* 2010;36(11):1925-1933.

Muñoz G, Albarrán-Diego C, Sakla HF, Javaloy J. Increased risk for flap dislocation with perioperative brimonidine use in femtosecond laser in situ keratomileusis. *J Cataract Refract Surg.* 2009;35(8):1338-1342.

Rodríguez-Galietero A, Martínez JV, Del Buey A, Bescós JA. Use of brimonidine before LASIK with femtosecond laser-created flaps for the correction of myopia: a contralateral eye study. *J Refract Surg.* 2010;26(1):28-32.

—Case 24—

A 34-year-old female presents on day 2 after bilateral myopic LASIK with increasing foreign body sensation in both eyes and blurred vision in the right eye. The patient had mild foreign body sensation on postoperative day 1, but it has worsened slightly.

Current medications: Topical antibiotic and a topical steroid 4 times daily in both eyes and frequent artificial tear use.

Case History		
	Right Eye	**Left Eye**
Present correction method	None	None
Manifest refraction	Plano	Plano
UCVA	$20/20^{-2}$	20/20
Physical examination	See Figure	Normal

Questions

1. Given the patient's presentation and clinical appearance, what is the most likely diagnosis?
2. What, if any, other conditions are in your differential diagnosis?
3. What elements of this case are most important in helping you to differentiate between the possible etiologies of this patient's symptoms?
4. What is the best course of treatment at this juncture for this patient's problem?
5. What is the next intervention if your first treatment is not successful?
6. What is the primary concern for this patient if she is not treated appropriately?

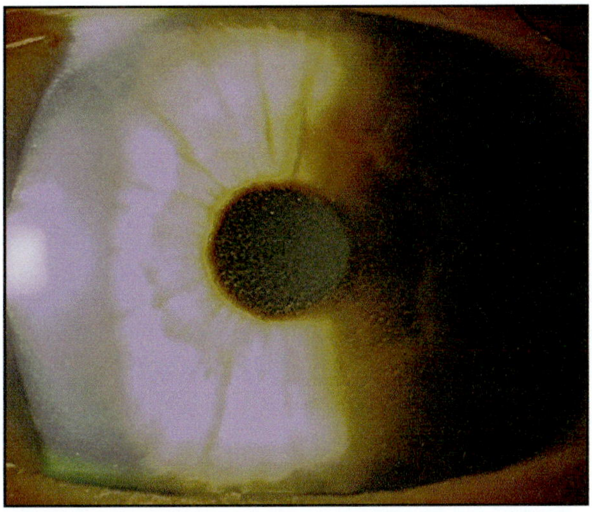

—Case 24—
Diffuse Lamellar Keratitis

Diffuse lamellar keratitis (DLK) is an idiopathic inflammatory response in the LASIK interface to a variety of stimuli, with a typical white blood cell build-up in the interface that coalesces as the condition advances. DLK typically presents in the first few days after LASIK, typically within the first 1 to 4 days, and usually is associated with increased foreign body sensation and subtle, diffuse, granular interface opacity but with minimal visual changes. If left untreated, DLK can increase in severity and progress to a dense, coalesced, focal scar with significant visual loss.

Case Analysis

- Case Figure shows a slit-lamp image demonstrating a fine, diffuse, granular opacity. Although the level cannot be determined by this image, the opacity is confined to the LASIK interface.

Pearl: *DLK is the most common symptomatic interface finding and must be managed aggressively and appropriately to prevent vision loss!*

Questions

1. Given the patient's presentation and clinical appearance, what is the most likely diagnosis?

   The most likely diagnosis is DLK, stage 2 to 3.

2. What, if any, other conditions are in your differential diagnosis?

   Infectious keratitis and benign interface debris are both possible differential diagnoses. The patient's presentation is not central toxic keratopathy (CTK), and it is too early postoperatively for pressure-induced stromal keratopathy (PISK) to have developed.

3. What elements of this case are most important in helping you to differentiate between the possible etiologies of this patient's symptoms?

   The most important elements are timing, presentation at onset, and symptoms. Central toxic keratopathy presents immediately, appearing as stage 4 DLK within the first 2 to 7 postoperative days, whereas DLK goes through stages of evolution prior to reaching stage 4. Further, almost all DLK cases are associated with foreign body sensation at initial presentation, opposed to CTK and PISK, which are frequently less symptomatic, or infectious keratitis, which is frequently more symptomatic and associated with conjunctival erythema.

4. What is the best course of treatment at this juncture for this patient's problem?

   The best course of treatment is aggressive administration of topical steroids, with the addition of oral steroids if the patient does not improve over the ensuing 24 hours.

5. What is the next intervention if your first treatment is not successful?

   Flap lift and irrigation should be performed if the patient does not improve with topical and oral steroid treatment for stage 2 DLK, and at initial presentation of stage 3 DLK. Late flap lift is controversial and may be contraindicated if the patient has evolved to stage 4 DLK, so all efforts must be undertaken to prevent this progression.

6. What is the primary concern for this patient if she is not treated appropriately?

   The primary concern would be flap necrosis with permanent, visually significant scarring.

Diffuse Lamellar Keratitis Etiology

Certain conditions are known to stimulate interface inflammation, including epithelial defects and heme under the flap. Although the appearance and management are the same for these causes and for idiopathic DLK, the obvious causes do not necessitate a search for the inciting factor. DLK has been associated with a variety of other potential inflammatory stimuli, including meibomian gland secretions, some surgical gloves, and marking pens; however, the most important source is bacterial endotoxin, which frequently originates from sterilization reservoir biofilms or unfiltered water sources. Thus, when a case of idiopathic DLK presents, other cases may soon follow, and steps should be taken to identify the source of contamination and eliminate it quickly.

Diffuse Lamellar Keratitis Staging

DLK is typically classified clinically into 4 stages. Stage 1 denotes inflammatory cells in the far periphery only. Stage 2 denotes a diffuse infiltrate frequently involving the visual axis and periphery, but sparing the central axis. Stage 3 denotes a denser infiltrate involving the visual axis and frequently associated with decreased visual acuity. Stage 4 is defined by a more focal, coalesced dense haze and scarring, signifying flap necrosis, and it usually results in permanent corneal scarring, with visual acuity loss of varying severity.

Among the various interface complications, DLK tends to evolve, for better or worse, relatively quickly, usually over the course of days, rather than weeks, as may be the case for other interface disorders. During this evolution, DLK may mimic benign interface debris (stage 1), PISK (stage 2 to 3), or CTK (stage 4) (See Figure 5-6 from Chapter 5).

Distinguishing Diffuse Lamellar Keratitis From Other Possible Etiologies

Compared to stage 1 DLK, benign interface debris is asymptomatic and does not change over time, with or without steroid use. Pressure-induced stromal keratopathy takes 2 to 3 weeks to develop, compared with the early onset of DLK. Central toxic keratopathy presents with a stage 4 DLK-like appearance within the first few days after surgery, opposed to DLK, which takes longer to evolve to this appearance.

Diffuse Lamellar Keratitis Related to Femtosecond Laser Flap Creation

DLK and transient light sensitivity were reported to occur at a higher rate with earlier generation femtosecond lasers than with mechanical microkeratomes. However, modern femtosecond lasers appear to have lowered this incidence significantly. The severity of femtosecond laser-specific DLK appears similar to stage 1 to 2 cases, with generally rapid resolution without major sequelae. Diffuse lamellar keratitis can still occur in more severe forms in femtosecond laser cases; however, the etiology in these cases is unlikely to be the femtosecond laser itself.

Diffuse Lamellar Keratitis Management

Diffuse lamellar keratitis is highly sensitive to steroids and responsive to aggressive topical steroids for mild cases, frequently up to every-hour administration, and a combination of topical and oral steroids in moderate cases. Many surgeons advocate using oral steroids for stages 2 and 3 DLK, with flap lift and irrigation for stage 2 cases that are not responding rapidly to treatment and for all stage 3 cases. If any confusion persists regarding the diagnosis of DLK, cultures can be obtained at the time of flap lift. For stage 4, aggressive steroid regimens to minimize scar density are warranted and may be partially effective; however, flap lift should be avoided to prevent tissue loss. It is imperative to monitor intraocular pressure during treatment for DLK, as some patients may have a significant steroid response.

Diffuse Lamellar Keratitis Visual Outcomes

Reported visual acuity after DLK resolves is generally quite good; however, this may be slightly misleading, as DLK appears to affect visual quality and contrast sensitivity more than absolute Snellen acuity measurements. Diffuse lamellar keratitis frequently induces a mild-to-moderate hyperopic shift after resolution, with potentially both regular and irregular astigmatism, especially in stage 4 cases. If significant ametropia persists, patients may undergo retreatment without increased risk of developing DLK a second time, as long as the inciting issue has been resolved (ie, elimination of the endotoxin). For stage 4 cases, retreatment may still be warranted if the refractive error is regular. Surface ablation is a better option than flap relift for the aforementioned reasons.

Bibliography

Beer SM, Campos M, Lopes PT, Andre JA Jr, Schor P. Ocular wavefront aberrations in patients after diffuse lamellar keratitis. *Cornea*. 2007;26(1):6-8.

Buhren J, Baumeister M, Cichocki M, Kohnen T. Confocal microscopic characteristics of stage 1 to 4 diffuse lamellar keratitis after laser in situ keratomileusis. *J Cataract Refract Surg*. 2002;28(8):1390-1399.

Buhren J, Baumeister M, Kohnen T. Diffuse lamellar keratitis after laser in situ keratomileusis imaged by confocal microscopy. *Ophthalmology*. 2001;108(6):1075-1081.

Chen S, Feng Y, Stojanovic A, Jankov MR II, Wang Q. IntraLase femtosecond laser vs mechanical microkeratomes in LASIK for myopia: a systematic review and meta-analysis. *J Refract Surg*. 2012;28(1):15-24.

Choe CH, Guss C, Musch DC, Niziol LM, Shtein RM. Incidence of diffuse lamellar keratitis after LASIK with 15 KHz, 30 KHz, and 60 KHz femtosecond laser flap creation. *J Cataract Refract Surg*. 2010;36(11):1912-1918.

Dada T, Pangtey MS, Sharma N, Vajpayee RB, Jhanji V, Sethi HS. Hyeropic shift after LASIK induced diffuse lamellar keratitis. *BMC Ophthalmol*. 2006;6:19.

De Rojas Silva MV, Abraldes MJ, Diez-Feijoo E, Yanez PM, Javaloy J, Sanchez-Salorio M.. Confocal microscopy and histopathological examination of diffuse lamellar keratitis in an experimental animal model. *J Refract Surg*. 2007;23(3):299-304.

De Rojas Silva MV, Diez-Feijoo E, Rodriguez-Ares MT, Sanchez-Salorio M. Confocal microscopy of stage 4 diffuse lamellar keratitis with spontaneous resolution. *J Refract Surg*. 2004;20(4):391-396.

Gil-Cazorla R, Teus MA, de Benito-Llopis L, Fuentes I. Incidence of diffuse lamellar keratitis after laser in situ keratomileusis associated with the IntraLase 15 kHz femtosecond laser and Moria M2 microkeratome. *J Cataract Refract Surg*. 2008;34(1):28-31.

Hazin R, Daoud YJ, Khalifa YM. What is Central Toxic Keratopathy Syndrome if it is not diffuse lamellar keratitis Grade IV? *Middle East Afr J Ophthalmol*. 2010;17(1):60-2.

Hoffman RS, Fine IH, Packer M. Incidence and outcomes of LASIK with diffuse lamellar keratitis treated with topical and oral corticosteroids. *J Cataract Refract Surg*. 2003;29(3):451-456.

Holland SP, Mathias RG, Morck DW, Chiu J, Slade SG. Diffuse lamellar keratitis related to endotoxins released from sterilizer reservoir biofilms. *Ophthalmology*. 2000;107(7):1227-1233; discussion 1233-1234.

Javaloy J, Alio JL, El Kady B, Munoz G. Barraquer RI, Maldonado MJ. Refractive outcomes and quality of vision related to an outbreak of diffuse lamellar keratitis. *J Refract Surg*. 2011;27(11):804-810.

Javaloy J, Alio JL, Rodriguez A, Gonzalez A, Perez-Santonja JJ. Epidemiological analysis of an outbreak of diffuse lamellar keratitis. *J Refract Surg.* 2011;27(11):796-803.

Javaloy J, Artola A, Vidal MT, Munoz G, De Rojas V, Alio JL. Severe diffuse lamellar keratitis after femtosecond lamellar keratectomy. *Br J Ophthalmol.* 2007;91(5):699.

Linebarger EJ, Hardten DR, Lindstrom RL. Diffuse lamellar keratitis: diagnosis and management. *J Cataract Refract Surg.* 2000;26(7):1072-1077.

Michieletto P, Balestrazzi A, Balestrazzi A, Alegente M, Boccassini B. Stage 4 diffuse lamellar keratitis after laser in situ keratomileusis. Clinical, topographical, and pachymetry resolution 5 years later. *J Cataract Refract Surg.* 2006;32(2):353-356.

Peters NT, Iskander NG, Anderson Penno EE, Woods DE, Moore RA, Gimbel HV. Diffuse lamellar keratitis: isolation of endotoxin and demonstration of the inflammatory potential in a rabbit laser in situ keratomileusis model. *J Cataract Refract Surg.* 2001;27(6):917-923.

Smith RJ, Maloney RK. Diffuse lamellar keratitis. A new syndrome in lamellar refractive surgery. *Ophthalmology.* 1998;105(9):1721-1726.

Stulting RD, Randleman JB, Couser JM, Thompson KP. The epidemiology of diffuse lamellar keratitis. *Cornea.* 2004;23(7):680-688.

—CASE 25—

A 24-year-old male presents 3 weeks after bilateral myopic LASIK, with painless, blurred vision in the right eye only. The patient reports initially good vision in both eyes, with gradual decrease in visual acuity in the right eye over the past week. He is otherwise asymptomatic, denying foreign body sensation or any trouble with his left eye.

Current medications: Topical steroid 4 times daily in right eye, frequent artificial tear use in both eyes.

CASE HISTORY		
	Right Eye	**Left Eye**
Present correction method	None	None
Manifest refraction	Plano	Plano
UCVA	20/100	20/20
CDVA	Not obtained	Not obtained
Physical examination	See Figure	Normal

QUESTIONS

1. What additional information would you like to have on this patient to aid in making the correct diagnosis?
2. What entities are in your differential diagnosis?
3. What elements of the case are most important in helping you differentiate between the possible etiologies of this patient's symptoms?
4. What is the best course of treatment at this juncture for this patient's problem?
5. What is your primary concern for this patient if he is not treated appropriately?

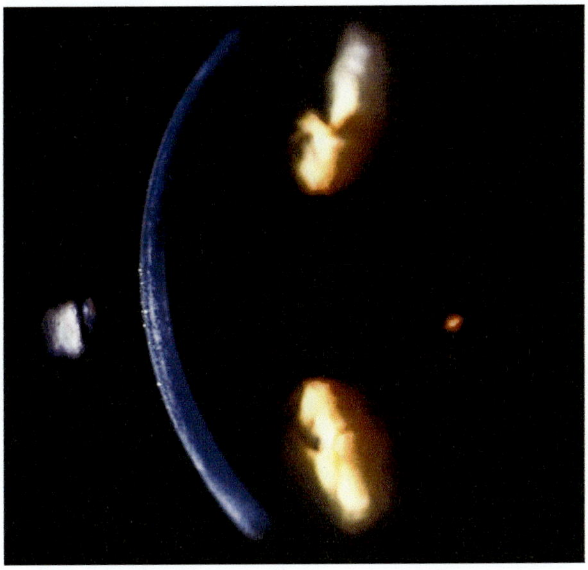

—Case 25—
Pressure-Induced Stromal Keratopathy

Pressure-induced stromal keratopathy (PISK) is a condition precipitated by steroid use, where the steroid response causes increased intraocular pressure (IOP), resulting in fluid accumulation in the LASIK interface. The result is a hazy, granular interface appearance, with decreased visual acuity. In some instances the fluid is easily appreciated with slit-lamp biomicroscopy; however, there are cases where no demonstrable fluid is visible. PISK resembles the early stages of diffuse lamellar keratitis (DLK); however, the treatment plans are opposite. DLK is an inflammatory condition that is sensitive to topical steroids, while PISK is a steroid response that is worsened by prolonged steroid use.

Case Analysis

- Case Figure shows a slit-lamp image depicting interface opacity notable in slit view. There is no definitive fluid cleft, but interface fluid is the mechanism causing this appearance.

Pearl: *ALWAYS measure IOP peripherally as well as centrally in patients on extended topical steroids, and reconsider the DLK diagnosis when the clinical course is atypical!*

Questions

1. What additional information would you like to have on this patient to aid in making the correct diagnosis?

   IOP readings are critical at this juncture. Steroid response must be ruled out in this patient who developed interface haze while on steroids.

2. What entities are in your differential diagnosis?

   Differential diagnoses include DLK, PISK, infectious keratitis, or benign interface debris (unlikely). Notably, central toxic keratopathy (CTK) does NOT present with this appearance.

3. What elements of the case are most important in helping you differentiate between the possible etiologies of this patient's symptoms?

   The most important elements of this case are time of onset, foreign body sensation symptoms, visual acuity, history of steroid use, and IOP.

4. What is the best course of treatment at this juncture for this patient's problem?

   Start topical glaucoma medications immediately and stop topical steroids with close observation. Close observation will allow one to confirm that the cornea is clearing as the IOP normalizes. If for some reason there is concomitant interface inflammation (DLK) with increased IOP, judicious use of steroids may be necessary, along with aggressive glaucoma medications and potentially even oral acetazolamide.

5. What is your primary concern for this patient he is not treated appropriately?

   The primary concern would be glaucomatous optic nerve atrophy resulting from high IOP. Although uncommon in the short-term, if this condition is not recognized and appropriate treatment started, permanent visual loss can occur.

Pressure-Induced Stromal Keratopathy

It is essential to differentiate PISK from DLK early in the course of the evaluation to appropriately treat the patient and avoid serious optic nerve damage. This can be done based on time of onset, the patient's symptoms, the severity of vision loss, the clinical course, and the response to steroids. Diffuse lamellar keratitis begins within the first 1 to 4 postoperative days, and almost always is associated with foreign body sensation at least equal to visual loss at presentation. In contrast, PISK usually presents after the first 2 to 3 weeks postoperatively in patients taking continual tropical steroids; at presentation, visual symptoms are usually worse, whereas most patients experience little, if any, foreign body sensation. Further, DLK will evolve over a short period of time, for better or worse, but will not remain stable, whereas PISK may maintain a similar appearance for some time if steroids are not stopped and IOP is unchanged. Any patient with the presumptive diagnosis of DLK, which is unchanged after 1 to 2 weeks of treatment, should have the diagnosis reconsidered and therapy changed.

It is critical to routinely measure IOP, even in the early postoperative period, for any patient on chronic topical steroids after LASIK, and recognize that even a small amount of interface fluid, which is not easily detectable as a fluid pocket, may falsely lower IOP. LASIK lowers IOP through corneal thickness reduction and flap creation; thus, any patient with IOP measurements higher than their preoperative values should be considered to have elevated IOP, even if the absolute numbers are not particularly high. For instance, if a moderately myopic individual has an IOP in the mid-teens before LASIK and his or her IOP is in the mid 20s postoperatively, increased IOP should be addressed because the "true" IOP is likely much higher. Peripheral corneal IOP measurements with all devices are more accurate than central measurements in PISK cases.

Bibliography

Belin MW, Hannush SB, Yau CW, Schultze RL. Elevated intraocular pressure-induced interlamellar stromal keratitis. *Ophthalmology.* 2002;109(10):1929-1933.

Davidson RS, Brandt JD, Mannis MJ. Intraocular pressure-induced interlamellar keratitis after LASIK surgery. *J Glaucoma.* 2003;12(1):23-26.

Dawson DG, Schmack I, Holley GP, Waring GO III, Grossniklaus HE, Edelhauser HF. Interface fluid syndrome in human eye bank corneas after LASIK: causes and pathogenesis. *Ophthalmology.* 2007;114(10):1848-1859.

Galal A, Artola A, Belda J, et al. Interface corneal edema secondary to steroid-induced elevation of intraocular pressure simulating diffuse lamellar keratitis. *J Refract Surg.* 2006;22(5):441-447.

Hamilton DR, Manche EE, Rich LF, Maloney RK. Steroid-induced glaucoma after laser in situ keratomileusis associated with interface fluid. *Ophthalmology.* 2002;109(4):659-665.

Nordlund ML, Grimm S, Lane S, Holland EJ. Pressure-induced interface keratitis: a late complication following LASIK. *Cornea.* 2004;23(3):225-234.

Randleman JB, Lesser GR. Glaucomatous damage from pressure- induced stromal keratopathy after LASIK. *J Refract Surg.* 2012;28(6):378-379.

Randleman JB, Shah RD. LASIK interface complications: etiology, management, & outcomes. *J Refract Surg.* 2012;28(8):575-588.

Tourtas T, Kopsachilis N, Meiller R, Kruse FE, Cursiefen C. Pressure-induced interlamellar stromal keratitis after laser in situ keratomileusis. *Cornea.* 2011;30(8):920-923.

Wheeldon CE, Hadden OB, Niederer RL, McGhee CN. Presumed late diffuse lamellar keratitis progressing to interface fluid syndrome. *J Cataract Refract Surg.* 2008;34(2):322-326.

—Case 26—

A 29-year-old female presents on day 3 after bilateral myopic LASIK with blurred vision in both eyes, right worse than left, and moderate photophobia in both eyes. The patient reported good visual acuity with only mild foreign body sensation on postoperative day 1. UDVA on day 1 was 20/20 in the right eye and 20/15 in the left eye.

Current medications: Topical antibiotic and topical steroids 4 times daily in both eyes and frequent artificial tear use.

CASE HISTORY		
	Right Eye	**Left Eye**
UCVA	20/50	20/60
Manifest refraction	Plano	Plano
CDVA	20/50	20/60
Physical examination	See Figure	See Figure

Questions

1. Given the patient's presentation, what is the most likely diagnosis?
2. What other conditions are included in your differential diagnoses?
3. What clinical factors are most critical in differentiating this entity from the others on your list?
4. What is the most effective prudent therapy at this juncture?
5. What is the likely clinical outcome, and what are reasonable treatment strategies to improve unaided visual acuity?

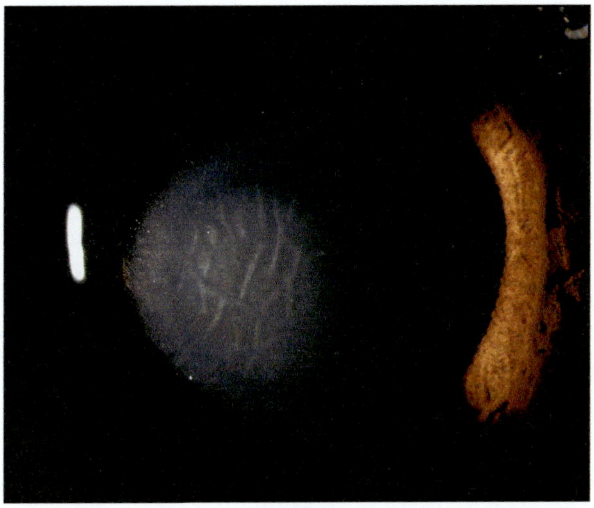

A

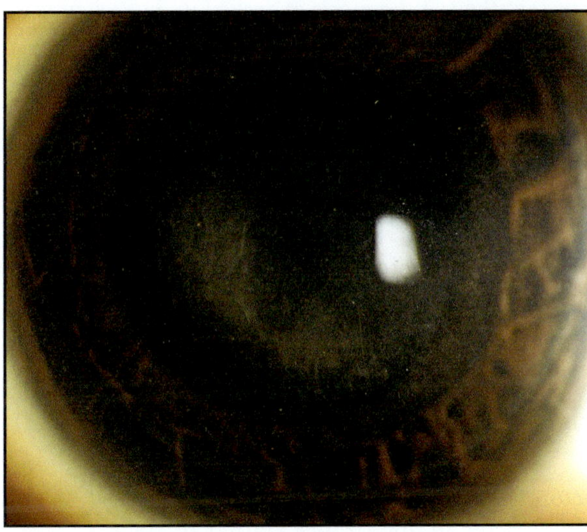

B

—Case 26—
Central Toxic Keratopathy

Central toxic keratopathy (CTK) is a noninflammatory central corneal opacification that can occur within days after uneventful LASIK or photorefractive keratectomy. The etiology is unknown, but it may be related to enzymatic degradation of keratocytes. Central toxic keratopathy is self-limited, and treatment is not warranted. In fact, flap lift and irrigation may worsen the final outcome. Most individuals recover well after a variable clinical course; however, most patients retain some faint corneal haze and some have a visually significant, persistent hyperopic shift.

Case Analysis

- Case Figures show slit-lamp images of the (A) right and (B) left eyes demonstrating a focal, clearly defined opacity with multiple crack-like lines running through the opacity.

Pearl: *Central toxic keratopathy is a diagnosis of exclusion, but when it is made, observation is the most appropriate course!*

Questions

1. Given the patient's presentation, what is the most likely diagnosis?

   The most likely diagnosis is CTK.

2. What other conditions are included in your differential diagnoses?

   Other conditions may be diffuse lamellar keratitis (DLK) stage 4 or infectious keratitis.

3. What clinical factors are most critical in differentiating this entity from the others on your list?

   Critical factors are timing and presentation at onset. Central toxic keratopathy immediately presents in appearance similar to stage 4 DLK within the first 2 to 7 postoperative days, whereas DLK passes through stages of evolution prior to reaching stage 4.

4. What is the most effective, prudent therapy at this juncture?

   The most prudent therapy is observation. Although steroid administration is unlikely to cause any harm, it is also unlikely to help. Flap lift and irrigation are contraindicated.

5. What is the likely clinical outcome, and what are reasonable treatment strategies to improve unaided visual acuity?

   The most likely outcome is resolution with a relatively normal postoperative outcome. In cases of persistent hyperopia, retreatment may be warranted, and could be undertaken with surface ablation or flap relift.

Central Toxic Keratopathy

CTK can be confused with stage 4 DLK and occasionally with infectious keratitis. However, infection can quickly be ruled out based on the clinical examination over the first few days. Key differentiators between CTK and stage 4 DLK is the clinical course and time of onset. Clinically, CTK closely resembles stage 4 DLK; however, this stage 4-like appearance in CTK occurs within the first few days after surgery as the immediate clinical presentation, whereas stage 4 DLK usually takes weeks to develop and is always preceded by a more diffuse appearance (see Chapter 5 for a more complete discussion).

Topographic findings are highly variable and can demonstrate pronounced focal irregularity corresponding to the area of opacity, even after the opacity has diminished clinically (Case Figure 26-1).

There is no specific treatment for CTK. Topical and oral steroids do not appear effective; however, neither appears to have any deleterious effects, so, if in doubt, it is reasonable to continue steroid use with close observation and intraocular pressure checks. The treatment of stage 4 DLK should not include flap lift or irrigation, nor should they be included in the treatment of CTK; therefore, in many instances, the initial management of these different conditions can overlap without clinical consequence.

Although the occurrence of CTK appears to be quite rare, it is important for the practitioner to be aware of this condition and recognize it if it does occur. With appropriate diagnosis, treatment, and differentiation from stage 4 DLK, CTK can have good outcomes. However, if misdiagnosed and incorrectly treated, the results can be poor.

Bibliography

Hainline BC, Price MO, Choi DM, Price FW Jr. Central flap necrosis after LASIK with microkeratome and femtosecond laser created flaps. *J Refract Surg.* 2007;23(3):233-242.

Liu A, Manche EE. Anterior segment optical coherence tomography imaging of central toxic keratopathy. *Ophthalmic Surg Lasers Imaging.* 2010;Apr 2:1-3. doi:10.3928/15428877-20100325-10

Lyle WA, Jin GJ. Central lamellar keratitis. *J Cataract Refract Surg.* 2001;27(4):487-490.

Moshirfar M, Hazin R, Khalifa YM. Central toxic keratopathy. *Curr Opin Ophthalmol.* 2010;21(4):274-29.

Neira W, Holopainen JM, Tervo TM. Long-term outcome of central toxic keratopathy after photorefractive keratectomy. *Cornea.* 2011;30(11):1207-1212.

Randleman JB, Shah RD. LASIK interface complications: etiology, management, & outcomes. *J Refract Surg.* 2012;28(8):575-588.

Sikder S, Khalifa YM, Neuffer MC, Moshirfar M. Tomographic corneal profile analysis of central toxic keratopathy after LASIK. *Cornea.* 2012;31(1):48-51.

Sonmez B, Maloney RK. Central toxic keratopathy: description of a syndrome in laser refractive surgery. *Am J Ophthalmol.* 2007;143(3):420-427.

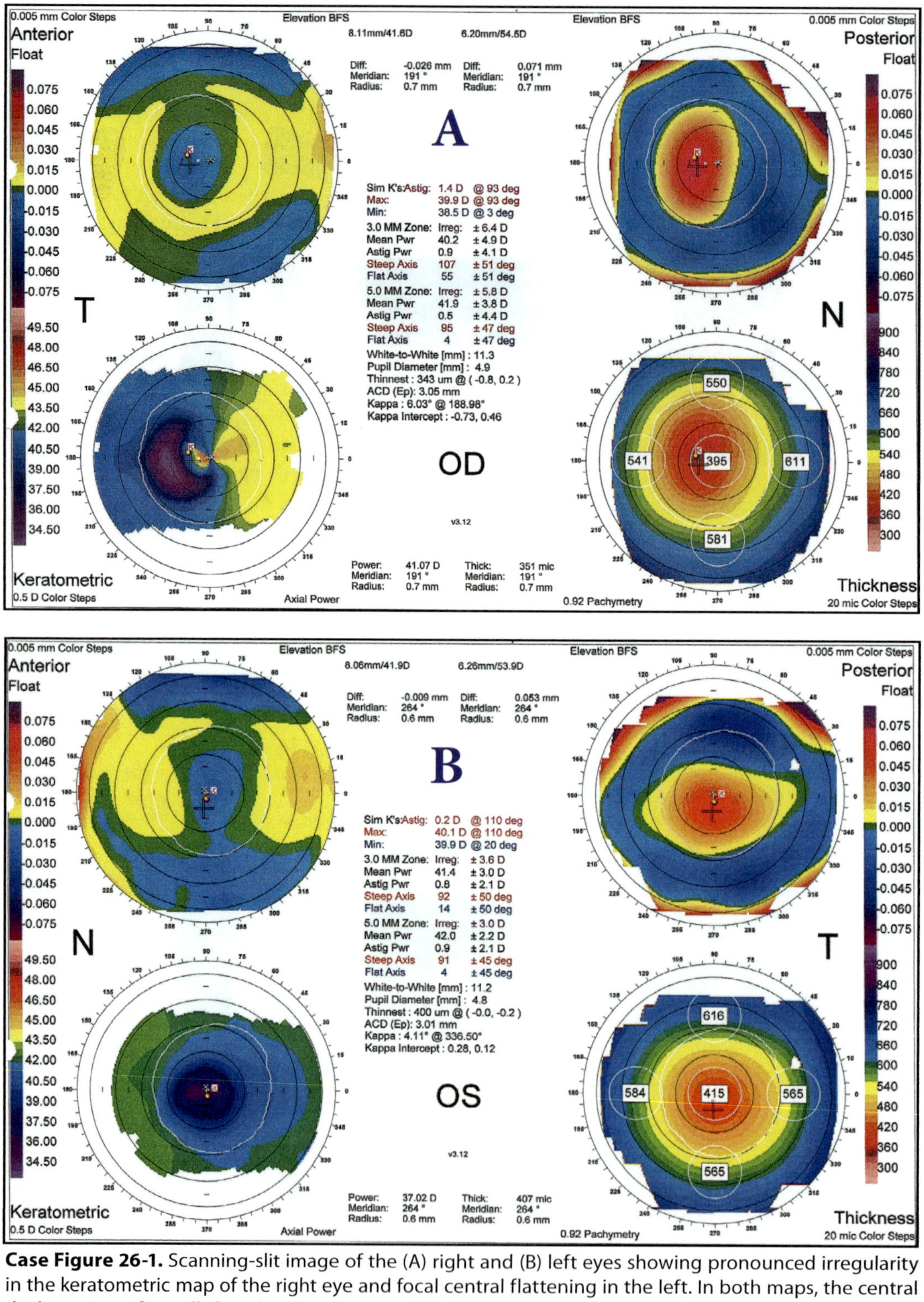

Case Figure 26-1. Scanning-slit image of the (A) right and (B) left eyes showing pronounced irregularity in the keratometric map of the right eye and focal central flattening in the left. In both maps, the central thickness is artifactually low due to opacity.

—Case 27—

A 36-year-old male presents 10 days after LASIK retreatment on his right eye with blurred vision, foreign body sensation, and photophobia. UCVA in the right eye prior to retreatment was 20/25, with manifest refraction: -0.75 +0.25 x 084 = 20/15.

Current medications: None. The patient finished a routine 1-week course of topical antibiotics and steroids 3 days prior to presentation.

CASE HISTORY		
	Right Eye	**Left Eye**
Present correction method	None	None
Manifest refraction	Plano	-0.50 sphere
UCVA	20/40	20/20
Central corneal thickness	Not obtained	Not obtained
Intraocular pressure	Not obtained	Not obtained
Physical examination	See Figure	

Questions

1. Given the patient's presentation and clinical appearance, what is the most likely diagnosis?
2. What other conditions are included in your differential diagnosis?
3. What elements of the case are most important in helping you differentiate between the possible etiologies of this patient's symptoms?
4. What is the best course of action at this juncture to diagnose and treat this patient's problem?
5. What is the next intervention if your first treatment is not successful?

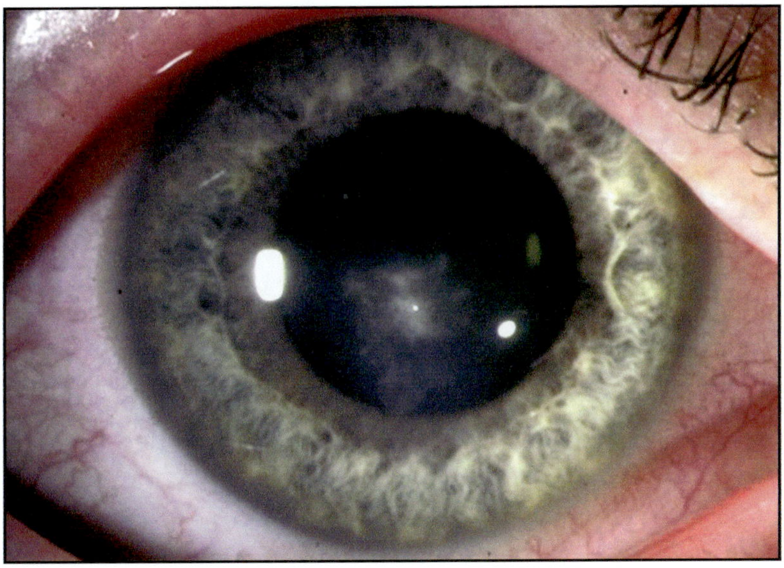

—Case 27—
Infectious Keratitis After Laser Vision Correction

Infectious keratitis occurs rarely after surface ablation or LASIK, but it can have serious visual consequences if it does occur. A variety of organisms can cause postoperative keratitis, including viruses (Adenovirus and herpes simplex virus [HSV]), bacteria (*Staphylococcus* species and *Pseudomonas*), atypical mycobacteria, fungi, and *Acanthamoeba*. The incidence of nonviral infectious keratitis is estimated to range from 0.02% to 0.2% with surface ablation and 0.03% to 0.1% with LASIK, thus, infectious keratitis is less common than DLK (0.1% to 1%) occurrence in the early postoperative period.

Case Analysis

- Case Figure shows a slit-lamp photo of the right eye exhibiting a paracentral infiltrate with relatively well-defined borders and focal density, with moderate conjunctival reaction.

Pearl: *Infectious keratitis is more challenging to treat under a LASIK flap; the causative organisms can be predicted from the time of onset postoperatively!*

Questions

1. Given the patient's presentation and clinical appearance, what is the most likely diagnosis?

   The most likely diagnosis is nonviral infectious keratitis, probably bacterial.

2. What other conditions are included in your differential diagnosis?

   The differential diagnosis includes diffuse lamellar keratitis (DLK) and central toxic keratopathy (CTK), although neither is likely based on appearance. This patient's presentation is too focal in nature to be considered as pressure-induced stromal keratopathy (PISK).

3. What elements of the case are most important in helping you to differentiate between the possible etiologies of this patient's symptoms?

   The important elements include timing, presentation at onset, and symptoms. DLK and CTK generally both present earlier in the postoperative course, whereas PISK would not usually present by 10 days. Further, the more focal nature of the interface haze and the patient's increased, progressively worsening symptoms would be highly atypical for any etiology other than infection.

4. What is the best course of action at this juncture to diagnose and treat this patient's problem?

   The best course of action is flap lift, with cultures and antibiotic irrigation, followed by topical fortified antibiotics.

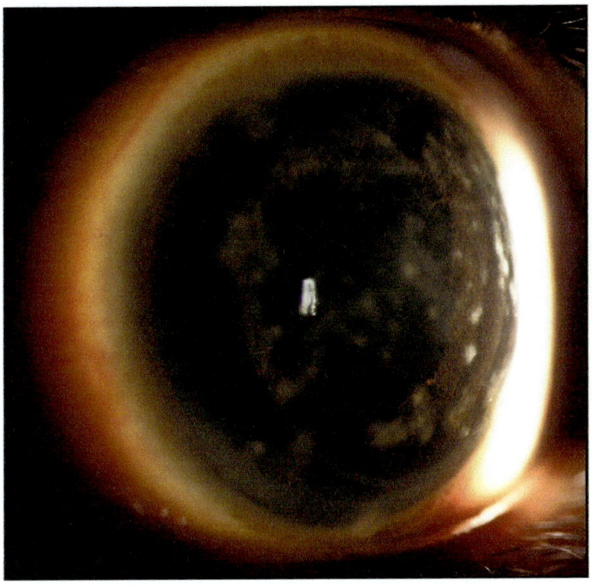

Case Figure 27-1. Slit-lamp image taken at an oblique angle to highlight the multiple scattered focal opacities throughout the cornea in a case with reactivation of adenoviral subepithelial infiltrates after LASIK. (Reprinted from Randleman JB. Etiology and clinical presentations of irregular astigmatism after keratorefractive surgery. In: Wang M, ed. *Irregular Astigmatism: Diagnosis and Treatment.* Thorofare, NJ: SLACK Incorporated; 2007:79-90.)

5. What is the next intervention if your first treatment is not successful?

   The next intervention would be to change the patient's antibiotic regimen, based on culture results. If the patient continues to worsen despite maximal therapy, flap amputation may be necessary to resolve the infection.

Viral Keratitis After Laser Vision Correction

Viral keratitis is usually caused by Adenovirus or HSV after LASIK or surface ablation. Adenovirus usually has a relatively benign course, with ultimately good visual acuity. Some controversy exists in the literature about the effects of surface ablation for patients with a history of Adenovirus, as flares can certainly occur (Case Figure 27-1). HSV frequently leads to loss of best visual acuity after surface ablation or LASIK and is a relative contraindication for excimer laser ablation, as the ultraviolet light spectrum appears to stimulate herpes viral activation.

Nonviral Infectious Keratitis After Laser Vision Correction

In the past, the most common causative organism for post-LASIK infectious keratitis was atypical *Mycobacterium*, usually presenting within the first 2 to 3 weeks after surgery. However, fourth-generation fluoroquinolones appear to have increased efficacy against this organism prophylactically, and in recent surveys and reports, the incidence of Mycobacterium infections has decreased significantly, and the most common organism is now *Staphylococcus aureus* (Case Figure 27-2). Comparatively, Staphylococcus generally presents earlier—within the first 2 to 5 days postoperatively—compared with *Mycobacterium*, fungal infections, and *Acanthamoeba*, which all generally present later.

Most cases of infectious keratitis appear related to normal bacterial flora, but instrument contamination should be considered, especially with the presence of *Mycobacterium*, which is more prone to be present in outbreaks than other organisms. Some evidence exists that contact lens

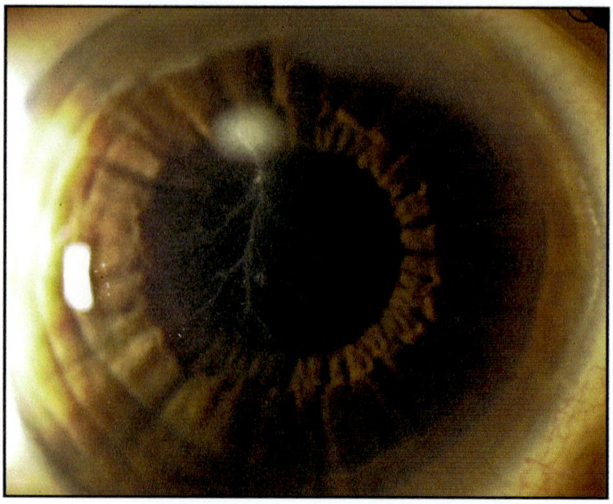

Case Figure 27-2. Slit-lamp image of infectious keratitis after PRK. In this case, MRSA caused a focal infiltrate 5 days after PRK.

wearers may have altered conjunctival flora and that health care workers are especially prone to carrying methicillin resistant strains of *S aureus* (MRSA).

Any patients with epithelial defects at the time of surgery, or those who wear contact lenses in the initial postoperative period, are at increased risk for infectious keratitis, which accounts for the increased risk with surface ablation as compared with LASIK.

Diagnosis and Management of Infectious Keratitis

Because of its rare presentation, but serious consequences, practitioners must have a high level of suspicion for any interface haze and infiltrates with even a moderately focal appearance presenting within the first 2 weeks postoperatively. DLK is more common and the most likely entity to be confused with infectious keratitis. Most infections do have interface inflammation, but with a more focal infiltrate. Interface debris, CTK, and PISK do not resemble interface infections and should be easily differentiated. Although the use of fluoroquinolones has reduced the incidence of *Mycobacterium* infections, they may have influenced the course of MRSA strains, as fluoroquinolone-resistant MRSA appears to be increasing in frequency.

In the initial phase of treatment, LASIK flaps should be lifted, cultures taken, and the flap bed irrigated with fortified antibiotics. Broad-spectrum topical antibiotics should be started, based on timing of onset; within the first week, and appropriate coverage includes agents that are active against gram positive (vancomycin or cefazolin) and gram negative (tobramycin and gentamycin) organisms. After 2 weeks, it may be appropriate to also use amikacin to treat for any atypical organisms. If the infection does not respond to treatment, flap amputation may be necessary to allow for better antibiotic penetration and to debulk the infection. With more aggressive organisms, corneal perforation can occur and may necessitate treatment with therapeutic penetrating keratoplasty. Management of infections after PRK is similar to routine corneal ulcer management, as no flap exists to act as a barrier to antibiotic penetration.

Infectious Keratitis Outcomes

Most adenoviral cases resolve with limited sequelae. With all other organisms, mild to moderate loss of best corrected visual acuity frequently occurs based on scar location. Some patients may have a relatively insignificant opacity but may have significant accompanying irregular astigmatism.

Bibliography

Amayem A, Ali AT, Waring GO, 3rd, Ibrahim O. Bacterial keratitis after photorefractive keratectomy. *J Refract Surg.* 1996;12(5):642-644.

de Rojas V, Llovet F, Martinez M, et al. Infectious keratitis in 18,651 laser surface ablation procedures. *J Cataract Refract Surg.* 2011;37(10):1822-1831.

Donnenfeld ED, Kim T, Holland EJ, et al. ASCRS White Paper: Management of infectious keratitis following laser in situ keratomileusis. *J Cataract Refract Surg.* 2005;31(10):2008-2011.

Dunphy D, Andrews D, Seamone C, Ramsey M. Fungal keratitis following excimer laser photorefractive keratectomy. *Can J Ophthalmol.* 1999;34(5):286-289.

Hofling-Lima AL, de Freitas D, Sampaio JL, Leao SC, Contarini P. In vitro activity of fluoroquinolones against Mycobacterium abscessus and Mycobacterium chelonae causing infectious keratitis after LASIK in Brazil. *Cornea.* 2005;24(6):730-734.

Javadi MA, Kanavi MR, Zarei-Ghanavati S, et al. Outbreak of Nocardia keratitis after photorefractive keratectomy: clinical, microbiological, histopathological, and confocal scan study. *J Cataract Refract Surg.* 2009;35(2):393-398.

Kaldawy RM, Sutphin JE, Wagoner MD. Acanthamoeba keratitis after photorefractive keratectomy. *J Cataract Refract Surg.* 2002;28(2):364-368.

Karimian F, Baradaran-Rafii A, Javadi MA, Nazari R, Rabei HM, Jafarinasab MR. Bilateral bacterial keratitis in three patients following photorefractive keratectomy. *J Refract Surg.* 2007;23(3):312-315.

Karp CL, Tuli SS, Yoo SH, et al. Infectious keratitis after LASIK. *Ophthalmology.* 2003;110(3):503-510.

Leccisotti A, Bartolomei A, Greco G, Manetti C. Incidence of bacterial keratitis after photorefractive keratectomy. *J Refract Surg.* 2005;21(1):96.

Llovet F, de Rojas V, Interlandi E, et al. Infectious keratitis in 204 586 LASIK procedures. *Ophthalmology.* 2010;117(2):232-238. e1-4.

Moshirfar M, Welling JD, Feiz V, Holz H, Clinch TE. Infectious and noninfectious keratitis after laser in situ keratomileusis. Occurrence, management, and visual outcomes. *J Cataract Refract Surg.* 2007;33(3):474-483.

Mozayan A, Madu A, Channa P. Laser in-situ keratomileusis infection: review and update of current practices. *Curr Opin Ophthalmol.* 2011;22(4):233-237.

Solomon R, Donnenfeld ED, Perry HD, Biser S. Bilateral methicillin-resistant staphylococcus aureus keratitis in a medical resident following an uneventful bilateral photorefractive keratectomy. *Eye Contact Lens.* 2003;29(3):187-189.

Woodward M, Randleman JB. Bilateral methicillin-resistant Staphylococcus aureus keratitis after photorefractive keratectomy. *J Cataract Refract Surg.* 2007;33(2):316-319.

Wroblewski KJ, Pasternak JF, Bower KS, et al. Infectious keratitis after photorefractive keratectomy in the United States army and navy. *Ophthalmology.* 2006;113(4):520-5.

—Case 28—

A 48-year-old female returns to clinic complaining of progressively blurred vision in the left eye and requests surgical correction. She had LASIK bilaterally 9 months earlier and bilateral enhancement 3 months prior to her current visit. The vision in her right eye is good after enhancement and is stable per her report.

CASE HISTORY		
	Right Eye	**Left Eye**
UDVA	20/25	20/40
Manifest refraction	+0.50 sphere	+0.50 +0.75 x 077
CDVA (current)	20/20	20/30
CNVA (current)	20/20	20/30
Near add	+2.00	+1.75
Central corneal thickness	416 µm	408 µm
Physical examination	Normal	See Figure
Estimated ablation depth	15 µm	20 µm

Questions

1. Is this patient a candidate for refractive surgical retreatment? If so, what treatment options are available?
2. What are the most likely causes for the patient's refractive error at this time point?
3. Considering all factors, what is the most effective, prudent therapy at this juncture and why?
4. What is the likely clinical outcome, and what are reasonable treatment strategies to improve unaided visual acuity?
5. If the patient decides she desires observation only, what, if any, concerns do you have?

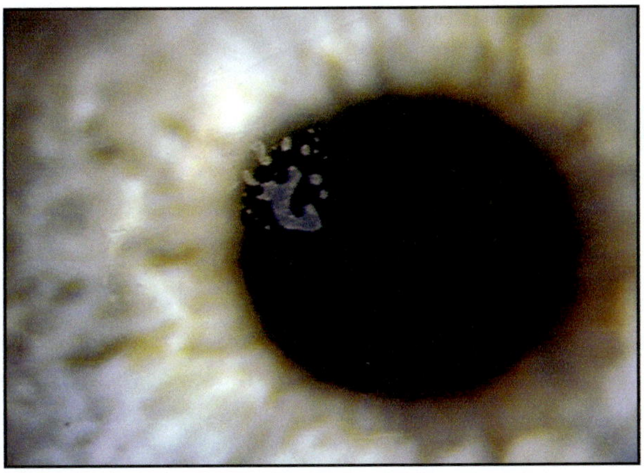

A

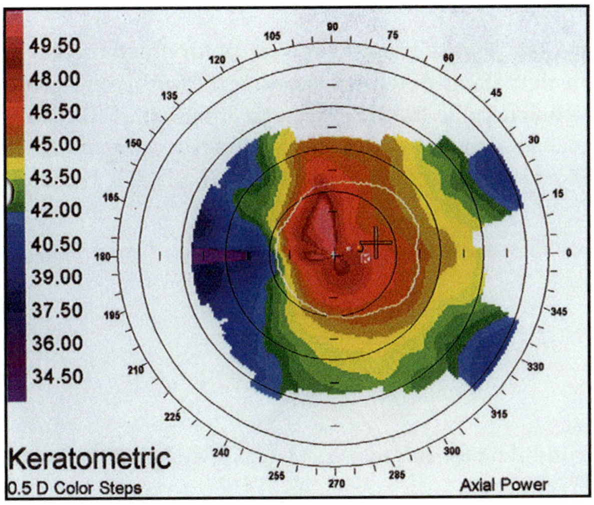
49.50
48.00
46.50
45.00
43.50
42.00
40.50
39.00
37.50
36.00
34.50
Keratometric
0.5 D Color Steps
Axial Power

B

—CASE 28—

Epith eli al Ingrowth After LASIK

Epithelial ingrowth occurs when a fistula develops under the flap, allowing epithelial cell growth into the interface. This disorder usually occurs weeks to months after LASIK, more commonly after flap lift retreatment, and occurs more commonly at the peripheral LASIK flap edges, but it occurs occasionally near enough to the visual axis to be visually significant. Appropriate management includes flap lift and epithelial cell removal. For recurrent cases flap fixation is necessary.

Case Analysis

- Case Figures show (A) focal area of epithelial ingrowth noted on slit-lamp examination with (B) focal irregular astigmatism noted on topography, with the steepest area corresponding to the region of epithelial cells. (Reprinted from Randleman JB. Etiology and clinical presentations of irregular astigmatism after keratorefractive surgery. In: Wang M, ed. *Irregular Astigmatism: Diagnosis and Treatment*. Thorofare, NJ: SLACK Incorporated; 2007:79-90.)

Pearl: *Epithelial ingrowth occurs from fistula formation, and treatment MUST include fistula closure for recurrent cases!*

QUESTIONS

1. Is this patient a candidate for refractive surgical retreatment? If so, what treatment options are available?

    No, this patient is not currently a candidate for further excimer laser ablation, as the current refraction is affected by the presence of epithelial cells under the flap.

2. What are the most likely causes for the patient's refractive error at this time point?

    The most likely cause is irregular astigmatism resulting from flap elevation, which corresponds to the focal area of epithelial ingrowth.

3. Considering all factors, what is the most effective, prudent therapy at this juncture and why?

    The most prudent therapy is flap lift, combined with epithelial cell removal (scraping) and flap repositioning with or without sutures or tissue sealant.

4. What is the likely clinical outcome, and what are reasonable treatment strategies to improve unaided visual acuity?

    Treatment is likely to be successful with an improvement of UDVA. However, the patient is at increased risk for recurrent epithelial ingrowth. If the patient has stable residual refractive error after epithelial cell removal and follow-up, she may be a candidate for surface ablation retreatment, but she would not be an ideal candidate for further flap relift.

5. If the patient decides she desires observation only, what, if any, concerns do you have?

   The patient is at risk for worsening irregular astigmatism if the epithelial cells are left without treatment and flap melt if they worsen. This could result in scarring, permanent irregular astigmatism, and vision loss.

Epithelial Ingrowth

Most cases of epithelial ingrowth are mild, clinically insignificant, and can be managed with observation only. However, irregular astigmatism, with or without flap melt, and scarring can develop, requiring intervention. The distinct appearance of epithelial ingrowth is usually not confused with other interface disorders (see Chapter 5), but it has been related in the literature to atypical diffuse lamellar keratitis and pressure-induced stromal keratopathy.

For LASIK retreatment, the increased incidence of epithelial ingrowth is associated with flap lift retreatment performed 3 or more years after primary LASIK, and possibly associated with the use of contact lenses after retreatment, although this is not conclusive. Femtosecond laser flap creation reduces the incidence of visually significant epithelial ingrowth.

The initial surgical treatment for epithelial ingrowth is performed with flap lift, removal of epithelial cells from the posterior surface of the flap and the stromal bed with a blade or similar instrument, and replacement of the flap, usually without sutures or tissue glue. With recurrent episodes of ingrowth, additional measures are typically taken, including flap suture, fibrin glue, or neodymium-doped yttrium aluminum garnet (Nd:YAG) laser treatment underneath the flap to disrupt the epithelial cell nests. A fistula extending from outside the flap is generally present, and this must be closed to prevent recurrence. Severe cases with flap melt result in scarring and irregular astigmatism and are not amenable to further LASIK flap lifts (Case Figure 28-1), but, in some instances, they may be treated with surface ablation.

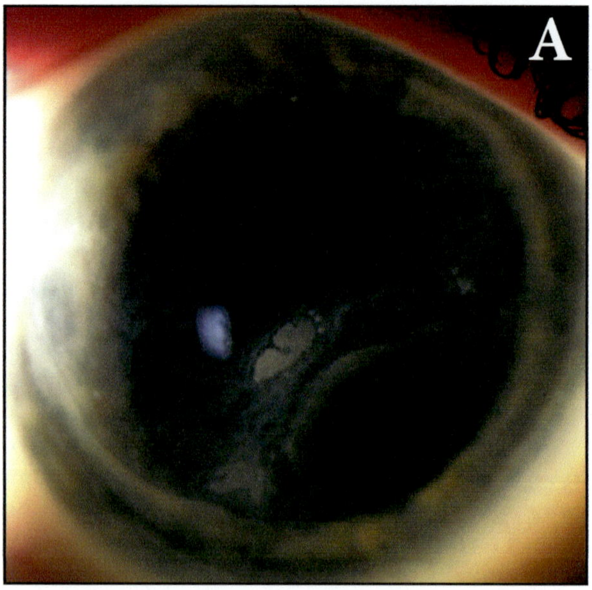

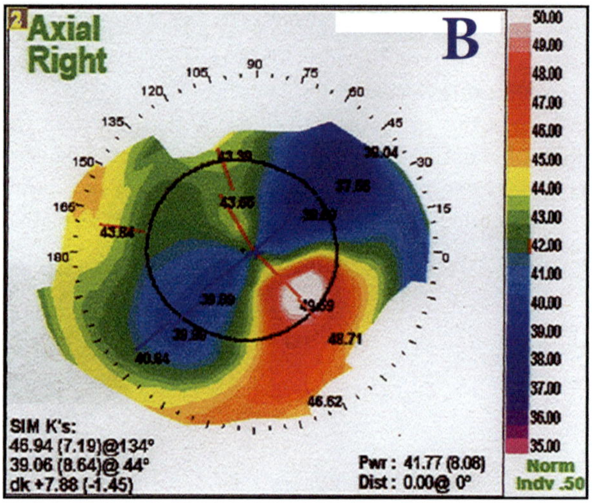

Case Figure 28-1. (A) Severe epithelial ingrowth resulting in flap melt, with resulting scarring in the visual axis and irregular astigmatism demonstrated on (B) corneal topography. This patient had significant visual improvement after surface ablation to correct astigmatism, but still suffered loss of best acuity from persistent irregular astigmatism. (Reprinted from Randleman JB. Etiology and clinical presentations of irregular astigmatism after keratorefractive surgery. In: Wang M, ed. *Irregular Astigmatism: Diagnosis and Treatment*. Thorofare, NJ: SLACK Incorporated; 2007:79-90.)

Bibliography

Anderson NJ, Hardten DR. Fibrin glue for the prevention of epithelial ingrowth after laser in situ keratomileusis. *J Cataract Refract Surg*. 2003;29(7):1425-1429.

Asano-Kato N, Toda I, Hori-Komai Y, Takano Y, Tsubota K. Epithelial ingrowth after laser in situ keratomileusis: clinical features and possible mechanisms. *Am J Ophthalmol*. 2002;134(6):801-807.

Ayala MJ, Alió JL, Mulet ME, De La Hoz F. Treatment of laser in situ keratomileusis interface epithelial ingrowth with neodymium:yytrium-aluminum-garnet laser. *Am J Ophthalmol*. 2008;145(4):630-634.

Beerthuizen JJ, Siebelt E. Surface ablation after laser in situ keratomileusis: retreatment on the flap. *J Cataract Refract Surg*. 2007;33(8):1376-13780.

Caster AI, Friess DW, Schwendeman FJ. Incidence of epithelial ingrowth in primary and retreatment laser in situ keratomileusis. *J Cataract Refract Surg*. 2010;36(1):97 101.

Chan CC, Boxer Wachler BS. Comparison of the effects of LASIK retreatment techniques on epithelial ingrowth rates. *Ophthalmology*. 2007;114(4):640-642.

Coskunseven E, Kymionis GD, Grentzelos MA, Portaliou DM, Kolli S, Jankov MR II. Femtosecond LASIK retreatment using side cutting only. *J Refract Surg*. 2012;28(1):37-41.

Dawson DG, Kramer TR, Grossniklaus HE, Waring GO III, Edelhauser HF. Histologic, ultrastructural, and immunofluorescent evaluation of human laser-assisted in situ keratomileusis corneal wounds. *Arch Ophthalmol.* 2005;123(6):741-756.

Henry CR, Canto AP, Galor A, Vaddavalli PK, Culbertson WW, Yoo SH. Epithelial ingrowth after LASIK: clinical characteristics, risk factors, and visual outcomes in patients requiring flap lift. *J Refract Surg.* 2012;28(7):488-492.

Jabbur NS, Chicani CF, Kuo IC, O'Brien TP. Risk factors in interface epithelialization after laser in situ keratomileusis. *J Refract Surg.* 2004;20(4):343-348.

Kamburoğlu G, Ertan A. Epithelial ingrowth after femtosecond laser-assisted in situ keratomileusis. *Cornea.* 2008;27(10):1122-1125.

Letko E, Price MO, Price FW Jr. Influence of original flap creation method on incidence of epithelial ingrowth after LASIK retreatment. *J Refract Surg.* 2009;25(11):1039-1041.

McAlinden C, Moore JE. Retreatment of residual refractive errors with flap lift laser in situ keratomileusis. *Eur J Ophthalmol.* 2011;21(1):5-11.

Mohamed TA, Hoffman RS, Fine IH, Packer M. Post-laser assisted in situ keratomileusis epithelial ingrowth and its relation to pretreatment refractive error. *Cornea.* 2011;30(5):550-552.

Randleman JB, Banning CS, Stulting RD. Persistent epithelial ingrowth. *Ophthalmology.* 2006;113(8):1468.

Randleman JB, Shah RD. LASIK interface complications: etiology, management, and outcomes. *J Refract Surg.* 2012;28:575-588.

Rapuano CJ. Management of epithelial ingrowth after laser in situ keratomileusis on a tertiary care cornea service. *Cornea.* 2010;29(3):307-313.

Rojas MC, Lumba JD, Manche EE. Treatment of epithelial ingrowth after laser in situ keratomileusis with mechanical debridement and flap suturing. *Arch Ophthalmol.* 2004;122(7):997-1001.

Spanggord HM, Epstein RJ, Lane HA, et al. Flap suturing with proparacaine for recurrent epithelial ingrowth following laser in situ keratomileusis surgery. *J Cataract Refract Surg.* 2005;31(5):916-921.

Wang MY, Maloney RK. Epithelial ingrowth after laser in situ keratomileusis. *Am J Ophthalmol.* 2000;129(6):746-751.

—Case 29—

A 39-year-old male complains of blurred vision bilaterally, left much worse than right, for the past 2 years. He had bilateral LASIK 5 years ago, with an original prescription of approximately -6.00 diopters in both eyes, and reported good visual acuity initially, but he experienced a gradual progressive blur approximately 1 year after LASIK. He is otherwise asymptomatic. The patient desires further refractive surgical correction, if possible.

CASE HISTORY		
	Right Eye	**Left Eye**
UDVA	20/100	20/400
Manifest refraction	-2.75 +1.00 x 145	-4.75 +1.25 x 040
CDVA (current)	20/40	20/60
Near acuity (current)	20/40	20/60
Ocular alignment	Orthophoric	Orthophoric
Keratometry		
Flat K	38.6 @ 040	39.25 @ 130
Steep K	40.2 @ 130	40.7 @ 040
Pupil size (bright)	4.7 mm	4.0 mm
Pupil size (dim)	6.8 mm	6.9 mm
Central corneal thickness	455 µm	460 µm
Physical examination	See Figure	See Figure
Estimated ablation depth	50 µm	75 µm

Questions

1. What is the most likely cause for the patient's decreased visual acuity?
2. Is this patient a candidate for further refractive surgery? If so, what treatment options are available?
3. Considering all factors, what treatment would you recommend and why?
4. What additional treatment might you recommend, in addition to your primary choice?
5. What is the likely clinical outcome, and what are reasonable treatment strategies to improve unaided visual acuity?

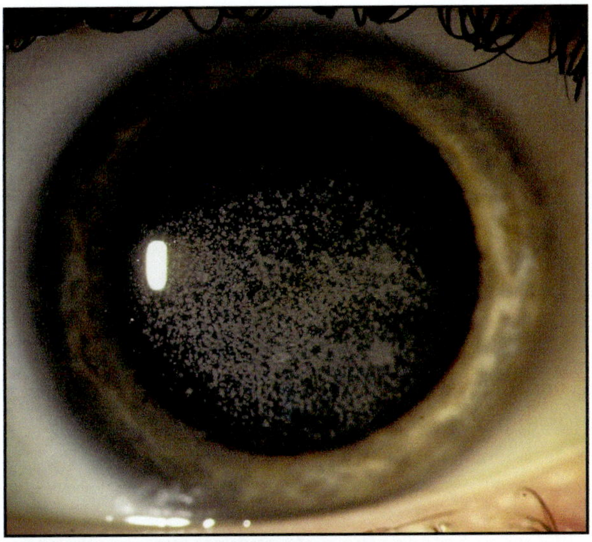

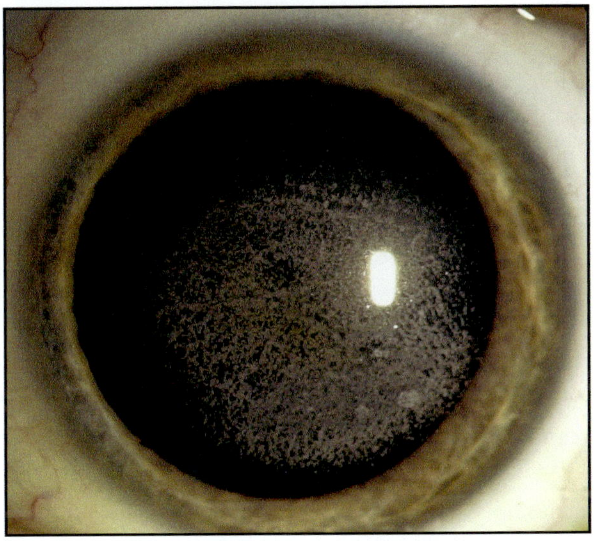

—CASE 29—
Treatment Options for Corneal Stromal Dystrophy Exacerbation After LASIK

When patients with stromal corneal dystrophies undergo LASIK, their condition usually worsens at an accelerated pace, causing significant visual disturbance that often requires aggressive management for visual rehabilitation.

Case Analysis

- Case Figures show slit-lamp photos of the right and left eyes, exhibiting dense, localized opacities in both eyes within the region of the LASIK flaps.

Pearl: *Flap amputation may improve visual acuity after corneal stromal dystrophy exacerbation: phototherapeutic keratectomy (PTK) may also be indicated, but the use of mitomycin C (MMC) is controversial!*

QUESTIONS

1. What is the most likely cause for the patient's decreased visual acuity?

   This patient exhibits findings that are consistent with a stromal corneal dystrophy (granular or Avellino variants), which is a contraindication to laser vision correction.

2. Is this patient a candidate for further refractive surgery? If so, what treatment options are available?

   No, further laser vision correction is unlikely to have any significant effect in the short-term and will likely further exacerbate the corneal opacity in the long-term for this patient.

3. Considering all factors, what treatment would you recommend and why?

   Due to the density and location of the opacity, the most logical initial step is flap amputation to debulk the opacity.

4. What additional treatment might you recommend, in addition to your primary choice?

   After flap amputation, therapeutic excimer laser ablation could be performed with or without MMC application, in an attempt to further clear the visual axis and delay the need for keratoplasty.

5. What is the likely clinical outcome, and what are reasonable treatment strategies to improve unaided visual acuity?

   The UDVA is unlikely to significantly improve, regardless of the treatment chosen. Ultimately, keratoplasty may be necessary for visual rehabilitation, but sufficient visual acuity may be obtained with the less invasive techniques mentioned previously accompanied by spectacle or contact lens wear.

Treatment Options for Stromal Corneal Dystrophy Exacerbation After Laser Vision Correction

The BIGH3 corneal stromal dystrophies are exacerbated by excimer laser ablation and are contraindications for laser vision correction (LVC); however, some patients inadvertently have had LVC and experience worsening of their visual acuity. Patients may also experience photophobia and corneal erosions from more superficial deposits. Treatment options are relatively limited when this occurs, and ultimately, keratoplasty is frequently indicated for visual rehabilitation.

Prior to keratoplasty, flap amputation with or without adjunctive PTK may improve acuity. The role of MMC is controversial in these cases. There are reports of successful treatment and reduced recurrence with MMC use; however, recent evidence suggests that functioning keratocytes are necessary to reduce keratoepithelin deposition and thereby maximize corneal clarity. Topical transforming growth factor beta antibody solutions are under investigation and may be indicated to suppress recurrence.

In the case presented herein, flap amputation with subsequent PTK left a residual stromal bed thickness < 250 μm; however, as the alternative is keratoplasty, the development of ectasia would not be as significant a complication as it otherwise might be.

Bibliography

Dogru M, Katakami C, Nishida T, Yamanaka A. Alteration of the ocular surface with recurrence of granular/avellino dystrophy after phototherapeutic keratectomy: report of five cases and literature review. *Ophthalmology.* 2001;108(4):810-817.

Han KE, Kim TI, Chung WS, Choi SI, Kim BY, Kim EK. Clinical findings and treatments of granular corneal dystrophy type 2 (Avellino corneal dystrophy): a review of the literature. *Eye Contact Lens.* 2010;36(5):296-299.

Inoue T, Watanabe H, Yamamoto S, et al. Different recurrence patterns after phototherapeutic keratectomy in the corneal dystrophy resulting from homozygous and heterozygous R124H BIG-H3 mutation. *Am J Ophthalmol.* 2001;132(2):255-257.

Kim TI, Pak JH, Chae JB, Kim EK, Tchah H. Mitomycin C inhibits recurrent Avellino dystrophy after phototherapeutic keratectomy. *Cornea.* 2006;25(2):220-223.

Lee ES, Kim EK. Surgical do's and don'ts of corneal dystrophies. Curr Opin Ophthalmol. 2003;14(4):186-191.

Moon JW, Kim SW, Kim TI, Cristol SM, Chung ES, Kim EK. Homozygous granular corneal dystrophy type II (Avellino corneal dystrophy): natural history and progression after treatment. *Cornea.* 2007;26(9):1095-1100.

—Case 30—

A 24-year-old male presents seeking options to improve his visual acuity. He had photorefractive keratectomy in both eyes 8 months earlier for approximately -8.00 diopters in both eyes. Surface ablation was performed because his "corneas weren't thick enough," per the patient. He reports initially good vision in both eyes after a few weeks of healing but gradually experienced increased blur, left worse than right. He denies pain, irritation, or other nonvisual symptoms since surgery.

CASE HISTORY		
	Right Eye	**Left Eye**
UDVA	20/100	20/400
Manifest refraction	-2.75 +1.50 x 100	-3.50 +0.75 x 095
CDVA	20/25	20/20
Cycloplegic refraction	-2.25 +1.50 x 100	-3.00 +0.75 x 095
Cycloplegic CDVA	20/25	20/20
Keratometry		
Flat K	41.75 @ 005	42.50 @ 015
Steep K	42.75 @ 095	43.75 @ 105
Central corneal thickness	450 µm	465 µm
Physical examination	See Figure	See Figure
Estimated ablation depth	45 µm	55 µm

Questions

1. What is the most likely cause for the patient's refractive error at this time point?
2. Is this patient a candidate for refractive surgery retreatment? If so, what treatment options are available?
3. Considering all factors, what treatment would you recommend and why?
4. What is the likely clinical outcome, and what are reasonable treatment strategies to improve unaided visual acuity?

A

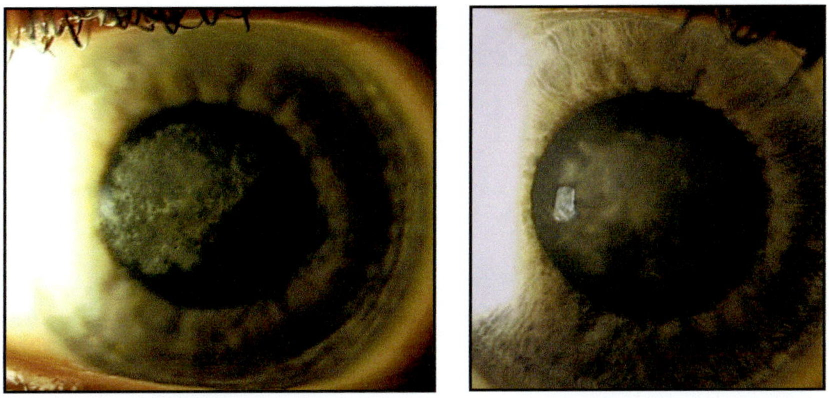

B

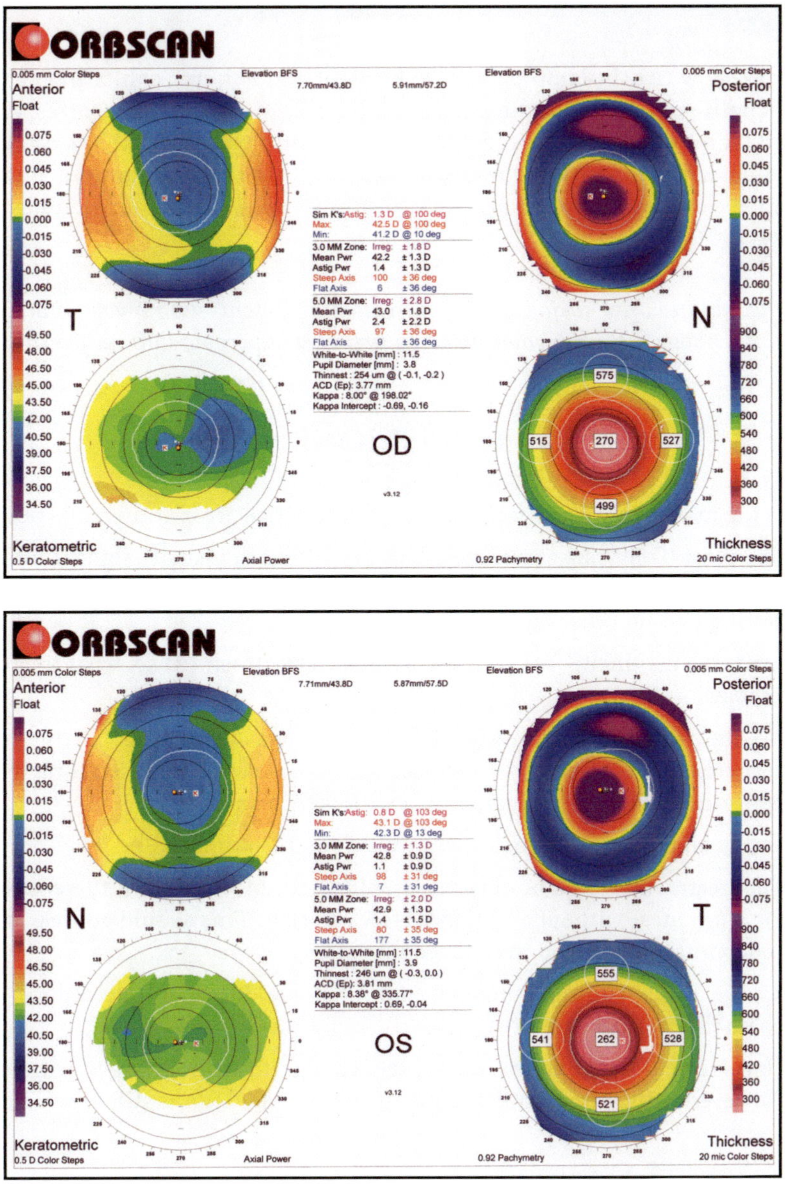
ORBSCAN
0.005 mm Color Steps
Anterior
Float
Elevation BFS
7.70mm/43.8D
5.91mm/57.2D
Elevation BFS
0.005 mm Color Steps
Posterior
Float
Sim K's:Astig: 1.3 D @ 100 deg
Max: 42.5 D @ 100 deg
Min: 41.2 D @ 10 deg
3.0 MM Zone: Irreg: ± 1.8 D
Mean Pwr 42.2 ± 1.3 D
Astig Pwr 1.4 ± 1.3 D
Steep Axis 100 ± 36 deg
Flat Axis 6 ± 36 deg
5.0 MM Zone: Irreg: ± 2.8 D
Mean Pwr 43.0 ± 1.8 D
Astig Pwr 2.4 ± 2.2 D
Steep Axis 97 ± 36 deg
Flat Axis 9 ± 36 deg
White-to-White [mm] : 11.5
Pupil Diameter [mm] : 3.8
Thinnest : 254 um @ (-0.1, -0.2)
ACD (Ep): 3.77 mm
Kappa : 8.00° @ 198.02°
Kappa Intercept : -0.69, -0.16
T
N
OD
v3.12
575
515
270
527
499
Keratometric
0.5 D Color Steps
Axial Power
0.92 Pachymetry
Thickness
20 mic Color Steps
ORBSCAN
0.005 mm Color Steps
Anterior
Float
Elevation BFS
7.71mm/43.8D
5.87mm/57.5D
Elevation BFS
0.005 mm Color Steps
Posterior
Float
Sim K's:Astig: 0.8 D @ 103 deg
Max: 43.1 D @ 103 deg
Min: 42.3 D @ 13 deg
3.0 MM Zone: Irreg: ± 1.3 D
Mean Pwr 42.8 ± 0.9 D
Astig Pwr 1.1 ± 0.9 D
Steep Axis 98 ± 31 deg
Flat Axis 7 ± 31 deg
5.0 MM Zone: Irreg: ± 2.0 D
Mean Pwr 42.9 ± 1.3 D
Astig Pwr 1.4 ± 1.5 D
Steep Axis 80 ± 35 deg
Flat Axis 177 ± 35 deg
White-to-White [mm] : 11.5
Pupil Diameter [mm] : 3.9
Thinnest : 246 um @ (-0.3, 0.0)
ACD (Ep): 3.81 mm
Kappa : 8.38° @ 335.77°
Kappa Intercept : 0.69, -0.04
N
T
OS
v3.12
555
541
262
528
521
Keratometric
0.5 D Color Steps
Axial Power
0.92 Pachymetry
Thickness
20 mic Color Steps

—Case 30—
Corneal Haze After Surface Ablation

Visually significant corneal haze after surface ablation presents most frequently after deeper ablations, especially when mitomycin C (MMC) was not used at the time of surgery. It is slightly more common in younger patients, males, and in retreatments after incisional surgery (radial keratotomy) or surface ablation.

Case Analysis

- Case Figures show (A) slit-lamp photos of the right and left eyes exhibiting dense, localized opacities in both eyes, corresponding to haze in the area of ablation. (B) Corresponding topographies exhibit minimal curvature irregularity, suggesting most visual loss is related to opacity, rather than irregularity. Note the artifactual focal thinning and elevation on the thickness and posterior elevation maps, respectively, resulting from inaccurate readings through the corneal opacity.

Pearl: *Significant haze after surface ablation frequently presents with myopic shift; however, always treat haze without further myopic ablation first or a hyperopic shift may result!*

Questions

1. What is the most likely cause for the patient's refractive error at this time point?

   The most likely cause is corneal haze, resulting in visually significant opacity, with induced myopia. Topography is only minimally irregular and CDVA is good, suggesting that no other factors are involved.

2. Is this patient a candidate for refractive surgery retreatment? If so, what treatment options are available?

   No, the patient is not a candidate for retreatment at this time. Further refractive surgery treatment is unlikely to be necessary after haze resolution. If further ablation is performed now, induced hyperopia will likely result.

3. Considering all factors, what treatment would you recommend and why?

   The treatment should be corneal scraping with MMC applied therapeutically (0.05% for 2 minutes) without additional laser ablation. This should address the haze, with concomitant reduction in induced myopia.

4. What is the likely clinical outcome, and what are reasonable treatment strategies to improve unaided visual acuity?

   Uncorrected visual acuity is unlikely to significantly improve without treatment. However, with appropriate treatment, good final UDVA is still likely and anticipated.

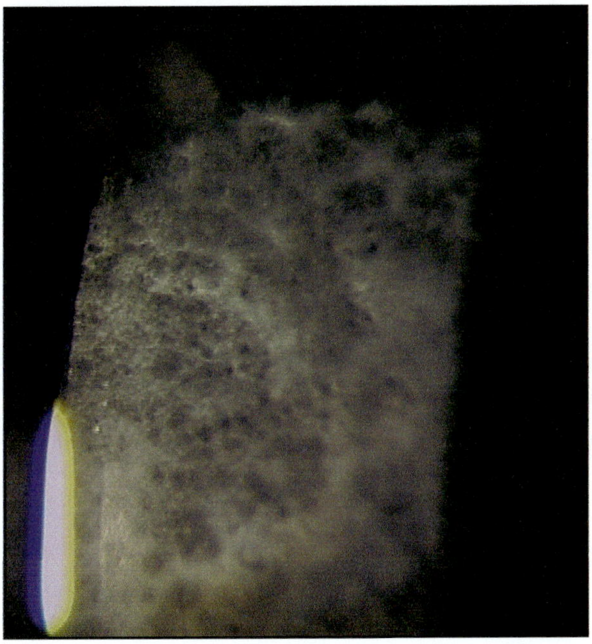

Case Figure 30-1. Slit-lamp image of the cornea under high magnification displaying typical reticulated opacification from fibroblast activity, resulting in clinically significant haze.

Corneal Haze After Surface Ablation: Etiology and Prevention

Corneal haze results from fibroblast activity after excimer laser ablation and exhibits a typical reticular pattern under high magnification (Case Figure 30-1). Subclinical haze is present in a significant number of eyes; however, most of these eyes are asymptomatic and have no measurable decrease in visual acuity. Most surgeons recommend prophylactic use of MMC for some patients undergoing surface ablation, and other surgeons use MMC for all cases, unless it is contraindicated. Time of application varies widely; the most commonly utilized dose for prophylaxis is 0.05% applied for 12 to 30 seconds. Some concerns for endothelial or limbal stem cell toxicity have been discussed, but to date there is no clear evidence that this low dose has any negative effect on the cornea or ocular surface. MMC at lower concentrations has been used, but they appear to be less effective in preventing haze development. Haze can present at any time point but is more common 3 to 9 months after surgery.

Corneal Haze: Management

Trace corneal haze is unlikely to be visually significant and does not warrant intervention. Significant haze should be treated with a therapeutic dose of MMC (usually 0.05% for 2 minutes) followed by copious irrigation of the corneal surface with balanced salt solution. Placement of a therapeutic bandage contact lens is optional. Most physicians use topical antibiotics and topical steroids postoperatively, often with an extended steroid taper. It is important to monitor intraocular pressure postoperatively.

Simultaneous ablation for myopia should not be performed, as most, if not all, haze-related myopia will resolve after treatment without ablation. If concurrent laser ablation is performed, induced hyperopia is likely to occur. After haze has resolved, and if myopia is still present, retreatment can be performed; however, the risk for recurrent haze is present. For recalcitrant cases, combined MMC and phototherapeutic keratectomy may be applied, but a resulting hyperopic shift is still likely.

Bibliography

Carones F, Vigo L, Scandola E, Vacchini L. Evaluation of the prophylactic use of mitomycin-C to inhibit haze formation after photorefractive keratectomy. *J Cataract Refract Surg.* 2002;28(12):2088-2095.

Gambato C, Ghirlando A, Moretto E, Busato F, Midena E. Mitomycin C modulation of corneal wound healing after photorefractive keratectomy in highly myopic eyes. *Ophthalmology.* 2005;112(2):208-218.

Goldsberry DH, Epstein RJ, Majmudar PA, et al. Effect of mitomycin C on the corneal endothelium when used for corneal subepithelial haze prophylaxis following photorefractive keratectomy. *J Refract Surg.* 2007;23(7):724-727.

Lee DH, Chung HS, Jeon YC, Boo SD, Yoon YD, Kim JG. Photorefractive keratectomy with intraoperative mitomycin-C application. *J Cataract Refract Surg.* 2005;31(12):2293-2298.

Majmudar PA, Forstot SL, Dennis RF, et al. Topical mitomycin-C for subepithelial fibrosis after refractive corneal surgery. *Ophthalmology.* 2000;107(1):89-94.

Nassaralla BA, McLeod SD, Nassaralla JJ Jr. Prophylactic mitomycin C to inhibit corneal haze after photorefractive keratectomy for residual myopia following radial keratotomy. *J Refract Surg.* 2007;23(3):226-232.

Porges Y, Ben-Haim O, Hirsh A, Levinger S. Phototherapeutic keratectomy with mitomycin C for corneal haze following photorefractive keratectomy for myopia. *J Refract Surg.* 2003;19(1):40-43.

Shalaby A, Kaye GB, Gimbel HV. Mitomycin C in photorefractive keratectomy. *J Refract Surg.* 2009;25:S93-7

Srinivasan S, Drake A, Herzig S. Photorefractive keratectomy with 0.02% mitomycin C for treatment of residual refractive errors after LASIK. *J Refract Surg.* 2008;24(1 Suppl):S64-S67.

Thornton I, Xu M, Krueger RR. Comparison of standard (0.02%) and low dose (0.002%) mitomycin C in the prevention of corneal haze following surface ablation for myopia. *J Refract Surg.* 2008;24(1 Suppl):S68-S.6

Virasch VV, Majmudar PA, Epstein RJ, Vaidya NS, Dennis RF. Reduced application time for prophylactic mitomycin C in photorefractive keratectomy. *Ophthalmology.* 2010;117(5):885-889.

—Case 31—

A 31-year-old female presents seeking options to improve visual acuity in her right eye. She had LASIK in both eyes 12 weeks prior for an original prescription of -6.25 +2.25 x 090 in the right eye and -6.00 +2.00 x 090 in the left eye. Surgery was performed with a mechanical microkeratome with a planned 120-μm flap and nasal hinge. She reports blurred vision in the right eye since surgery, improving over the first few weeks and then stabilizing to its current level. She reports no problems with the left eye.

CASE HISTORY		
	Right Eye	**Left Eye**
UDVA	20/30	20/20
Manifest refraction	-0.75 +0.75 x 005	Plano
CDVA	20/25	20/15
Cycloplegic refraction	-0.75 +0.75 x 005	Plano
Cycloplegic CDVA	20/25	20/15
Keratometry		
Flat K	37.75 @ 015	38.5 @ 005
Steep K	39.25 @ 105	39.0 @ 095
Central corneal thickness	460 μm	480 μm
Physical examination	Normal	Normal
Estimated ablation depth	15 μm	N/A

Questions

1. What are the most likely causes for this patient's refractive error at this time point?
2. Is this patient a candidate for refractive surgery retreatment? If so, what treatment options are available?
3. What is the best course of treatment at this juncture to improve this patient's vision?
4. What is the next intervention if your first treatment is not successful?
5. What is the primary concern for this patient if she is not treated appropriately?

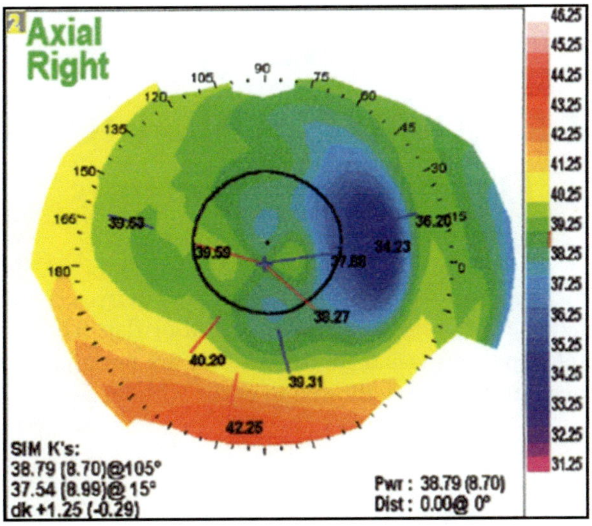
2
Axial
Right
SIM K's:
38.79 (8.70)@105°
37.54 (8.99)@ 15°
dk +1.25 (-0.29)
Pwr : 38.79 (8.70)
Dist : 0.00@ 0°
39.59
38.27
40.20
39.31
42.25
34.23
36.20
46.25
45.25
44.25
43.25
42.25
41.25
40.25
39.25
38.25
37.25
36.25
35.25
34.25
33.25
32.25
31.25

—Case 31—

Irregular Ablations

Decentered Ablations

Irregular astigmatism may result from irregular ablation patterns, especially when the ablation is functionally decentered in relation to the visual axis and/or flap. These irregular ablation patterns can have significant impact on visual acuity, but they are nonprogressive and may partially resolve over time if corneal remodeling is allowed to occur without further ablation.

Case Analysis

- Case Figure shows corneal topography of the right eye, demonstrating significant focal irregularity with peripheral flattening at the 3-o'clock meridian and a central bowtie pattern.

Pearl: *Irregular astigmatism may arise from decentered ablations or functionally decentered flaps, even with modern tracking device; therefore, surgeon-directed patient centering is key!*

Questions

1. What are the most likely causes for this patient's refractive error at this time point?

   This patient has predominantly irregular astigmatism resulting in reduced UDVA and CDVA, despite minimal refractive error.

2. Is this patient a candidate for refractive surgery retreatment? If so, what treatment options are available?

   No, the patient is not a candidate for refractive surgery treatment at this time. Irregular astigmatism is not amenable to treatment with conventional, optimized, or wavefront-guided ablation algorithms, and early in the postoperative course, natural corneal remodeling may minimize the ultimate irregularity.

3. What is the best course of treatment at this juncture to improve this patient's vision?

   Observation is the best course of action to allow for remodeling.

4. What is the next intervention if your first treatment is not successful?

   Depending on the patient's final status, topography-guided ablation may be of some benefit in regularizing the corneal curvature, thereby improving CDVA and possibly UDVA.

5. What is primary concern for this patient if she is not treated appropriately?

   Because this patient's problem represents a nonprogressive irregular astigmatism, there is no added long-term concern with or without intervention. However, if repeat ablation is performed too early in the postoperative course increased irregular astigmatism may result.

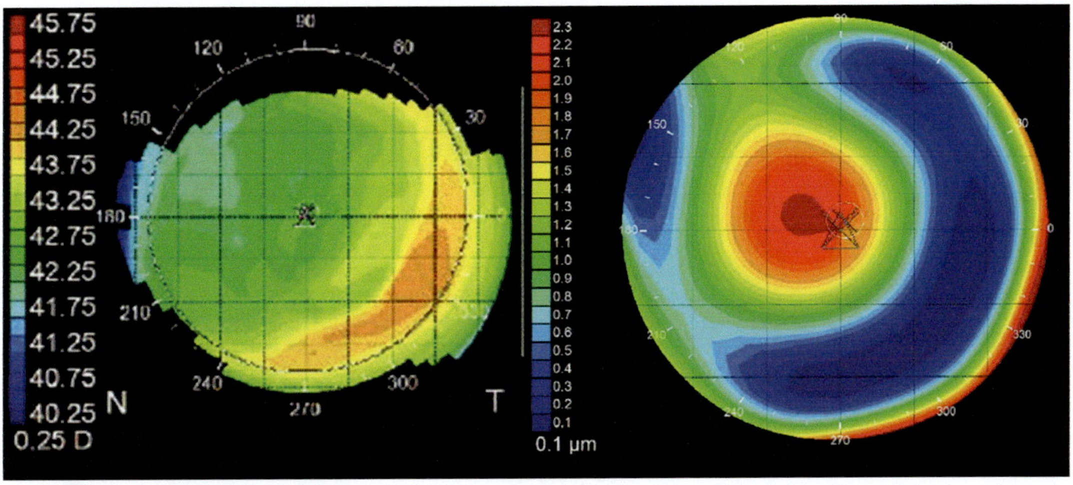

Case Figure 31-1. Composite image showing topography (left) and wavefront profile (right) maps demonstrating an arc of paracentral steepening from the 2-o'clock to the 7-o'clock meridians, with corresponding alterations to the wavefront profile.

Irregular Astigmatism After Laser Vision Correction

Irregular ablation patterns can occur if the patient's centration is suboptimal, even with modern laser tracking systems. Irregular ablations can also occur with well-centered ablations if the flaps are decentered, causing the ablation to either fall outside of the exposed stromal bed onto the epithelium (which will ultimately heal and reverse any ablation performed on it) (Case Figure 31-1) or, if the backside of the flap is ablated, usually around the hinge, resulting in a double ablation to that specific area (flap underside and exposed stroma) (see Case Figure). With well-centered flaps, hyperopic and astigmatic ablations are more likely to result in flap hinge ablation, as these ablations are peripheral in nature. Hyperopic treatments (Case Figure 31-2) are more sensitive to decentration, as the functional optical zone is smaller than after myopic treatment (Case Figure 31-3).

Decentered ablations from the aforementioned causes can result in monocular diplopia, or they can increase higher-order aberrations and reduce functional visual acuity, even when Snellen acuity is unaffected.

When the flap is involved or if treatment has occurred on the epithelium, subsequent treatment should be delayed until steady, consistent topographic findings and refractions are obtained, as the effect of the ablation will vary over time (and usually improve) until all remodeling is complete.

Topography-guided ablation is still being investigated in terms of its utility in improving subtle curvature irregularities, such as the case presented here. Other patterns, including optical zone decentration, small optical zones, and subtle central island patterns, may be appropriate for topography-guided treatment. If significant irregularity persists, rigid contact lenses may be needed for best visual acuity.

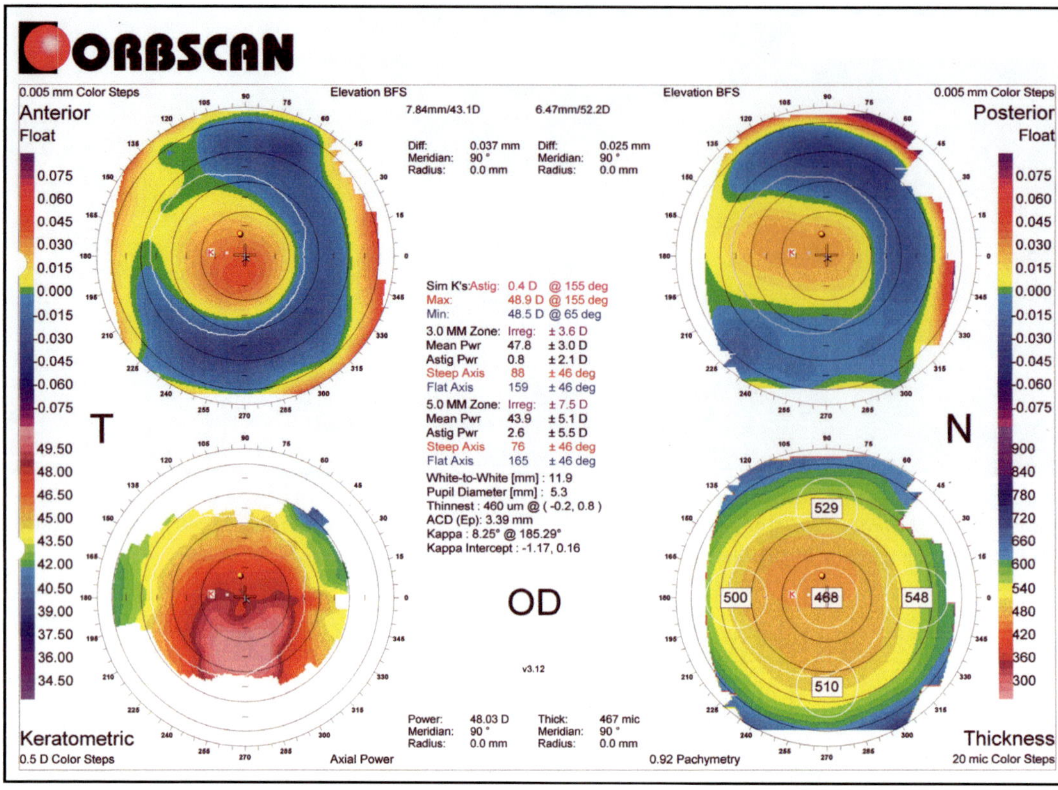

Case Figure 31-2. Topography after hyperopic ablation. The steepest point is marginally decentered, but the effect on visual acuity is dramatic due to the functionally small optical zone.

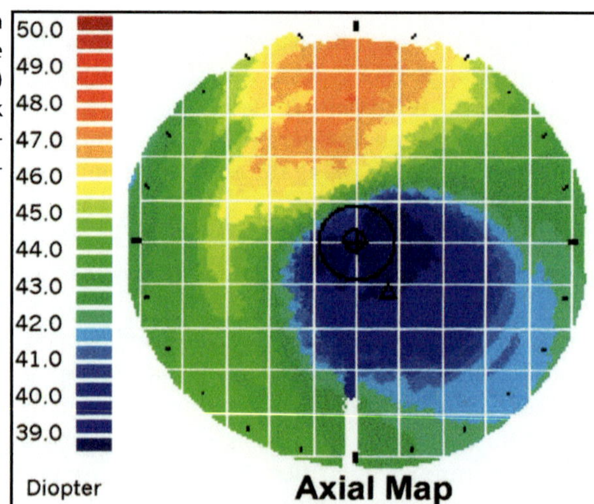

Case Figure 31-3. Topography showing an area of area of flattening, extending from the upper edge of the measured pupil (black circle) toward the paracentral cornea in the 4-o'clock meridian, corresponding to a mildly decentered myopic ablation. The patient had minimal symptoms from this decentration.

Bibliography

Chalita MR, Chavala S, Xu M, Krueger RR. Wavefront analysis in post-LASIK eyes and its correlation with visual symptoms, refraction, and topography. *Ophthalmology.* 2004;111(3):447-153.

Chalita MR, Roth AS, Krueger RR. Wavefront-guided surface ablation with prophylactic use of mitomycin C after a buttonhole laser in situ keratomileusis flap. *J Refract Surg.* 2004;20(2):176-181.

Chalita MR, Xu M, Krueger RR. Correlation of aberrations with visual symptoms using wavefront analysis in eyes after laser in situ keratomileusis. *J Refract Surg.* 2003;19(6):S682-S686.

Gatinel D, Bains HS. Treatment of highly aberrated eyes using the NIDEK CXIII excimer laser. *J Refract Surg.* 2010;26(6):453-457.

Jankov MR II, Panagopoulou SI, Tsiklis NS, Hajitanasis GC, Aslanides M, Pallikaris G. Topography-guided treatment of irregular astigmatism with the wavelight excimer laser. *J Refract Surg.* 2006;22(4):335-344.

Melamud A, Chalita MR, Krueger RR, Lee MS. Comatic aberration as a cause of monocular diplopia. *J Cataract Refract Surg.* 2006;32(3):529-532.

Mrochen M, Krueger RR, Bueeler M, Seiler T. Aberration-sensing and wavefront-guided laser in situ keratomileusis: management of decentered ablation. *J Refract Surg.* 2002;18(4):418-429.

Randleman JB. Etiology and clinical presentations of irregular astigmatism after keratorefractive surgery. In: Wang M, ed. *Irregular Astigmatism: Diagnosis and Treatment.* Thorofare, NJ:. SLACK Incorporated; 2007:79-90.

Takei K, Sano Y, Achiron LR, et al. Monocular diplopia related to asymmetric corneal topography after laser in situ keratomileusis. *J Refract Surg.* 2001;17(6):652-657.

Tan G, Chen X, Xie RZ, et al. Reverse geometry rigid gas permeable contact lens wear reduces high-order aberrations and the associated symptoms in post-LASIK patients. *Curr Eye Res.* 2010;35(1):9-16.

—Case 32—

A 42-year-old male presents seeking options to improve his visual acuity. He had LASIK in both eyes 1 year prior for an original prescription of -6.25 +0.50 x 010 in the right eye and -5.75 sphere in the left eye. Surgery was performed using a femtosecond laser for flap creation, with a planned 110-µm flap with a superior hinge and a wavefront-guided ablation. He reports blurred vision in both eyes from the first postoperative day, which has changed little over time. He denies pain, irritation, or other nonvisual symptoms since surgery.

Case History		
	Right Eye	**Left Eye**
UDVA	20/70	20/60
Manifest refraction	-1.50 +0.50 x 075	-1.00 +0.75 x 010
CDVA	20/40	20/30
Cycloplegic refraction	-1.50 +0.50 x 075	-1.00 +0.75 x 010
Cycloplegic CDVA	20/40	20/30
Keratometry		
Flat K	40.0 @ 020	39.5 @ 015
Steep K	41.25 @ 110	40.5 @ 105
Central corneal thickness	470 µm	460 µm
Physical examination	Normal	Normal
Estimated ablation depth	30 µm	30 µm

Questions

1. What is the most likely cause for the patient's refractive error at this time point?
2. Is this patient a candidate for refractive surgery retreatment? If so, what treatment options are available?
3. What additional testing may be useful to help determine your course of action?
4. What is the best course of treatment at this juncture to improve this patient's vision?
5. What is primary concern for this patient if he is not treated appropriately?

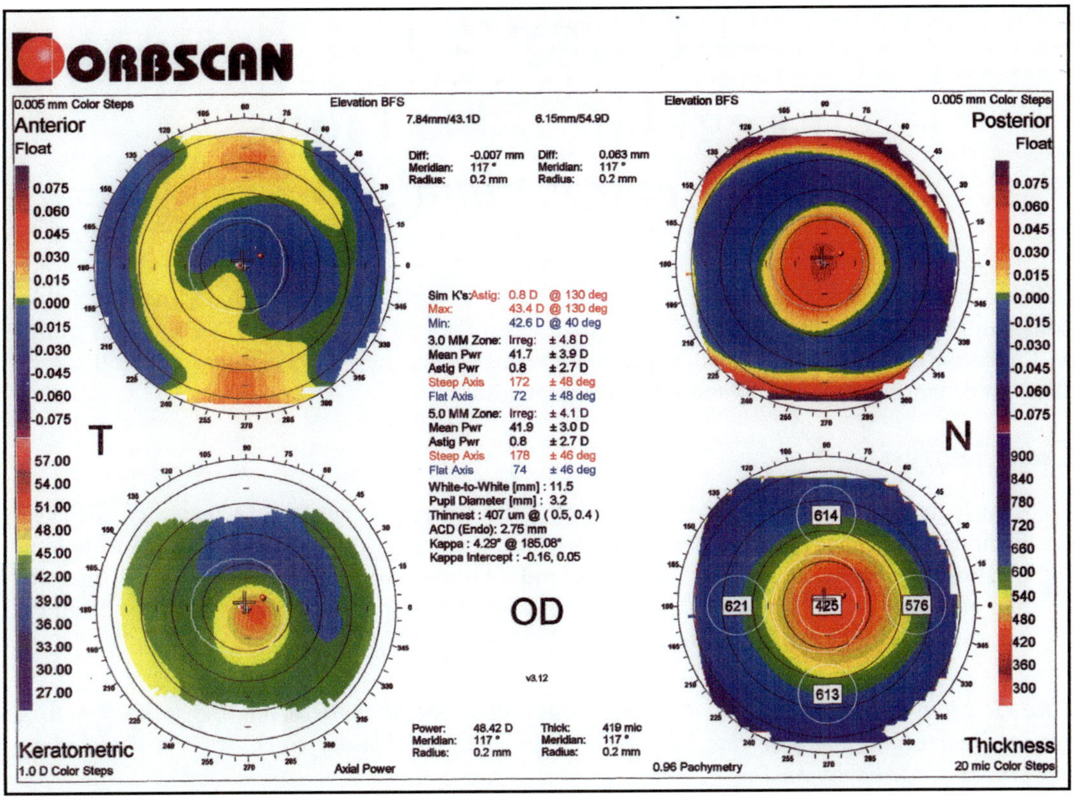
ORBSCAN
0.005 mm Color Steps
Anterior
Float
Elevation BFS
7.84mm/43.1D
6.15mm/54.9D
Elevation BFS
0.005 mm Color Steps
Posterior
Float
Diff: -0.007 mm
Meridian: 117°
Radius: 0.2 mm
Diff: 0.063 mm
Meridian: 117°
Radius: 0.2 mm
Sim K's:Astig: 0.8 D @ 130 deg
Max: 43.4 D @ 130 deg
Min: 42.6 D @ 40 deg
3.0 MM Zone: Irreg: ± 4.8 D
Mean Pwr 41.7 ± 3.9 D
Astig Pwr 0.8 ± 2.7 D
Steep Axis 172 ± 48 deg
Flat Axis 72 ± 48 deg
5.0 MM Zone: Irreg: ± 4.1 D
Mean Pwr 41.9 ± 3.0 D
Astig Pwr 0.8 ± 2.7 D
Steep Axis 178 ± 46 deg
Flat Axis 74 ± 46 deg
White-to-White [mm] : 11.5
Pupil Diameter [mm] : 3.2
Thinnest : 407 um @ (0.5, 0.4)
ACD (Endo): 2.75 mm
Kappa : 4.29° @ 185.08°
Kappa Intercept : -0.16, 0.05
T
N
OD
614
621
425
576
613
v3.12
Power: 48.42 D
Meridian: 117°
Radius: 0.2 mm
Thick: 419 mic
Meridian: 117°
Radius: 0.2 mm
Keratometric
1.0 D Color Steps
Axial Power
0.96 Pachymetry
Thickness
20 mic Color Steps

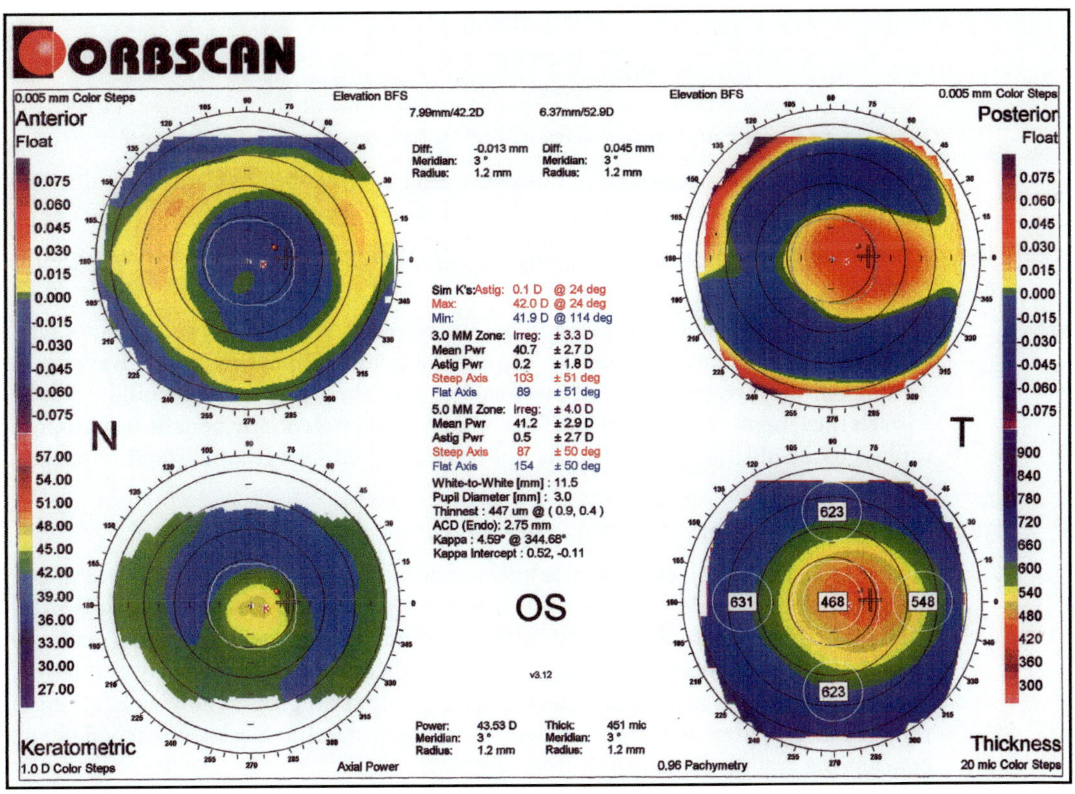
ORBSCAN
0.005 mm Color Steps
Anterior
Float
Elevation BFS
7.99mm/42.2D
6.37mm/52.9D
Elevation BFS
0.005 mm Color Steps
Posterior
Float
Diff: -0.013 mm
Meridian: 3°
Radius: 1.2 mm
Diff: 0.045 mm
Meridian: 3°
Radius: 1.2 mm
Sim K's:Astig: 0.1 D @ 24 deg
Max: 42.0 D @ 24 deg
Min: 41.9 D @ 114 deg
3.0 MM Zone: Irreg: ± 3.3 D
Mean Pwr 40.7 ± 2.7 D
Astig Pwr 0.2 ± 1.8 D
Steep Axis 103 ± 51 deg
Flat Axis 89 ± 51 deg
5.0 MM Zone: Irreg: ± 4.0 D
Mean Pwr 41.2 ± 2.9 D
Astig Pwr 0.5 ± 2.7 D
Steep Axis 87 ± 50 deg
Flat Axis 154 ± 50 deg
White-to-White [mm] : 11.5
Pupil Diameter [mm] : 3.0
Thinnest : 447 um @ (0.9, 0.4)
ACD (Endo): 2.75 mm
Kappa : 4.59° @ 344.68°
Kappa Intercept : 0.52, -0.11
N
T
OS
623
631
468
548
623
v3.12
Power: 43.53 D
Meridian: 3°
Radius: 1.2 mm
Thick: 451 mic
Meridian: 3°
Radius: 1.2 mm
Keratometric
1.0 D Color Steps
Axial Power
0.96 Pachymetry
Thickness
20 mic Color Steps

—Case 32—
Irregular Ablations
Central Islands

Fortunately, central islands are rare due to the use of modern flying spot excimer laser ablations, but they can be highly visually significant when they do occur. Central islands may mimic postoperative ectasia topographically on first appearance, but they are nonprogressive and carry a different prognosis and optimal management strategies.

Case Analysis

- Case Figures show scanning slit-beam topographic images of the right (OD) and left (OS) eyes demonstrating focal central steepening within a central region of flattening (from myopic ablation), resulting in a classic "central island" pattern. Note the artifactual focal thinning and elevation on the thickness and posterior elevation maps, respectively, resulting from the optical aberrations generated from the focal central steepening.

Pearl: *Many irregular patterns after laser vision correction are not ectasia; they indicate non-progressive irregular ablations that have different prognoses and management strategies, including topography-guided ablations!*

Questions

1. What is the most likely cause for the patient's refractive error at this time point?

   Central islands have occurred in both eyes after excimer laser ablation, resulting in significant irregular astigmatism.

2. Is this patient a candidate for refractive surgery retreatment? If so, what treatment options are available?

   This patient is probably not a candidate for retreatment. The irregular component of the refraction is not amenable to "regular" ablation with conventional, wavefront-optimized, or wavefront-guided approaches, and these approaches could actually worsen the irregular astigmatism. This patient could potentially benefit from topography-guided ablation in the future, but refractive and topographic stability need to be confirmed first.

3. What additional testing may be useful to help determine your course of action?

   Given the artifactual corneal thickness reading from the scanning-slit images, another method would be optimal to confirm that no significant thinning is present. This can be accomplished with ultrasound pachymetry measurements centrally and regionally or Scheimpflug imaging or optical coherence tomography evaluation. Serial topography is also useful, to both confirm that no progression is occurring if the diagnosis is in question and to determine when stability has been reached before considering any further surgical intervention.

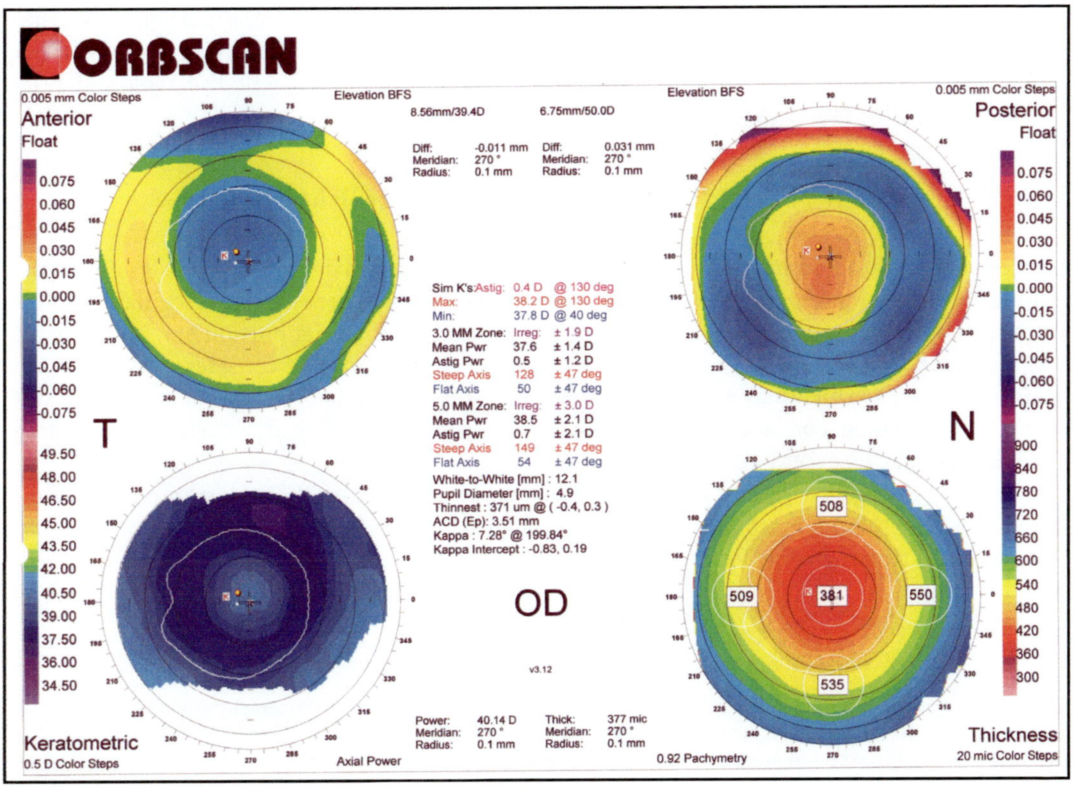

Case Figure 32-1. Scanning slit-beam image demonstrating focal central steepening within a central region of flattening (from myopic ablation), resulting in a "central island" pattern.

4. What is the best course of treatment at this juncture to improve this patient's vision?

   Because manifest refraction is minimally effectual in this case, fitting of rigid gas permeable contact lenses is the most likely option to improve visual acuity.

5. What is primary concern for this patient if he is not treated appropriately?

   Although the patient's visual acuity will not improve until he receives further treatment, there is no additional concern over a delay in treatment because the occurrence of central islands is a nonprogressive issue. However, if the patient is mistakenly diagnosed with postoperative corneal ectasia, visual acuity could worsen from incorrect intervention.

Central Islands: Etiology and Avoidance

Central island patterns (Case Figures and Case Figure 32-1) may occur secondary to use of broad-beam lasers treating in a nonhomogenous manner, central blockage of the laser treatment by laser plume, the central accumulation of fluid on the cornea, or, occasionally, as a result of substances on the laser head itself blocking the appropriate laser beam profile. The utilization of flying spot lasers and improved plume evacuation has significantly reduced the incidence of central island formation; however, they can still occur.

Avoidance is by far the best strategy for the management of central islands. To that end, surgeons must be diligent in ensuring proper functioning of the equipment they use, including paying careful attention to laser calibration and maintenance records. During surgery, careful attention must be paid to the surgical field and laser head at all times, ensuring that no fluid splash or other events alter the ablation pattern. Consistency in surgical technique will minimize variations that could affect outcomes through varying corneal hydration states, and it will also avoid potential fluid build up in the laser field during ablation.

Central Islands: Management

If central islands do occur, observation is a necessary first step to determine how significant the irregularity will ultimately be, as corneal remodeling may partially reverse the irregular topography. If significant refractive error occurs with central islands, the regular portion may be amenable to retreatment. In less steep islands, topography-guided ablation may be considered to regularize focal irregularities, which may improve uncorrected visual acuity, spectacle visual acuity, or soft contact lens tolerance. For more advanced irregularity, some form of rigid contact lens, including scleral lenses, may be necessary to restore visual acuity.

It bears repeating that central islands are in no way biomechanically similar to postoperative ectasia. Thus, there is no mechanistic basis to consider corneal collagen cross-linking or insertion of intracorneal ring segments for these cases.

Bibliography

Chen X, Stojanovic A, Zhou W, Utheim TP, Stojanovic F, Wang Q. Transepithelial, topography-guided ablation in the treatment of visual disturbances in LASIK flap or interface complications. *J Refract Surg.* 2012;28(2):120-126.

Cua IY, Pepose JS. Proper positioning of the plume evacuator in the VISX Star3 excimer laser minimizes central island formation in patients undergoing laser in situ keratomileusis. *J Refract Surg.* 2003;19(3):309-315.

Ghoreishi M, Naderi Beni A, Naderi Beni Z. Visual outcomes of topography-guided excimer laser surgery for treatment of patients with irregular astigmatism [published online ahead of print February 24, 2013]. *Lasers Med Sci.*

Hafezi F, Jankov M, Mrochen M, Wüllner C, Seiler T. Customized ablation algorithm for the treatment of steep central islands after refractive laser surgery. *J Cataract Refract Surg.* 2006;32(5):717-721.

Johnson JD, Azar DT. Surgically induced topographical abnormalities after LASIK: management of central islands, corneal ectasia, decentration, and irregular astigmatism. *Curr Opin Ophthalmol.* 2001;12(4):309-317.

Knorz MC, Jendritza B. Topographically-guided laser in situ keratomileusis to treat corneal irregularities. *Ophthalmology.* 2000;107(6):1138-1143.

McCormick GJ, Porter J, Cox IG, MacRae S. Higher-order aberrations in eyes with irregular corneas after laser refractive surgery. *Ophthalmology.* 2005;112(10):1699-1709.

Randleman JB. Etiology and clinical presentations of irregular astigmatism after keratorefractive surgery. In: Wang M, ed. *Irregular Astigmatism: Diagnosis and Treatment.* Thorofare, NJ: SLACK Incorporated; 2007:79-90.

Toda I, Yamamoto T, Ito M, Hori-Komai Y, Tsubota K. Topography-guided ablation for treatment of patients with irregular astigmatism. *J Refract Surg.* 2007;23(2):118-125.

—Case 33—

A 31-year-old male desires refractive surgical correction in his right eye. He had LASIK 2.5 years ago, with an original prescription of -7.50 +2.50 x 080 in the right eye and -6.75 +2.00 x 065 in the left eye. He reports good visual acuity in both eyes initially but experienced a gradual decrease in vision in the right eye for the past 6 months.

CASE HISTORY		
	Right Eye	**Left Eye**
UDVA	20/40	20/20
Manifest refraction	-2.00 +1.50 x 150	Plano
CDVA	20/25	20/20
Cycloplegic refraction	-2.00 +1.50 x 150	Plano
Cycloplegic CDVA	20/25	20/20
Keratometry		
Flat K	36.80 @ 045	37.2 @ 165
Steep K	38.9 @ 135	38.1 @ 075
Central corneal thickness	422 μm	425 μm
Physical examination	Normal	Normal
Estimated ablation depth	30 μm	N/A

Questions

1. What are the most likely causes for the patient's refractive error at this time point after LASIK?
2. Is this patient a candidate for refractive surgery retreatment? If so, what treatment options are available?
3. What additional testing may be useful to help determine your course of action?

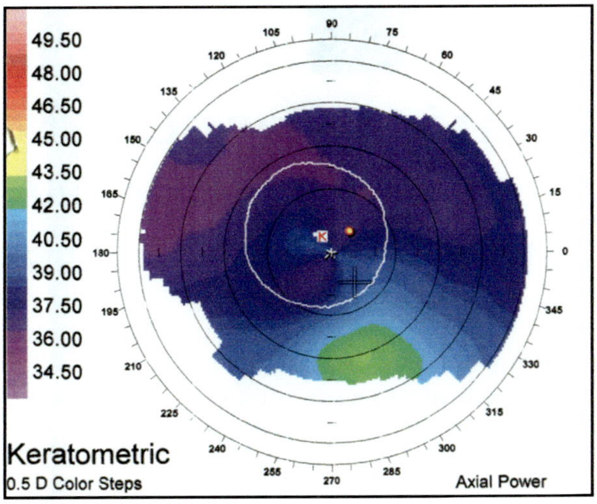
49.50
48.00
46.50
45.00
43.50
42.00
40.50
39.00
37.50
36.00
34.50
Keratometric
0.5 D Color Steps
Axial Power

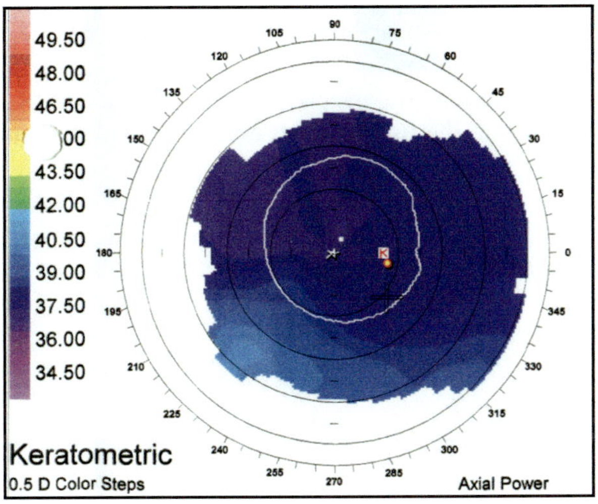
49.50
48.00
46.50
43.50
42.00
40.50
39.00
37.50
36.00
34.50
Keratometric
0.5 D Color Steps
Axial Power

—Case 33—

Postoperative Corneal Ectasia

Early Manifestations and Initial Management Considerations

Astigmatism after LASIK can be due to residual ametropia or, theoretically, can occur because of regression; however, this case is suspicious for postoperative corneal ectasia, especially when irregular astigmatism is noted, presenting clinically as reduced CDVA.

Case Analysis

- Estimated residual stromal bed thickness is approximately 270 μm in the right eye (assuming a flap of 120 μm).
- Case Figures show suspicious topographic patterns after myopic LASIK, with inferior steepening and skewed radial axis in the right eye and mild inferior steepening in the far periphery in the left eye.

Pearl: *Beware of early ectasia in patients presenting for retreatment after LASIK, especially in eyes with increasing astigmatism or eyes that do not correct to 20/20!*

Questions

1. What are the most likely causes for the patient's refractive error at this time point after LASIK?

    In young patients with normal corrected distance visual acuity, pachymetry, and topographic pattern, the change in refraction could indicate simple regression. In older patients, cataract formation could also induce these findings, including reduced best-corrected visual acuity. However, when these findings are accompanied by abnormal topography, postoperative ectasia must be ruled out before considering any further refractive surgery.

2. Is this patient a candidate for refractive surgery retreatment? If so, what treatment options are available for this patient?

    No, this patient is not a candidate for retreatment at this time. The patient has significant astigmatism, which has developed in the past few months per the patient's report, and does not correct to 20/20, signifying there is a component of irregular astigmatism. These findings and the accompanying topographic image with inferior steepening are suspicious for early postoperative ectasia.

3. What additional testing may be useful to help determine your course of action?

   Preoperative and, ideally, early postoperative records, especially topographies, would be helpful to determine the net change in pattern and to identify the cause for this change. With early ectatic changes, it is important to compare the steepest areas postoperatively with the preoperative maps to determine actual postoperative steepening, as opposed to "pseudosteepening" from mapping an area that was outside the laser ablation zone and thus has retained its preoperative curvature.

Distinguishing Postoperative Ectasia From Regression Before Retreatment

For all patients presenting for potential retreatment after laser vision correction, early postoperative corneal ectasia or other reasons for ametropia, other than refractive regression, including cataract development, must be first ruled out. Careful evaluation of postoperative corneal topography is necessary, as topographic patterns exhibiting steepening with corresponding thinning are concerning, and comparison to preoperative topographies is essential to determine the actual focal corneal shape changes in these eyes. Difference maps can be especially helpful when the data are available (Case Figures 33-1 and 33-2). If the initial surgery was performed elsewhere, some data files may be extracted to facilitate creating difference maps. In other cases, manual comparison of images will be necessary (Case Figure 33-3). In contrast, pseudosteepening patterns can appear concerning (Case Figure 33-4) until they are compared with preoperative topographies (Case Figure 33-5).

Postoperative Ectasia: Initial Management Considerations

In the past, postoperative ectasia was challenging to manage when it occurred, as the primary measures available included spectacles use or gas permeable contact lenses wear, followed by corneal transplantation when necessary. However, now there are numerous treatment strategies available. The primary goal is to halt the ectatic process and stabilize the cornea, to both prevent worsening and provide options for ultimate visual rehabilitation. Some authors have advocated the early use of intraocular pressure-lowering medications, but this has yet to be validated as successful in the long or short term.

Insertion of intracorneal ring segments is approved for use in the United States for keratoconus, and they have been used off-label for postoperative corneal ectasia. They may have some efficacy in stabilizing the cornea, and, in some instances, reduce refractive error. However, in cases where astigmatism is the primary refractive error, they are less useful.

The cornerstone of all future treatments for ectasia is corneal collagen cross-linking early on to prevent significant corneal warpage. If the patient does not opt for treatment at this time, close follow-up is warranted to monitor for any progression and to intervene as early as possible to prevent further corneal warpage.

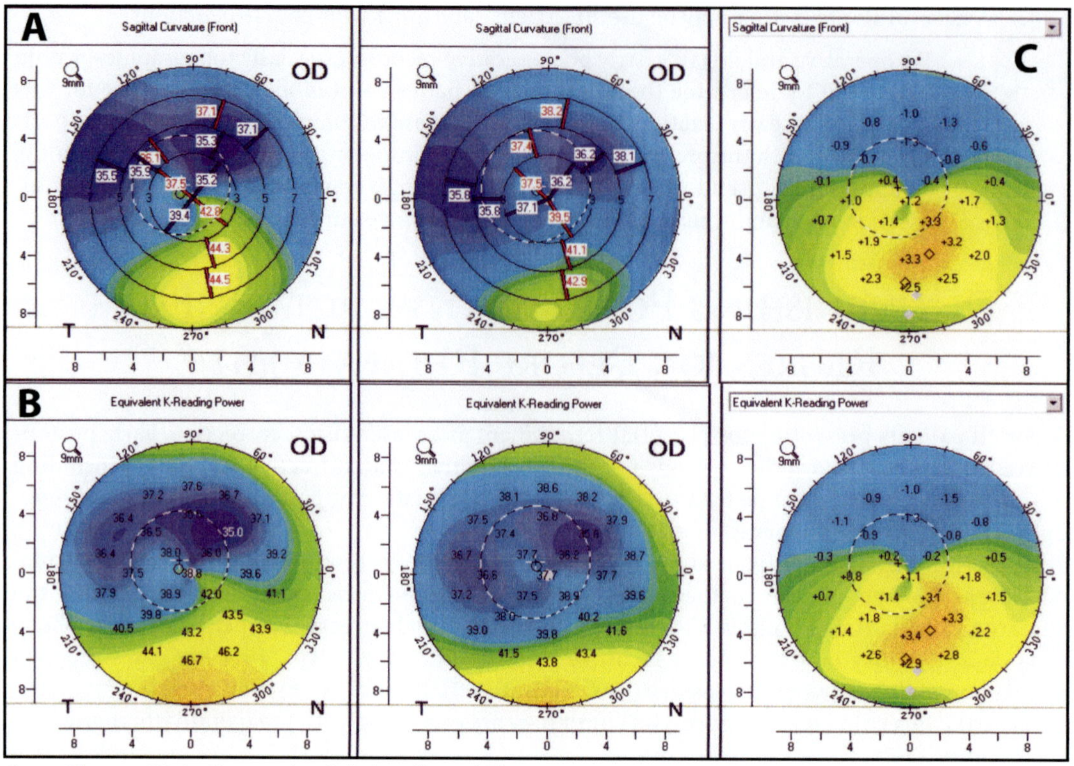

Case Figure 33-1. Composite Scheimpflug difference map image demonstrating increasing postoperative corneal curvature based on (A) sagittal curvature (upper images) and (B) equivalent keratometry powers (lower images). (C) Images on the far right of the image depict the difference map, demonstrating increasing steepening over time. (Modified and reprinted with permission from Randleman JB, Woodward MA. Evaluation and diagnosis of postoperative corneal ectasia. In: Hafezi F, Randleman JB [eds]. *Corneal Collagen Cross Linking*. Thorofare, NJ: SLACK Incorporated; 2013:31-38.)

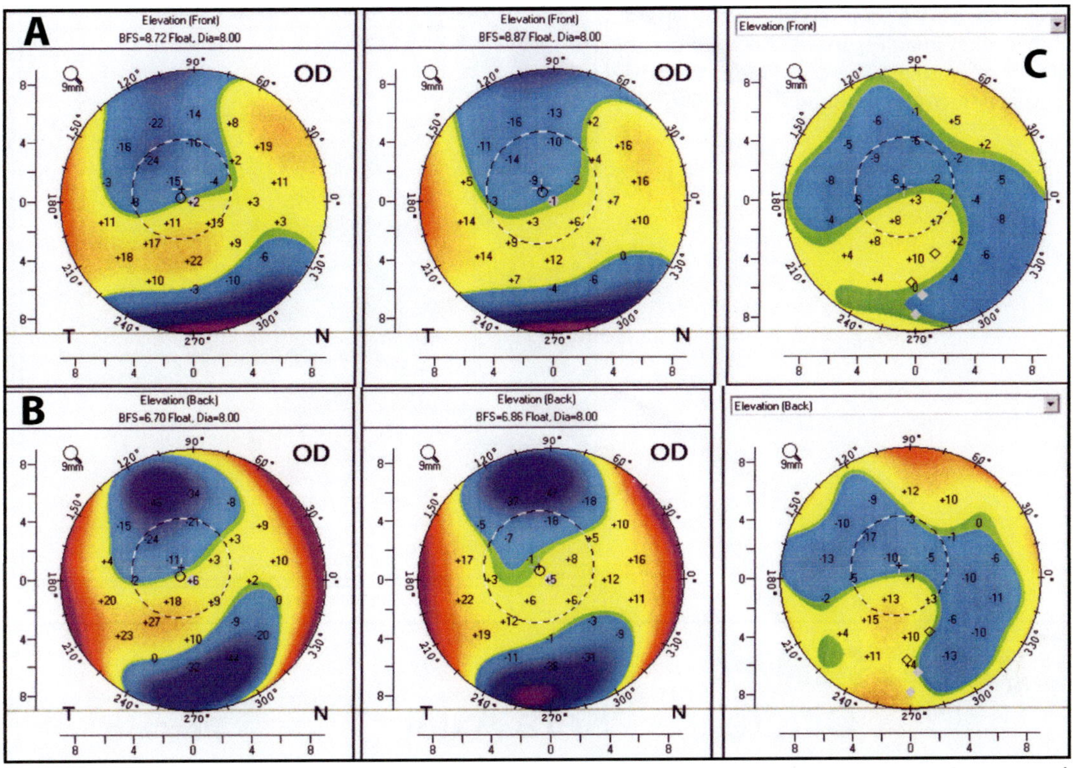

Case Figure 33-2. Composite Scheimpflug difference map image demonstrating increasing corneal elevation based on (A) front elevation (upper images) and (B) back elevation (lower images) maps. (C) Images on the far right of the image depict the difference map, demonstrating increasing focal front and back elevation over time. (Modified and reprinted with permission from Randleman JB, Woodward MA. Evaluation and diagnosis of postoperative corneal ectasia. In: Hafezi F, Randleman JB [eds]. *Corneal Collagen Cross Linking*. Thorofare, NJ: SLACK Incorporated; 2013:31-38.)

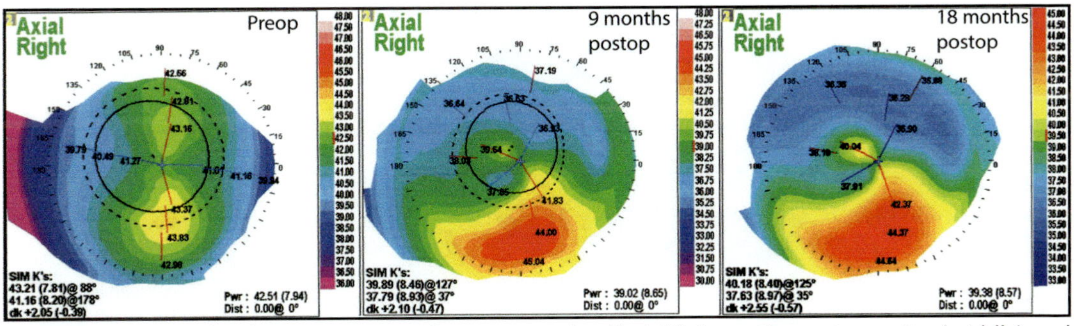

Case Figure 33-3. Placido images comparing preoperative (far left), 9 months postoperative (middle), and 18 months postoperative (far right) patterns. Note the increasing inferior steepening in the postoperative images, which are steeper than the corresponding region preoperatively and worsening over time.

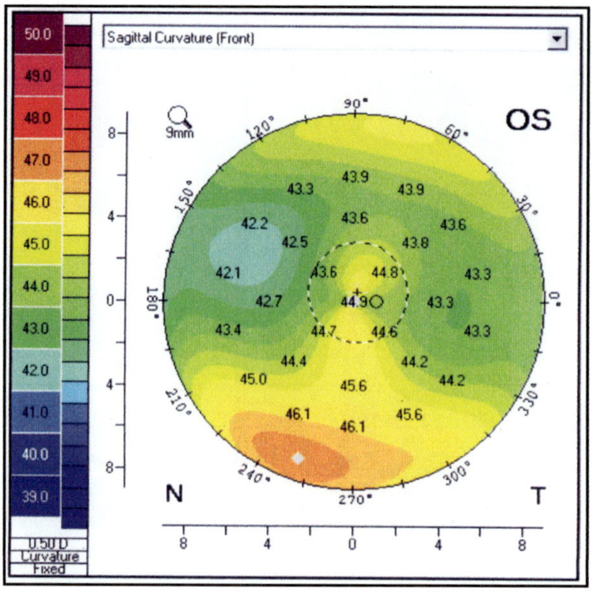

Case Figure 33-4. Sagittal curvature map from Scheimpflug imaging after LASIK with notable inferior steepening. This could indicate corneal ectasia, or it could be pseudosteepening.

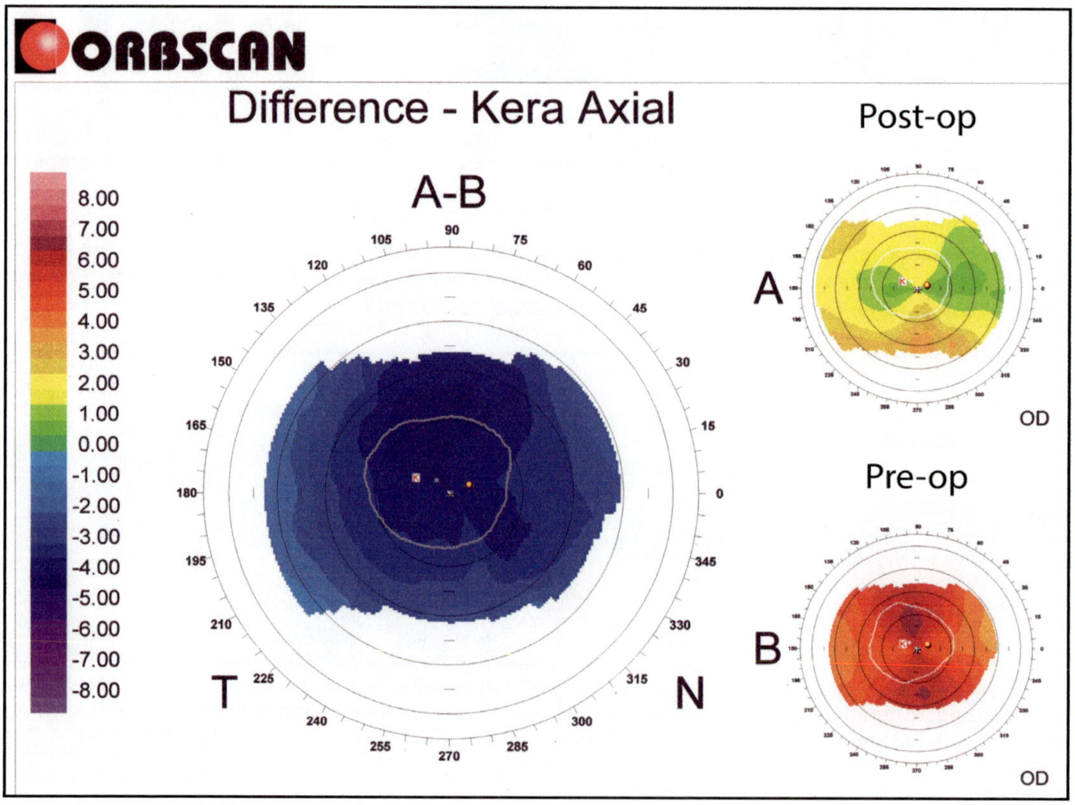

Case Figure 33-5. Difference map from the same eye as Case Figure 33-4 demonstrating actual flattening in the concerning area when compared directly with preoperative mapping. This indicates pseudosteepening without actual inferior steepening and not postoperative ectasia.

Bibliography

Bromley JG, Randleman JB. Treatment strategies for corneal ectasia. *Curr Opin Ophthalmol.* 2010;21(4):255-258.

Hafezi F, Mavrakanas N. Corneal collagen cross-linking for postoperative corneal ectasia. In Hafezi F, Randleman JB (eds). *Corneal Collagen Cross Linking.* Thorofare, NJ: SLACK Incorporated; 2013:75-80.

Hiatt JA, Wachler BS, Grant C. Reversal of laser in situ keratomileusis-induced ectasia with intraocular pressure reduction. *J Cataract Refract Surg.* 2005;31(8):1652-1655.

Randleman JB, Woodward MA. Evaluation and diagnosis of postoperative corneal ectasia. In Hafezi F, Randleman JB (eds). *Corneal Collagen Cross Linking.* Thorofare, NJ: SLACK Incorporated; 2013:31-38.

Woodward M, Randleman JB, Russell B, Lynn MJ, Ward MA, Stulting RD. Visual rehabilitation and outcomes for ectasia after corneal refractive surgery. *J Cataract Refract Surg.* 2008;34:383-388.

—Case 33 (Part 2)—

The patient elected observation after his initial consultation and did not notice any further significant change in his visual acuity for the next 9 months. However, he now presents with worsened visual acuity in both eyes for the past 6 months and wishes to explore treatment options for visual rehabilitation.

CASE HISTORY		
	Right Eye	**Left Eye**
UDVA	20/60	20/40
Manifest refraction	-3.25 +3.25 x 180	Plano +1.50 x 175
CDVA	20/30	20/25
Central corneal thickness	402 µm	405 µm
Physical examination	Normal	Normal
Estimated ablation depth	50 µm	15 µm

Questions

1. Is this patient a candidate for refractive surgery retreatment? If so, what treatment options are available?
2. What is the best course of treatment for the patient at this juncture?
3. What additional interventions are possible for this patient?
4. What is the primary concern for this patient if he is not treated appropriately?
5. What treatment option is ultimately most likely to maximize this patient's best visual acuity?

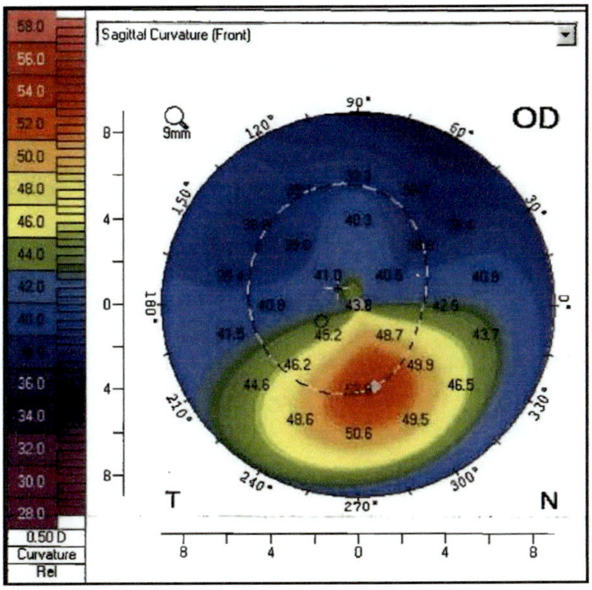
Sagittal Curvature (Front)
OD
9mm
T
N
0.50 D
Curvature
Rel

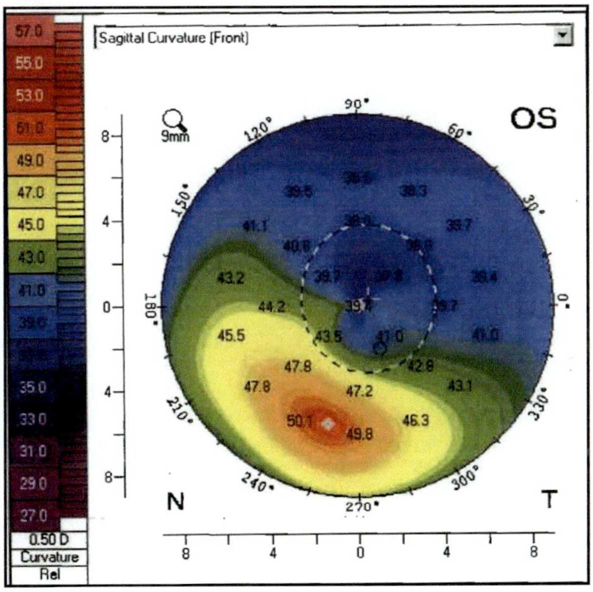
Sagittal Curvature (Front)
OS
9mm
N
T
0.50 D
Curvature
Rel

—Case 33 (Part 2)—

Postoperative Corneal Ectasia

Advanced Manifestations and Management Options

When postoperative corneal ectasia becomes manifest, effective alternatives for visual rehabilitation must address 3 fundamental principles:

1. Halt the ectatic process
2. Reduce corneal curvature irregularity
3. Correct residual refractive error

Case Analysis

- Case Figures show significant inferior corneal steepening in both eyes, which is classic for advanced postoperative corneal ectasia.

Pearl: *Consider corneal collagen cross-linking as early as possible to prevent uncorrectable corneal warpage, to expand treatment options, and to avoid keratoplasty!*

Questions

1. Is this patient a candidate for refractive surgery retreatment? If so, what treatment options are available?

   No, this patient is not a candidate for retreatment because he has postoperative corneal ectasia, which is a specific contraindication to further laser vision correction.

2. What is the best course of treatment for the patient at this juncture?

   Corneal collagen cross-linking (CXL) should be considered, as it is the only treatment available to halt, and in some cases partially reverse, the ectatic process. Corneal collagen cross-linking is currently available in the United States through clinical trials, but it is readily available in many countries outside of the United States.

3. What additional interventions are possible for this patient?

   Other minimally invasive treatments include insertion of intracorneal ring segments, which can be used adjunctively with CXL or in isolation, and contact lens fitting. For some patients, phakic intraocular lens (PIOL) implantation can be advantageous, but this patient does not have a refraction that would benefit from it. In the future, limited surface ablation may be utilized to regularize corneal curvature.

4. What is the primary concern for this patient if he is not treated effectively?

   If the patient continues to progress, he may ultimately require keratoplasty for visual recovery.

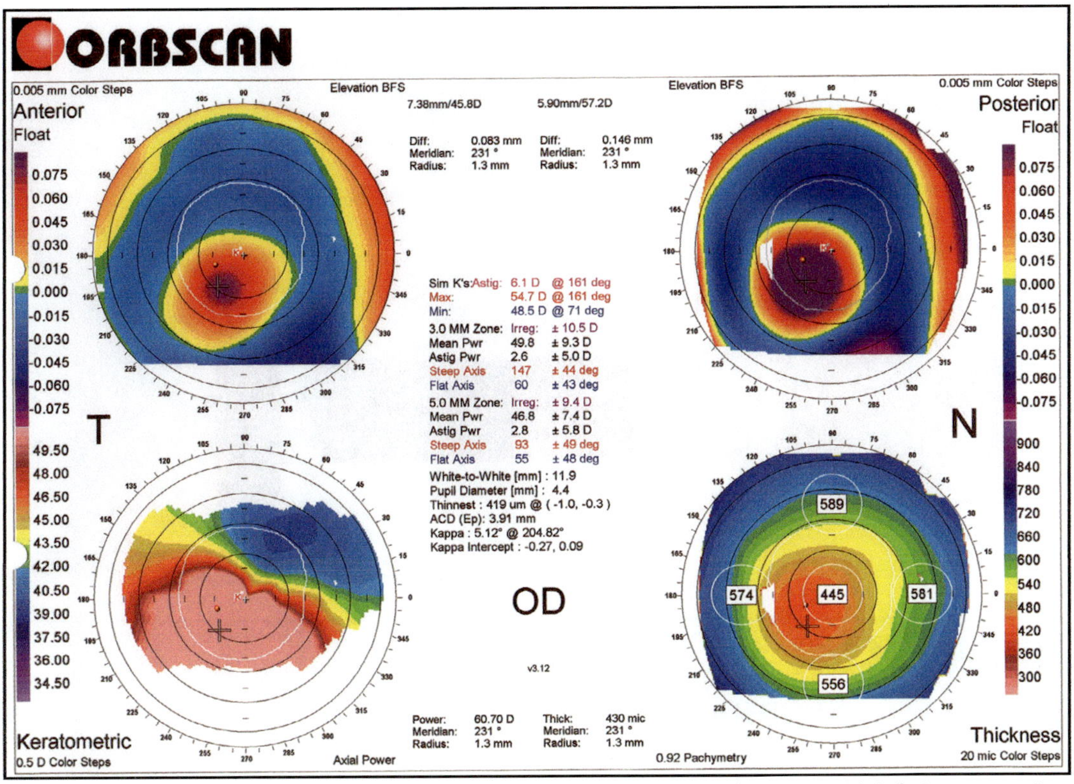

Case Figure 33-6. Typical topographic features of postoperative corneal ectasia, with inferior steepening and irregularity on the keratometric map and concomitant thinning and elevations on the thickness and float maps.

5. What treatment option is ultimately most likely to maximize this patient's final visual acuity?

   Regardless of the initial approach taken, this patient will most likely require rigid contact lenses, either traditional rigid gas permeable lenses or scleral lenses, for maximal visual rehabilitation. However, acceptable vision correction may be obtainable through spectacle use.

Postoperative Ectasia: Advanced Manifestations

In advanced stages, postoperative ectasia mimics keratoconus, both in appearance and biomechanically. Significant curvature alteration, with focal steepening and warpage, can be appreciated on topography (Case Figure 33-6), and focal thinning is evident in more advanced cases (Case Figure 33-7). Common slit-lamp findings of keratoconus, including Fleischer ring, striae, and apical scarring can also be present.

Postoperative Ectasia: Management Options

Visual rehabilitation can be accomplished through a variety, and possibly a combination, of treatments, including CXL (Case Figure 33-8), intracorneal stromal ring segments (Case Figure 33-9), PIOL implantation, and excimer laser ablation in specific cases after CXL.

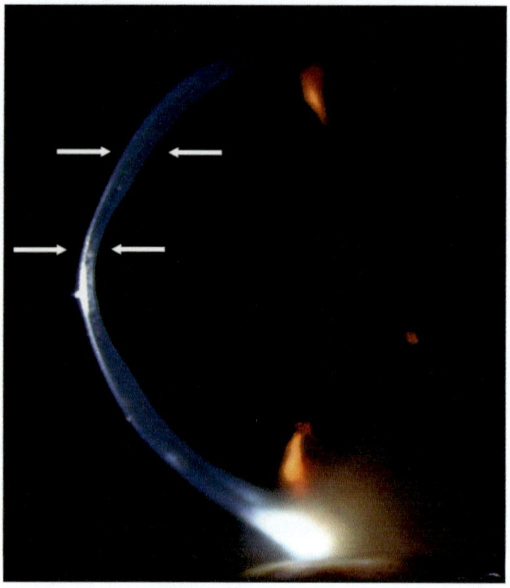

Case Figure 33-7. Slit-lamp features of postoperative corneal ectasia. Note the significant corneal thinning (lower white arrows) that has developed after LASIK, in comparison to the region with normal corneal thickness (upper white arrows). (Reprinted from Randleman JB. Clinical features of keratoectasia. In: Wang M, ed. *Keratoconus and Keratoectasia: Prevention, Diagnosis, and Treatment*. Thorofare, NJ: SLACK Incorporated; 2009:79-90.)

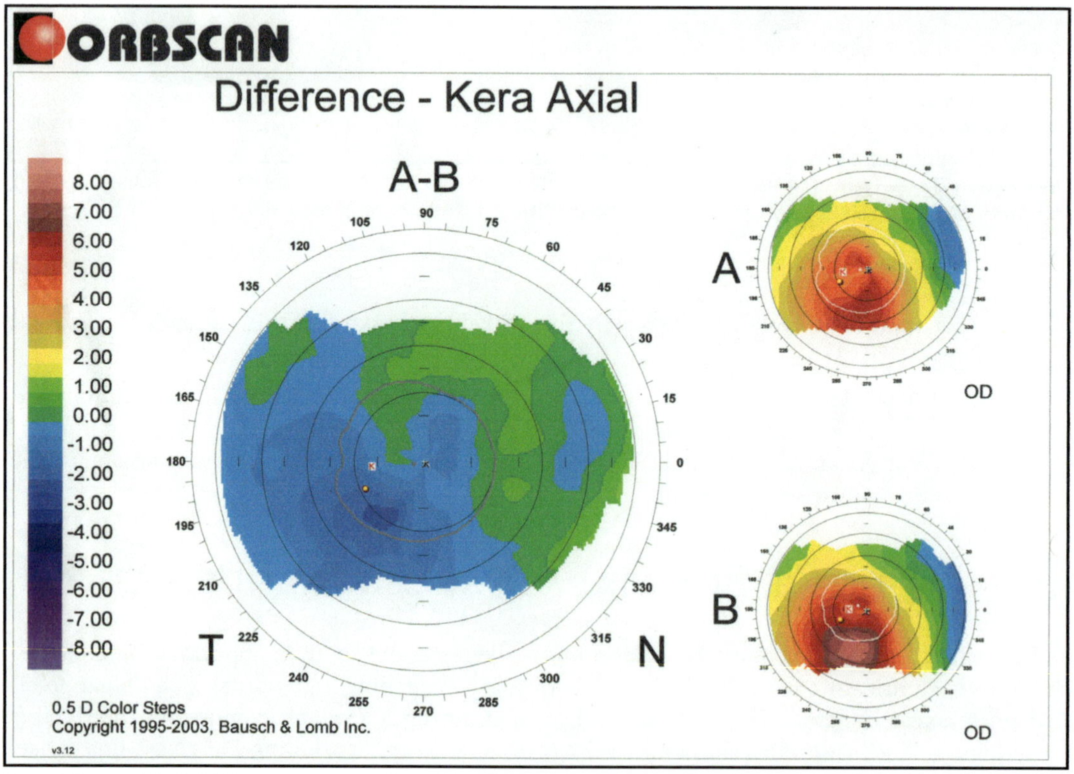

Case Figure 33-8. Difference maps after CXL, demonstrating notable flattening and improved corneal curvature regularity.

To date, many of the treatments advocated for postoperative ectasia have been used primarily for keratoconus; however, because these processes are equivalent biomechanically, the same treatment concepts should apply to both.

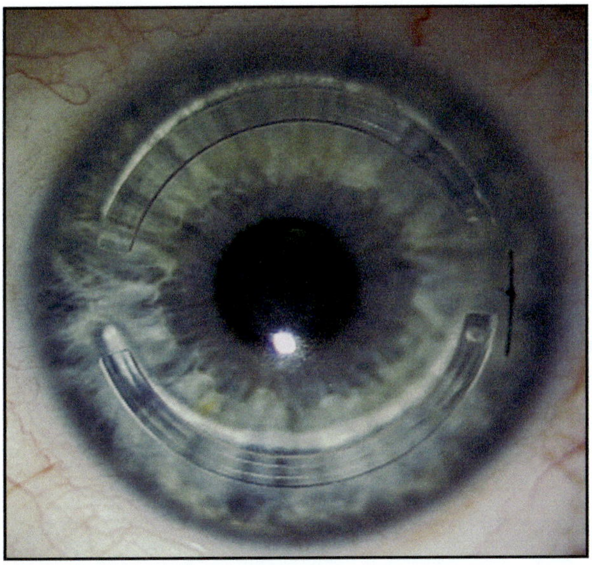

Case Figure 33-9. Intracorneal stromal ring segments (Intacs, Addition Technology) for ectasia.

Bibliography

Bromley JG, Randleman JB. Treatment strategies for corneal ectasia. *Curr Opin Ophthalmol.* 2010;21(4):255-258.

Colin J. European clinical evaluation: use of Intacs prescription inserts for the treatment of keratoconus. *J Cataract Refract Surg.* 2006;32(5):747-755.

Coskunseven E, Jankov MR II, Hafezi F, Atun S, Arslan E, Kymionis G. Effect of treatment sequence in combined intrastromal corneal rings and corneal collagen cross-linking for keratoconus. *J Cataract Refract Surg.* 2009;35(12):2084-2091.

Coskunseven E, Kymionis GD, Tsiklis NS, et al. One-year results of intrastromal corneal ring segment implantation (KeraRing) using femtosecond laser in patients with keratoconus. *Am J Ophthalmol.* 2008;145(5):775-779.

Ertan A, Karacal H, Kamburoglu G. Refractive and topographic results of transepithelial cross-linking treatment in eye with intacs. *Cornea.* 2009;28(7):719-723.

Güell JL, Morral M, Malecaze F, Gris O, Elies D, Manero F. Collagen crosslinking and toric iris-claw phakic intraocular lens for myopic astigmatism in progressive mild to moderate keratoconus. *J Cataract Refract Surg.* 2012;38(3):475-484.

Hafezi F, Kanellopoulos J, Wiltfang R, Seiler T. Corneal collagen crosslinking with riboflavin and ultraviolet A to treat induced keratectasia after laser in situ keratomileusis. *J Cataract Refract Surg.* 2007;33(12):2035-2040.

Hafezi F, Randleman JB (eds). *Corneal Collagen Cross Linking.* Thorofare, NJ: SLACK Incorporated; 2013.

Hersh PS, Greenstein SA, Fry KL. Corneal collagen crosslinking for keratoconus and corneal ectasia: one-year results. *J Cataract Refract Surg.* 2011;37(1):149-160.

Kamburoglu G, Ertan A. Intacs implantation with sequential collagen cross-linking treatment in postoperative LASIK ectasia. *J Refract Surg.* 2008;24(7):S726-S729.

Kanellopoulos AJ, Binder PS. Management of corneal ectasia after LASIK with combined, same-day, topography-guided partial transepithelial PRK and collagen cross-linking: the Athens protocol. *J Refract Surg.* 2011;27(5):323-331.

Kymionis GD, Portaliou DM, Kounis GA, Limnopoulou AN, Kontadakis GA, Grentzelos MA. Simultaneous topography-guided photorefractive keratectomy followed by corneal collagen cross-linking for keratoconus. *Am J Ophthalmol.* 2011;152(5):748-755.

Kymionis GD, Tsiklis NS, Pallikaris AI, et al. Long-term follow-up of Intacs for post-LASIK corneal ectasia. *Ophthalmology.* 2006;113(11):1909-1917.

Piñero DP, Alio JL, Uceda-Montanes A, El Kady B, Pascual I. Intracorneal ring segment implantation in corneas with post-laser in situ keratomileusis keratectasia. *Ophthalmology.* 2009;116(9):1665-1674.

Randleman JB. Ectasia after LASIK: new treatments, new hope. *J Refract Surg.* 2011;27(5):319.

Richoz O, Mavrakanas N, Pajic B, Hafezi F. Corneal collagen cross-linking for ectasia after refractive laser surgery: long-term results. *Ophthalmology.* 2013;120(7):1354-1359.

—Case 34—

A 43-year-old female presents seeking options to improve her visual acuity. She had LASIK in both eyes 5 months ago for an original prescription of -1.50 +1.25 x 165 in the right eye and -2.00 +1.75 x 010 in the left eye and was targeted for modified monovision (near in the left eye with a -1.00-diopter [D] target). Surgery was performed using a mechanical microkeratome and a conventional ablation pattern. She had retreatment performed in the right eye and reports some improvement from initial visual acuity, but her distance vision is still not as good as she had hoped. Her near visual acuity is good. She denies pain, irritation, or other nonvisual symptoms since surgery.

The patient brought with her the topographies from before (A) initial and (B) repeat surgery for your review. Today's topographies are shown as Figure C.

Case History		
	Right Eye	**Left Eye**
UDVA	20/70	20/60
Manifest refraction	-1.50 +1.25 x 075	-1.25 +0.50 x 120
CDVA	20/25	20/15
Cycloplegic refraction	-1.50 +1.25 x 075	-1.25 +0.50 x 110
Cycloplegic CDVA	20/25	20/15
Keratometry		
Flat K	44.7 @ 175	45.0 @ 130
Steep K	45.75 @ 085	45.5 @ 020
Central corneal thickness	520 µm	545 µm
Physical examination	Normal	Normal
Estimated ablation depth	25 µm	N/A

Questions

1. What is the most likely cause for this patient's refractive error at this time point?
2. Is this patient a candidate for refractive surgery retreatment? If so, what treatment options are available?
3. What additional information may be useful to help determine your course of action?
4. What is the best course of treatment at this juncture to improve this patient's vision?
5. What is the optimal timing for additional surgery for this patient, if warranted?

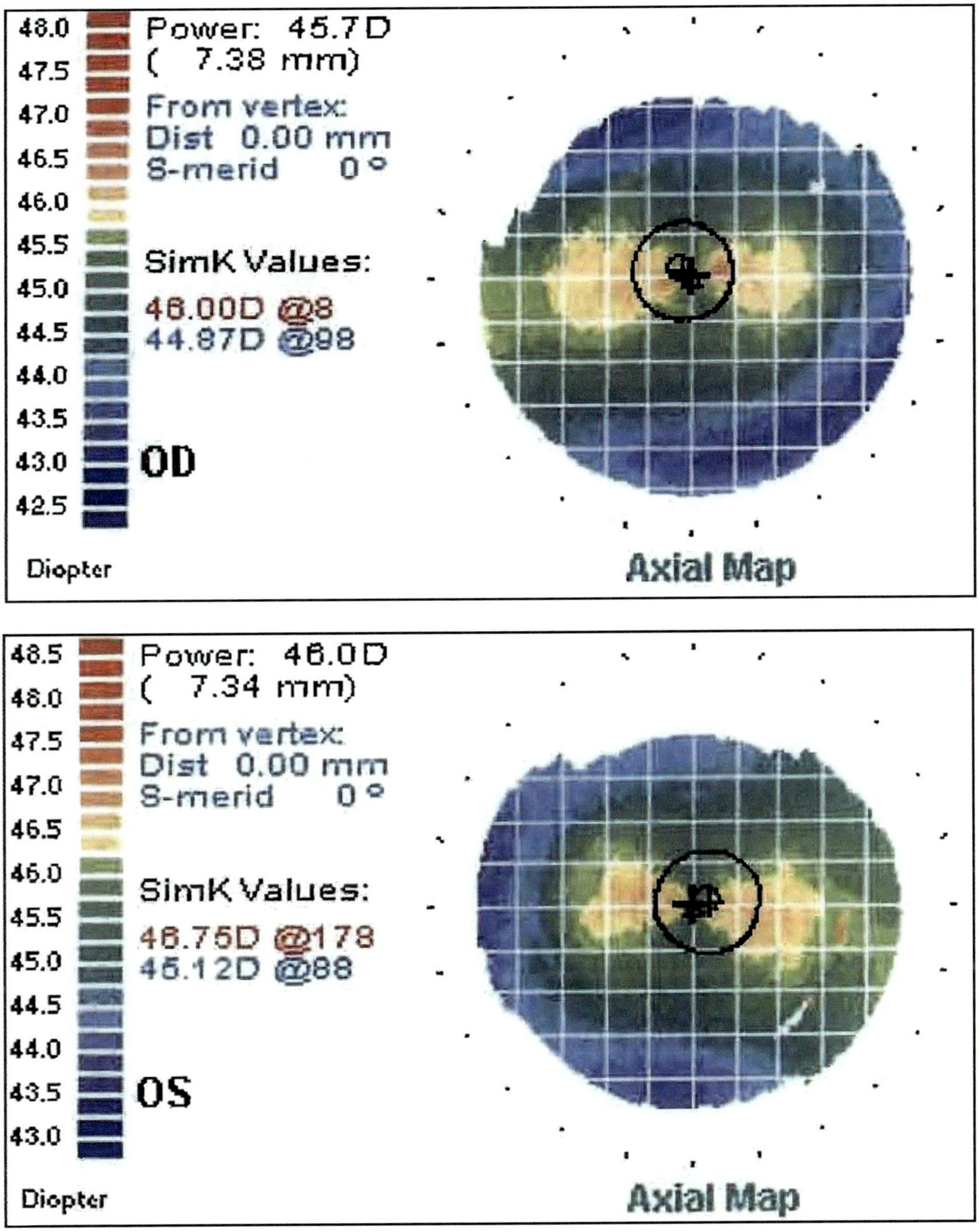
48.0
47.5
47.0
46.5
46.0
45.5
45.0
44.5
44.0
43.5
43.0
42.5
Diopter
Power: 45.7D
(7.38 mm)
From vertex:
Dist 0.00 mm
S-merid 0°
SimK Values:
46.00D @8
44.87D @98
OD
Axial Map
48.5
48.0
47.5
47.0
46.5
46.0
45.5
45.0
44.5
44.0
43.5
43.0
Diopter
Power: 46.0D
(7.34 mm)
From vertex:
Dist 0.00 mm
S-merid 0°
SimK Values:
46.75D @178
45.12D @88
OS
Axial Map

A

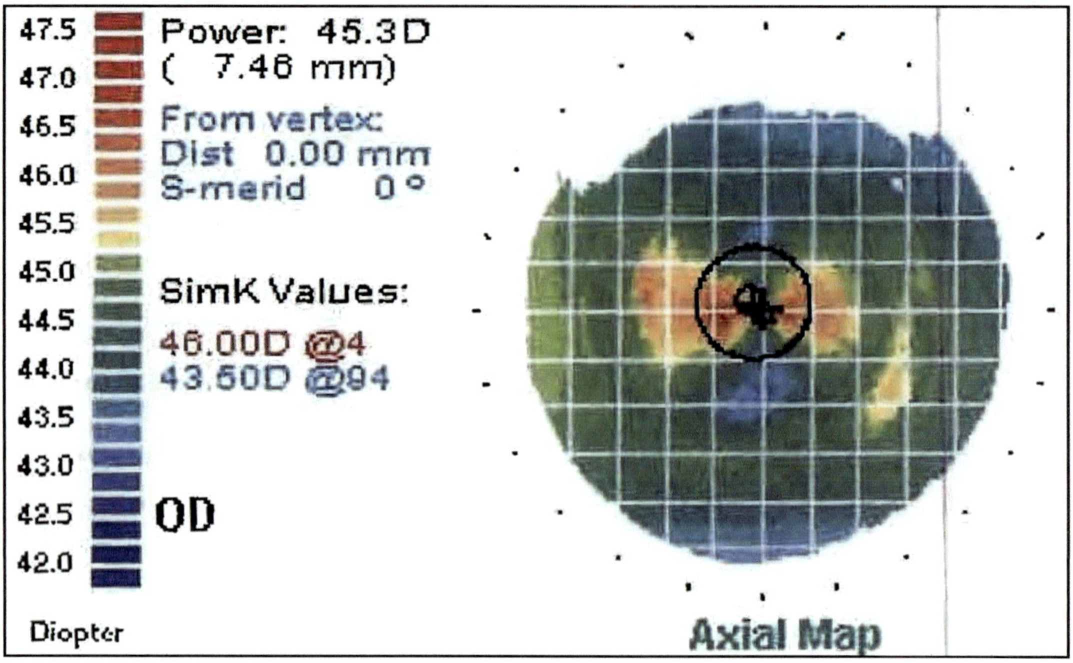
47.5
47.0
46.5
46.0
45.5
45.0
44.5
44.0
43.5
43.0
42.5
42.0
Diopter
Power: 45.3D
(7.46 mm)
From vertex:
Dist 0.00 mm
S-merid 0°
SimK Values:
46.00D @4
43.50D @94
OD
Axial Map

B

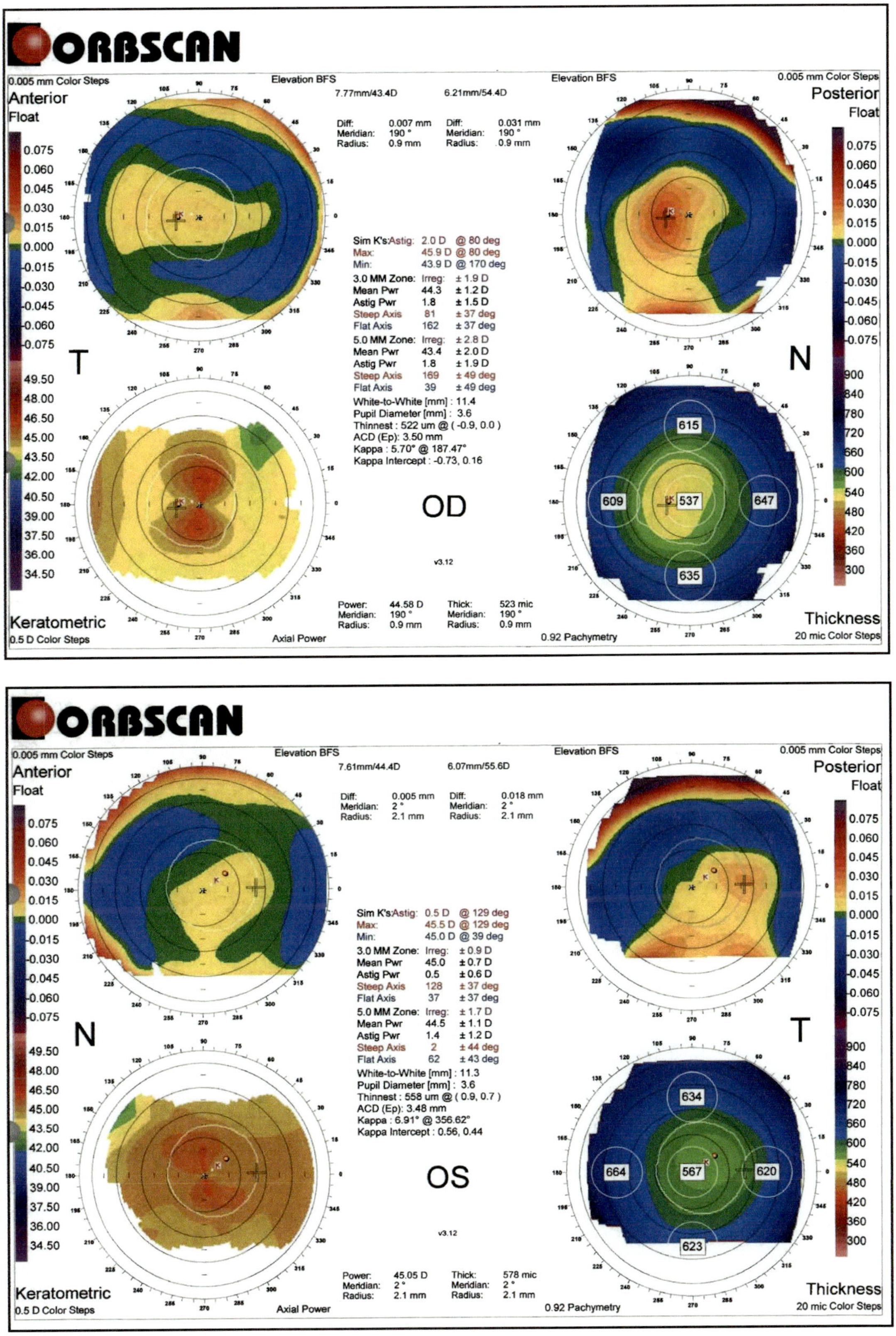
ORBSCAN
0.005 mm Color Steps
Anterior
Float
Elevation BFS
7.77mm/43.4D
6.21mm/54.4D
Elevation BFS
0.005 mm Color Steps
Posterior
Float
Diff: 0.007 mm
Meridian: 190 °
Radius: 0.9 mm
Diff: 0.031 mm
Meridian: 190 °
Radius: 0.9 mm
Sim K's:Astig: 2.0 D @ 80 deg
Max: 45.9 D @ 80 deg
Min: 43.9 D @ 170 deg
3.0 MM Zone: Irreg: ± 1.9 D
Mean Pwr 44.3 ± 1.2 D
Astig Pwr 1.8 ± 1.5 D
Steep Axis 81 ± 37 deg
Flat Axis 162 ± 37 deg
5.0 MM Zone: Irreg: ± 2.8 D
Mean Pwr 43.4 ± 2.0 D
Astig Pwr 1.8 ± 1.9 D
Steep Axis 169 ± 49 deg
Flat Axis 39 ± 49 deg
White-to-White [mm] : 11.4
Pupil Diameter [mm] : 3.6
Thinnest : 522 um @ (-0.9, 0.0)
ACD (Ep): 3.50 mm
Kappa : 5.70° @ 187.47°
Kappa Intercept : -0.73, 0.16
T
N
OD
v3.12
615
609
537
647
635
Power: 44.58 D
Meridian: 190 °
Radius: 0.9 mm
Thick: 523 mic
Meridian: 190 °
Radius: 0.9 mm
Keratometric
0.5 D Color Steps
Axial Power
0.92 Pachymetry
Thickness
20 mic Color Steps
ORBSCAN
0.005 mm Color Steps
Anterior
Float
Elevation BFS
7.61mm/44.4D
6.07mm/55.6D
Elevation BFS
0.005 mm Color Steps
Posterior
Float
Diff: 0.005 mm
Meridian: 2 °
Radius: 2.1 mm
Diff: 0.018 mm
Meridian: 2 °
Radius: 2.1 mm
Sim K's:Astig: 0.5 D @ 129 deg
Max: 45.5 D @ 129 deg
Min: 45.0 D @ 39 deg
3.0 MM Zone: Irreg: ± 0.9 D
Mean Pwr 45.0 ± 0.7 D
Astig Pwr 0.5 ± 0.6 D
Steep Axis 128 ± 37 deg
Flat Axis 37 ± 37 deg
5.0 MM Zone: Irreg: ± 1.7 D
Mean Pwr 44.5 ± 1.1 D
Astig Pwr 1.4 ± 1.2 D
Steep Axis 2 ± 44 deg
Flat Axis 62 ± 43 deg
White-to-White [mm] : 11.3
Pupil Diameter [mm] : 3.6
Thinnest : 558 um @ (0.9, 0.7)
ACD (Ep): 3.48 mm
Kappa : 6.91° @ 356.62°
Kappa Intercept : 0.56, 0.44
N
T
OS
v3.12
634
664
567
620
623
Power: 45.05 D
Meridian: 2 °
Radius: 2.1 mm
Thick: 578 mic
Meridian: 2 °
Radius: 2.1 mm
Keratometric
0.5 D Color Steps
Axial Power
0.92 Pachymetry
Thickness
20 mic Color Steps

C

—CASE 34—
Irregular Ablations
Incorrect Axis Ablation

Errors in laser programming can occur from a variety of sources but most commonly as a result of patient misidentification, data entry errors, or cylinder conversion (incorrect entry of the axis to be ablated). Fortunately, such errors are rare, but diligence is required at all steps of the surgical process to ensure safeguards are in place to avoid them. If errors do occur, the patient should be informed so that he or she can play an active role in determining the best course of treatment moving forward.

Case Analysis

- Case Figure A shows Placido topography of the right (OD) and left (OS) eyes, demonstrating symmetric bowtie patterns with 1.20 D (OD) and 1.50 D (OS) astigmatism oriented in the 180-degree meridian (against-the-rule astigmatism).
- Case Figure B shows Placido topography of the right eye, demonstrating symmetric bowtie patterns with 2.50 D astigmatism oriented in the 180-degree meridian (against-the-rule astigmatism). Note that the astigmatism is increased, not reduced, when compared with the preoperative topography, and the astigmatism is in the same orientation. This indicates that the astigmatism was effectively doubled, rather than reduced by the initial ablation.
- Case Figure C shows scanning slit-beam imaging of the right (OD) and left (OS) eyes, demonstrating a truncated symmetric bowtie pattern in the right eye with 2.00 D astigmatism oriented in the 90-degree meridian (with-the-rule), and a subtle symmetric bowtie pattern in the left eye with 0.50 D astigmatism. Thickness and float values are unremarkable in both eyes.

Pearl: *If a laser programming error results in incorrect axis treatment, many patients are ultimately able to be retreated, but refractive stability must be achieved before any retreatment is performed!*

QUESTIONS

1. What is the most likely cause for this patient's refractive error at this time point after LASIK?

   Induced astigmatism in the right eye likely resulted from repeat ablation too early in the postoperative period following initial incorrect axis treatment, which doubled, rather than treated, the astigmatism in the right eye.

2. Is this patient a candidate for refractive surgery retreatment? If so, what treatment options are available for this patient?

   Yes, the patient is most likely a candidate for further ablation, as the induced astigmatism is well within the available treatment parameters, and there are no other apparent biomechanical issues that preclude retreatment. LASIK flap relift and surface ablation are both possible options. In this time period, flap relift is likely the most advantageous treatment option, but the patient is at increased risk of epithelial ingrowth due to multiple flap lifts.

3. What additional information may be useful to help determine your course of action?

   Previous records, including laser ablation logs, would be especially useful in this case because there is some question about previous treatments, as well as the difference between the intended and obtained refractive outcome. Information about whether the patient is an under- or over-responder will be useful for subsequent treatment planning.

4. What is the best course of treatment at this juncture to improve this patient's vision?

   Treatment options include retreatment, spectacle use, or contact lens use for the right eye, as desired by the patient. All options should be equally efficacious, and the patient should be counseled about all of these options, given the challenging postoperative course she has had to date.

5. What is the optimal timing for additional surgery for this patient, if warranted?

   Retreatment must not be performed until refractive stability has been confirmed. Baseline measurements had been obtained at her initial visit, and from this juncture, a repeat evaluation in 4 to 6 weeks is warranted, along with continued observation and reevaluation until stability has been achieved. If the patient elects to wear a contact lens in the interim, she should remove the lens for up to 1 week prior to each subsequent stability visit.

Incorrect Axis Ablations: Avoidance and Recognition

Incorrect ablations are rare but can occur, resulting from a variety of mechanisms. The medicolegal implications of these errors are important, but they are outside the focus of this book. Attention should be given to minimizing the opportunity for errors to occur and identifying situations that are and are not amenable to further laser vision correction for rehabilitation.

Two primary issues related specifically to astigmatism correction include data entry errors and cylinder conversion errors when transposing data from clinical notes and refractions to laser programming data. Some excimer lasers require data input in a certain form (ie, minus cylinder or plus cylinder only), and it is important to identify how your laser accepts the data and confirms that the entry is correct. Data entry can also include an error in moving a decimal point, resulting in under- or overcorrection.

Developing a system of checks and balances, with both personnel and surgeon confirming data entry, will minimize opportunities for error. Confirming refractive data with topographic data provides an additional safeguard, although one must take lenticular astigmatism into account in these comparisons.

It is exceptionally uncommon to have large refractive errors, either residual or induced, after modern laser ablation, and most patients enjoy good uncorrected visual acuity early in their postoperative course. Any patients not seeing well postoperatively should have a full clinical examination and be refracted to establish a baseline, with the understanding that some shifts in prescription will likely occur during healing.

Incorrect Axis Ablations: Treatment Options

Treatment options will depend on the degree of the error, the biomechanical characteristics of the cornea, and the patient's desire and willingness to undergo further treatment. Induced astigmatism that does not exceed laser programming limits (approximately 6.00 D) should be treatable with subsequent ablation. The refractive error may not be fully correctable due to induced irregularity, and the patient should be counseled about this.

Prior to retreatment, it is critical that refractive stability be achieved as a treatment performed prior to this risks a suboptimal outcome and potentially can induce irregular astigmatism. Further, after LASIK, there is increased risk for epithelial ingrowth with each subsequent flap lift.

If irregular astigmatism has been induced through the ablation and healing processes, it is unlikely to fully respond to further ablation. If the degree of irregularity is mild, the patient may still benefit from repeat ablation; however, in cases where significant irregular astigmatism has occurred, these patients are more likely to benefit from gas permeable contact lens fitting than additional ablation.

Bibliography

Ivarsen A, Næser K, Hjortdal J. Laser in situ keratomileusis for high astigmatism in myopic and hyperopic eyes. *J Cataract Refract Surg*. 2013;39(1):74-80.

Karthikappallil J. Induced astigmatism after laser in situ keratomileusis. *J Cataract Refract Surg*. 2004;30(5):940-941.

Moshirfar M, Simpson RG, Dave SB, et al. Sources of medical error in refractive surgery. *J Refract Surg*. 2013;29(5):303-310.

—CASE 35—

A 52-year-old male and 51-year old female (husband and wife) present for an evaluation. Both had radial keratotomy (RK) performed approximately 20 years ago, both report good visual acuity for many years, and both have noted a decrease in visual acuity (distance and near) for the past several years. No preoperative records are available. Upon questioning, the husband has not noted any significant fluctuations in his visual acuity, whereas the wife says fluctuations have been significant for her from morning to evening and from day to day for many years.

Husband

CASE HISTORY		
	Right Eye	**Left Eye**
UDVA	20/40	20/60
Manifest refraction	+1.25 +1.00 x 105	+1.00 +2.00 x 040
CDVA	20/20	20/20
Keratometry		
Flat K	37.25 @ 175	35.5 @ 175
Steep K	38.25 @ 085	37.5 @ 085
Central corneal thickness	565 μm	565 μm
Physical examination	4-cut RK, otherwise unremarkable	4-cut RK, otherwise unremarkable
Estimated ablation depth	25 μm	25 μm

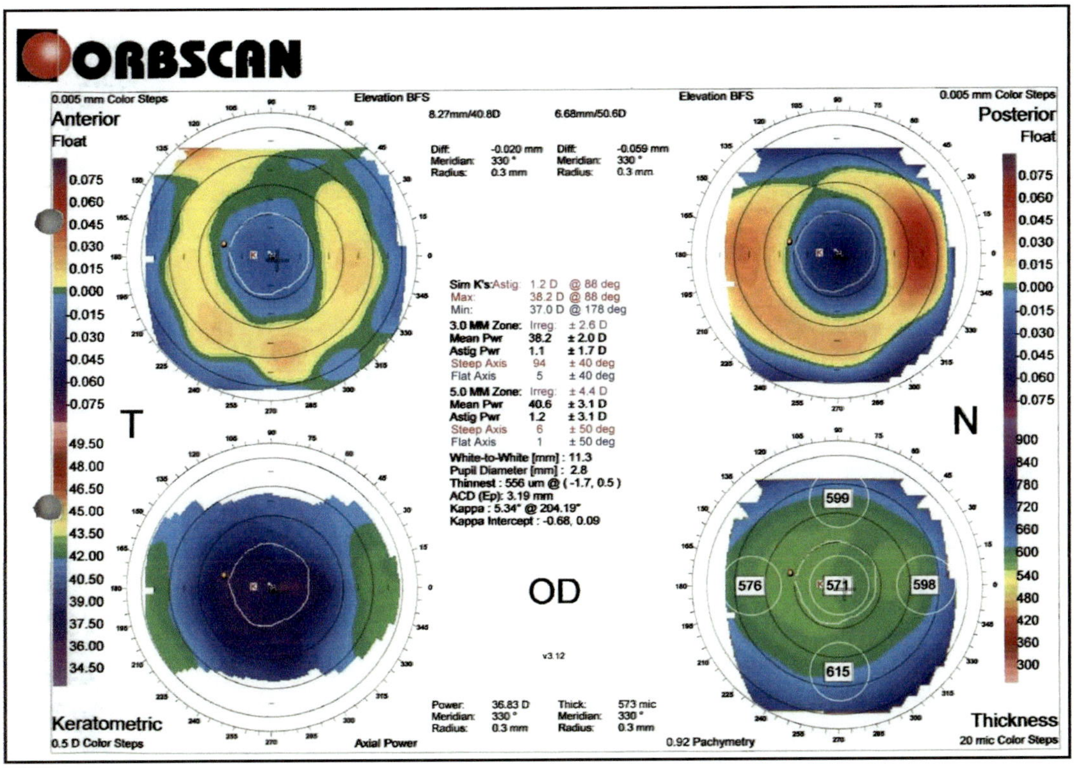

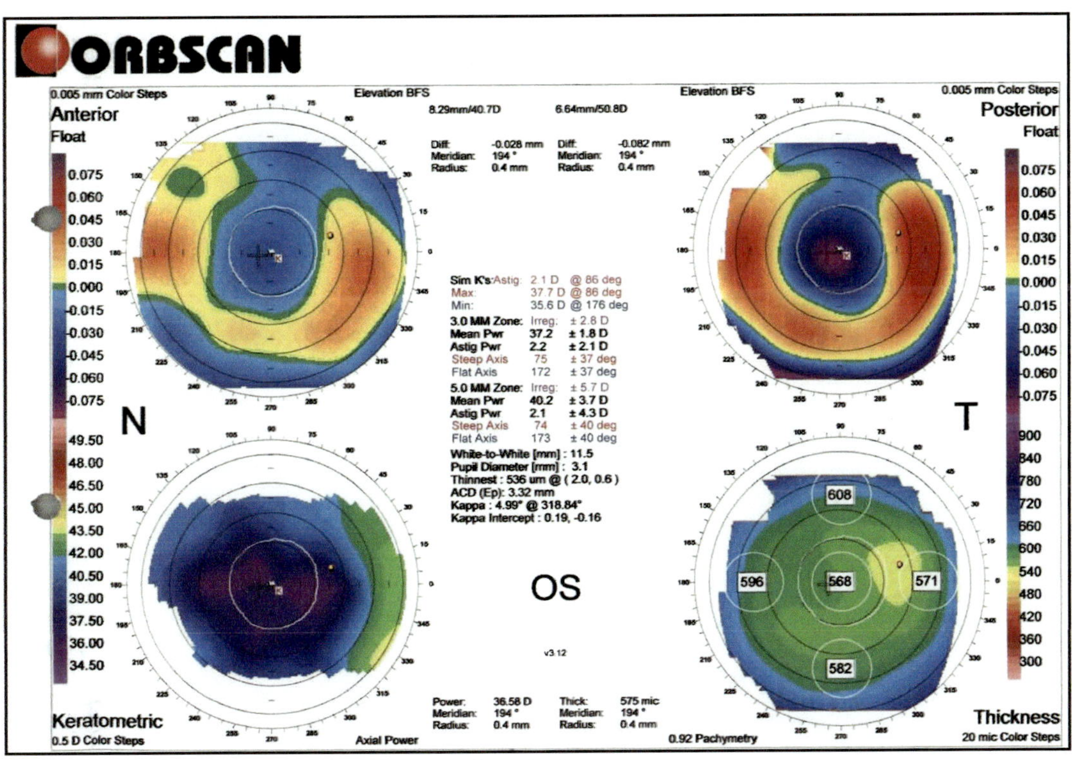

A: Husband's Topographies

Wife

CASE HISTORY		
	Right Eye	**Left Eye**
UDVA	20/60	20/30
Manifest refraction	+2.25 +0.50 x 050	+0.50 +0.75 x 090
CDVA	20/30	20/25
Keratometry		
Flat K	44.7 @ 175	45.0 @ 130
Steep K	45.75 @ 085	45.5 @ 020
Central corneal thickness	599 µm	591 µm
Physical examination	6-cut RK with 2 astigmatic keratotomies, otherwise unremarkable	6-cut RK with 2 astigmatic keratotomies, otherwise unremarkable
Estimated ablation depth	35 µm	15 µm

Questions

1. What is the most likely cause for this refractive error in each patient?
2. Is either patient a candidate for refractive surgery retreatment? If so, who (husband, wife, or both) and what treatment options are available?
3. What additional testing may be useful to help determine your course of action?
4. Considering all factors, what procedure would you recommend, for whom, and why?

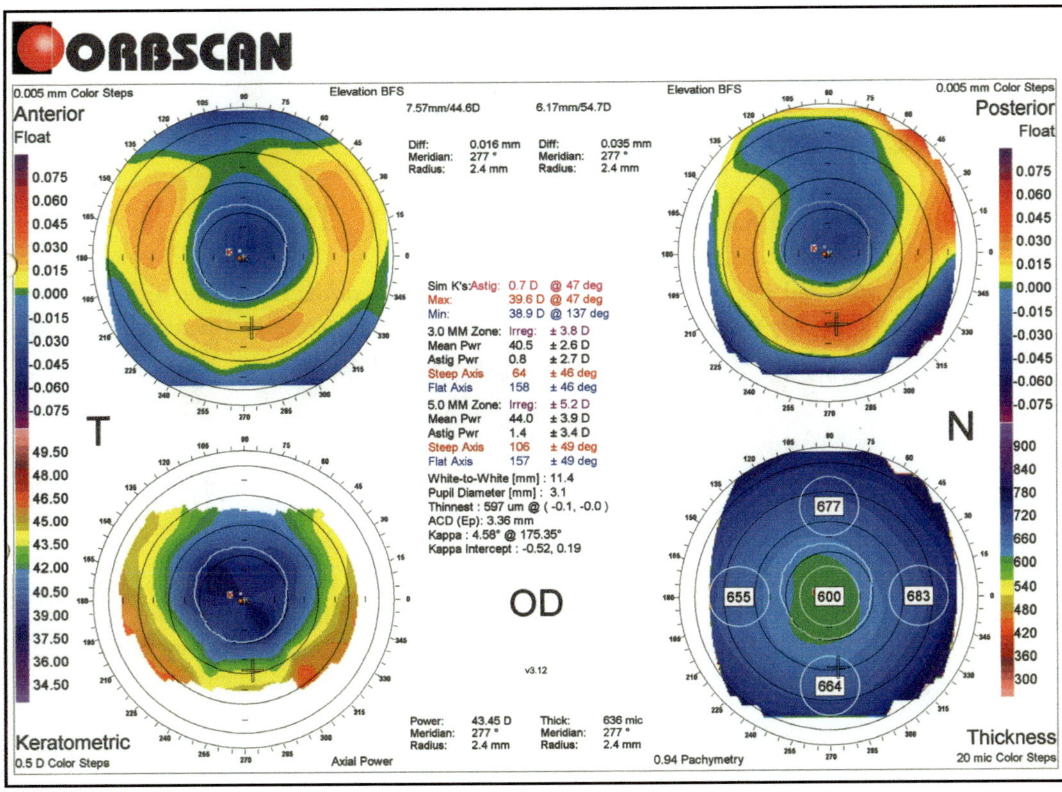

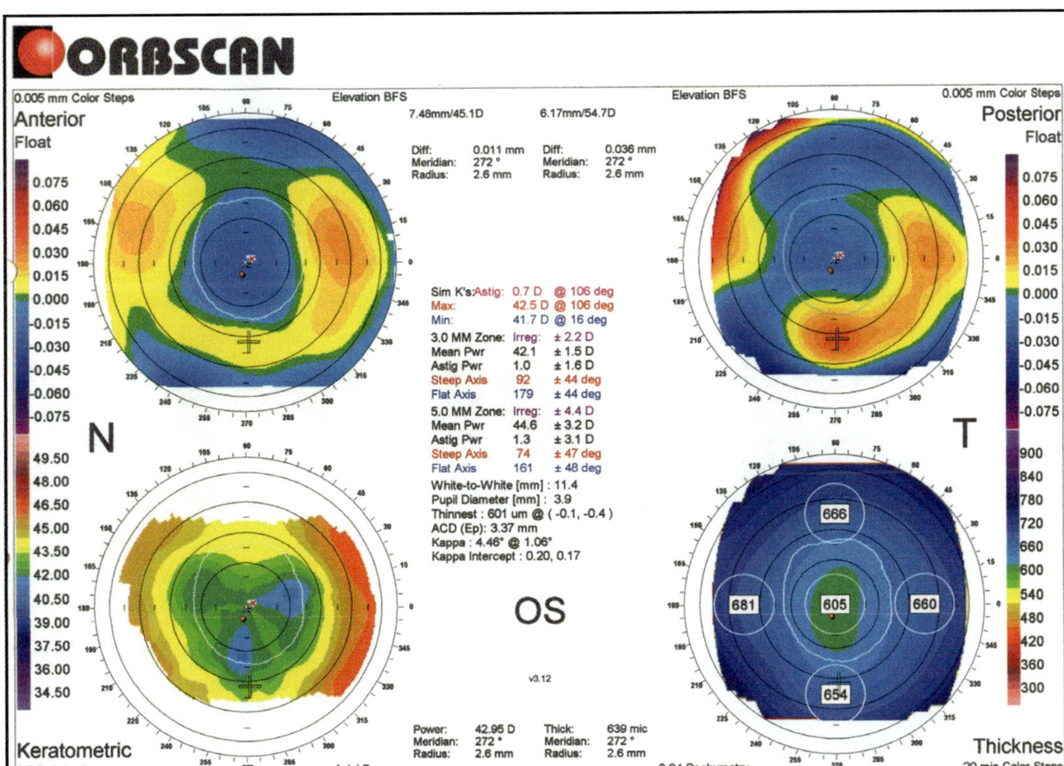

B: Wife's Topographies

—Case 35—
Retreatment Options After Radial Keratotomy

Many patients who had RK will present seeking options for retreatment after initially good visual acuity, often for many years. Some patients will be candidates for retreatment, whereas others will not. Clinical history is exceptionally important in these individuals.

Case Analysis

- Case Figures A show topography for the husband, demonstrating relatively uniform central flattening in both eyes indicative of prior myopic treatment. Corneal thickness is adequate in both eyes, and other measures are unremarkable.
- Case Figures B show topography for the wife, demonstrating relatively uniform central flattening in the right eye, indicative of prior myopic treatment, and a spoke-like or cloverleaf appearance of central irregularity in the left eye, which is characteristic for topographic images after RK. Corneal thickness and other measures are unremarkable in both eyes.

Pearl: *Seek out a history of diurnal fluctuations, day-to-day variations, and relative refractive stability before offering excimer laser treatment to patients who had RK!*

Questions

1. What is the most likely cause for this refractive error in each patient?

   Ametropia is a component for both patients (consecutive hyperopia with astigmatism). Ametropia is the major issue for the husband, whereas the wife has irregular astigmatism, which is equally of impact in her case.

2. Is either patient a candidate for refractive surgery retreatment? If so, who (husband, wife, or both) and what treatment options are available?

   The husband appears to be a reasonable candidate for laser vision correction, given a reasonable refractive error and good correctable visual acuity. The wife is not a good candidate, as most of her visual limitation comes from irregular astigmatism. Theoretically, both LASIK and surface ablation are options; however, LASIK has a higher incidence of complications after RK, so surface ablation would be the preferred approach.

3. What additional testing may be useful to help determine your course of action?

   For patients with a questionable history of diurnal or daily fluctuations, repeat refraction on separate days and times may be useful to establish the amount of fluctuation and whether is the fluctuations are too great to recommend further treatment. Recent past refractions may also be beneficial to establish relative refractive consistency. If a patient is undergoing a progressive refractive shift, he or she may not be an optimal candidate for further treatment.

4. Considering all factors, what procedure would you recommend, for whom, and why?

   If the husband is interested in improving distance visual acuity, is comfortable with reading spectacles, and is motivated for surgery, he could have surface ablation performed. For the wife, if she is motivated to improve her visual quality, rigid gas permeable contact lens fitting is indicated.

Treatment Considerations After Radial Keratotomy

Treatment options depend on the corneal anatomy, curvature, biomechanical profile, target refraction, refractive stability and symptoms, and patient age. Progressive hyperopic shift is common after RK, and many of these patients present after years or decades of good uncorrected visual acuity looking for additional treatment to avoid the use of spectacles or contact lenses. Patients with good corrected visual acuity and with low hyperopia, low astigmatism, or low myopia from regression are the best candidates for treatment. In contrast, patients with complaints that are not readily correctable with spectacles are not good surgical candidates. The common complaints in this category include diurnal fluctuations, severe starbursts, day-to-day fluctuations, or irregular astigmatism manifesting as less than optimal correctable visual acuity.

It is important to distinguish between patients who feel their visual acuity is adequate but are seeking a surgical alternative to spectacles or contact lenses (usually achievable with surgery) and those who desire better visual quality than they are able to achieve with spectacles or contact lenses (usually not achievable with surgery). Corneal topography evaluation can be challenging after RK, as "normal" patterns may have varying degrees of topographic irregularity, and there is visual overlap between some normal cases that are amenable to surgery and cases with mild, but visually significant, irregular astigmatism that is not amenable to surgery.

Finally, most patients returning for potential treatment after RK are older than the average laser vision correction population, and cataract development should be ruled out before proceeding with any corneal refractive surgery.

Treatment Strategies After Radial Keratotomy

There has been controversy and debate regarding the optimal surgical approach after previous incisional surgery. Early photorefractive keratectomy had significant corneal haze and scarring associated with treatment after RK, but this concern has been largely mitigated by the use of mitomycin C. LASIK minimizes the risk of haze but carries a significant risk for recalcitrant epithelial ingrowth (Case Figure 35-1). Epithelium can grow through the RK cuts to reach the LASIK interface, and because these incisions are within the visual axis, they cannot be permanently closed. Therefore, surface ablation is preferable to LASIK after RK.

Some surgeons advocate using mitomycin C for a longer time period in patients who had previous RK than in patients with primary treatments, with times ranging from 12 to 60 seconds, depending on surgeon preference. Special care should be taken during epithelial removal to confirm that a smooth surface has been created for ablation; some eyes have developed epithelial plugs in the RK incisions that may be more difficult to remove to generate a smooth surface.

Conductive keratoplasty (CK) is a treatment option for low hyperopia in patients who have not undergone prior corneal surgery, but it is used infrequently due to significant regression of the refractive outcome. The treatment is generally safe for patients without prior surgery; however, CK should not be performed after RK, as the induced collagen shrinkage may cause splaying of the incisions, with persistent postoperative pain or perforation in extreme cases (Case Figure 35-2).

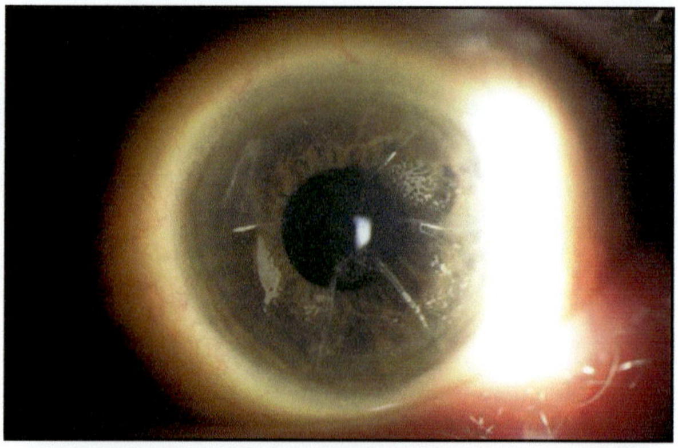

Case Figure 35-1. Epithelial ingrowth is seen through radial incisions in an eye with LASIK after RK. (Reprinted with permission from Randleman JB, Banning CS, Stulting RD. Persistent epithelial ingrowth. *Ophthalmology.* 2006;113(8):1468.e1-3.)

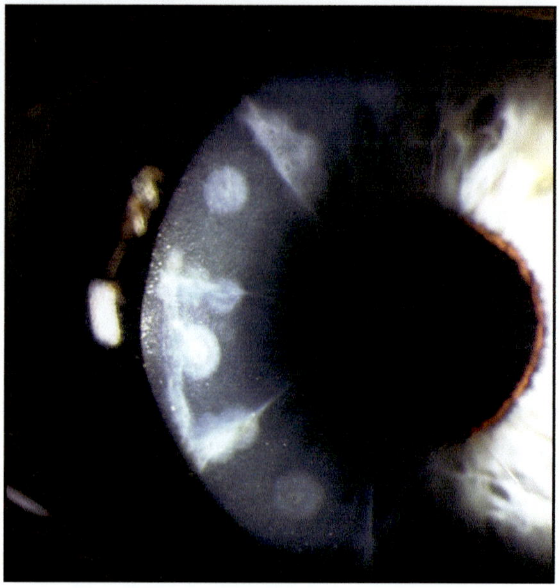

Case Figure 35-2. Conductive keratoplasty scars (peripheral round opacities) adjacent to RK and astigmatic keratotomy incisions (linear scars) in a patient who developed intractable pain after the CK procedure. (Reprinted with permission from Randleman JB. Etiology and clinical presentations of irregular astigmatism after keratorefractive surgery. In: Wang M, ed. *Irregular Astigmatism: Diagnosis and Treatment.* Thorofare, NJ: SLACK Incorporated; 2007:79-90.)

Bibliography

Francesconi CM, Nose RA, Nose W. Hyperopic laser-assisted in situ keratomileusis for radial keratotomy induced hyperopia. *Ophthalmology.* 2002;109(3):602605.

Gambato C, Ghirlando A, Moretto E, Busato F, Midena E. Mitomycin C modulation of corneal wound healing after photorefractive keratectomy in highly myopic eyes. *Ophthalmology.* 2005;112(2):208-218.

Kymionis GD, Titze P, Markomanolakis MM, Aslanides IM, Pallikaris IG. Corneal perforation after conductive keratoplasty with previous refractive surgery. *J Cataract Refract Surg.* 2003;29(12):2452-2454.

Majmudar PA, Forstot SL, Dennis RF, et al. Topical mitomycin-C for subepithelial fibrosis after refractive corneal surgery. *Ophthalmology.* 2000;107(1):89-94.

Oral D, Awwad ST, Seward MS, Bowman RW, McCulley JP, Cavanagh HD. Hyperopic laser in situ keratomileusis in eyes with previous radial keratotomy. *J Cataract Refract Surg.* 2005;31(8):1561-1568.

Randleman JB, Banning CS, Stulting RD. Persistent epithelial ingrowth. *Ophthalmology.* 2006;113(8):1468.e1-3.

Waring GO III, Lynn MJ, McDonnell PJ. Results of the Prospective Evaluation of Radial Keratotomy (PERK) Study 10 years after surgery. *Arch Ophthalmol.* 1994;112(10):1298-1308.

—Case 36—

A 53-year-old female complains of blurred vision in her left eye following refractive lens exchange (RLE) with multifocal intraocular lens (IOL) implant 9 months ago. The patient reports that vision "had never been good" following RLE. Specifically, she reports constant blur at all distances and significant glare and halos at night, and she is unable to perform her daily activities, specifically in low light or darkness. She cannot tell whether these symptoms have worsened over time, but she does not believe they have. Past ocular history is significant for bilateral photorefractive keratectomy performed 14 years ago for full distance correction in both eyes, with a good outcome in both eyes.

CASE HISTORY		
	Right Eye	**Left Eye**
UDVA	20/30	20/25
Present correction method	None	None
Manifest refraction	-0.75 +0.75 x 075	-0.25 +0.75 x 180
CDVA (current)	20/20	20/25
CNVA (current)	20/20	20/25
Add	+2.25	None
Dominant eye		Left
Pupil size (bright)	2.1	2.3
Pupil size (dim)	3.2	3.2
Slit Lamp Examination		
Cornea	Clear	Clear
Lens	2+NSC	Multifocal PCIOL—well centered
Capsule	Intact	Intact, trace opacification
Posterior Segment	Unremarkable	Unremarkable
Estimated ablation depth	N/A	10 µm

Questions

1. What are the most likely causes of the patient's visual symptoms in the left eye?
2. What treatment options are available for this patient?
3. Considering all factors, what treatment plan would you recommend and why?
4. What findings on examination are most useful in determining appropriate treatment options?
5. What are the most significant potential complications for the recommended treatment plan?

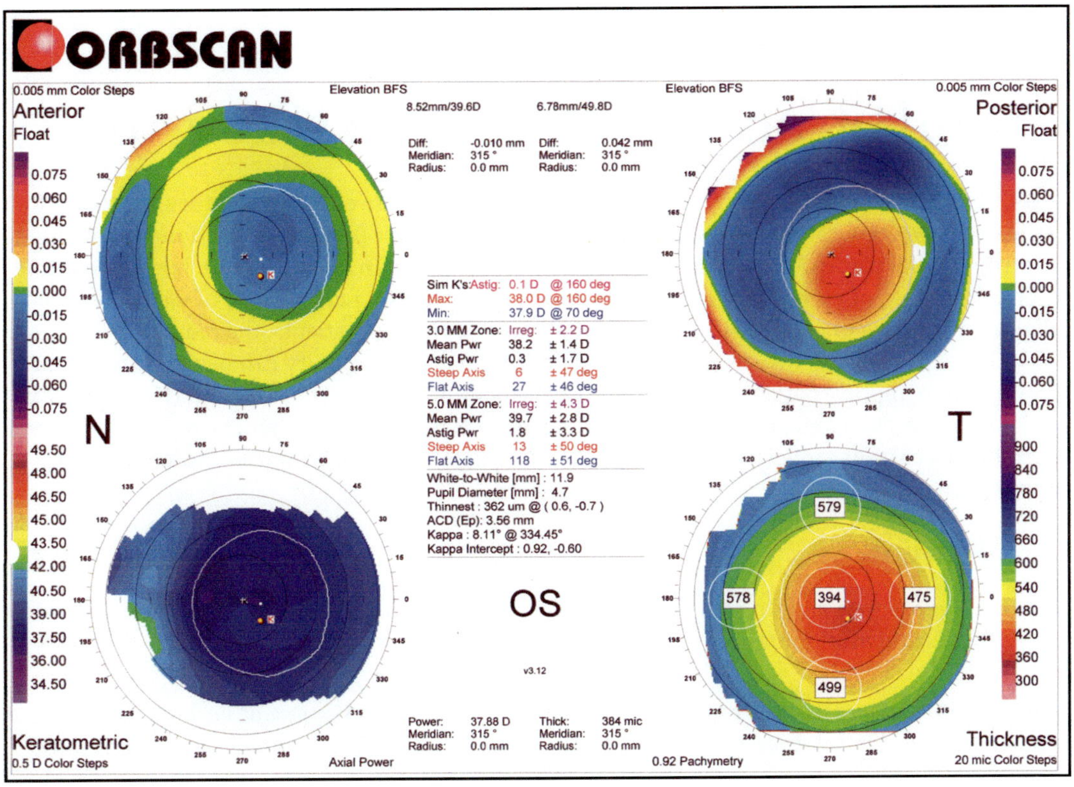
ORBSCAN
0.005 mm Color Steps
Anterior
Float
Elevation BFS
8.52mm/39.6D
6.78mm/49.8D
Diff: -0.010 mm
Meridian: 315°
Radius: 0.0 mm
Diff: 0.042 mm
Meridian: 315°
Radius: 0.0 mm
Elevation BFS
0.005 mm Color Steps
Posterior
Float
Sim K's:Astig: 0.1 D @ 160 deg
Max: 38.0 D @ 160 deg
Min: 37.9 D @ 70 deg
3.0 MM Zone: Irreg: ± 2.2 D
Mean Pwr 38.2 ± 1.4 D
Astig Pwr 0.3 ± 1.7 D
Steep Axis 6 ± 47 deg
Flat Axis 27 ± 46 deg
5.0 MM Zone: Irreg: ± 4.3 D
Mean Pwr 39.7 ± 2.8 D
Astig Pwr 1.8 ± 3.3 D
Steep Axis 13 ± 50 deg
Flat Axis 118 ± 51 deg
White-to-White [mm] : 11.9
Pupil Diameter [mm] : 4.7
Thinnest : 362 um @ (0.6, -0.7)
ACD (Ep): 3.56 mm
Kappa : 8.11° @ 334.45°
Kappa Intercept : 0.92, -0.60
N
T
OS
v3.12
579
578
394
475
499
Power: 37.88 D
Meridian: 315°
Radius: 0.0 mm
Thick: 384 mic
Meridian: 315°
Radius: 0.0 mm
Keratometric
0.5 D Color Steps
Axial Power
0.92 Pachymetry
Thickness
20 mic Color Steps

—CASE 36—
Mul tif oca l IOL Dissati sfacti on

Multifocal intraocular lenses (MFIOL) are currently the most effective intraocular option for presbyopia correction. These lenses, most of which are diffractive in design, functionally split light into various focal planes, thereby facilitating both near and distance acuity in each eye, providing the broadest range of vision. However, these lenses accomplish increased range of vision by potentially compromising quality of vision in any or all ranges. In most patients, the reduction in visual quality is not significant; however, in some individuals the visual quality can be poor and require intervention to improve patient functionality. In 1% to 5% of cases, intraocular lens (IOL) exchange may be necessary to alleviate patient symptoms. Newer IOL designs may reduce or alleviate these issues, but all current models appear susceptible to greater or lesser extent to the same potential complications.

Case Analysis

- Case Figure shows canning slit beam topographic image of the left eye demonstrating a mildly asymmetric central flattening pattern consistent with previous PRK.

Pearl: *ALL patients should be counseled about the possibility for significant visual aberrations with MFIOLs, and IOL exchange should be ruled out BEFORE Nd:YAG capsulotomy is performed!*

QUESTIONS

1. What are the most likely causes of the patient's visual symptoms in his left eye?

   Likely a combination of intrinsic multifocal IOL issues and posterior capsule opacification (PCO). Since the onset was nearly immediate after MFIOL implantation, intrinsic MFIOL issues are probably the primary issue.

2. What treatment options are available for this patient?

   The range of options include correction of residual refractive error, optimization of tear film, argon laser iridoplasty to improve relative IOL centration (if applicable), trial of pupil dilation to asses effect on night symptoms, cataract surgery in the right eye to improve binocular visual function, IOL exchange, or Nd:YAG capsulotomy.

3. Considering all factors, what treatment plan would you recommend and why?

   Given the patient's symptoms, time of onset, persistence over time, and effect on her activities, these issues are unlikely to resolve with anything less than IOL exchange.

4. What findings on examination are most useful in determining appropriate treatment options?

   Pupil size, corneal status, relative IOL position, and posterior capsule status are important when evaluating causes for visual dissatisfaction and treatment plans. Patients with small pupils are more likely to describe blur at some distances, as the full extent of the IOL multifocality may not functionally come into play. Any problems with corneal clarity or tear film will be magnified with MFIOLs. Relative pupil centration is important to maximize MFIOL function. MFIOLs are highly sensitive to PCO; however, the capsule should not be opened until IOL exchange has been ruled out, as an intact capsule greatly facilitates IOL exchange if it is necessary.

5. What are the most significant potential complications for the recommended treatment plan?

   IOL exchange carries increased risk, as compared to initial RLE, for posterior capsule rupture with vitreous loss, cystoid macular edema (CME), increased anterior segment inflammation, and corneal edema.

Multifocal IOL Complications

Complaints after MFIOL may be generally divided into two categories: blurred vision and photic phenomena. Patients may complain of one or the other category, or have issues with both general blur and photic phenomena. Blurred vision may be worse at a particular distance or similar through all distances.

Most diffractive IOLs have reduced efficacy in the mid-range, functionally about computer distance. Some patients describe their acuity as "waxy" or as "looking through water." Note that subjective blurred vision with MFIOLs often does not correlate with objective findings on Snellen acuity or manifest refraction. In fact, in past studies most patients with these complaints have had 20/30 or better uncorrected Snellen acuity and 0.5 D or less of spherical equivalent refractive error. Patients with MFIOLs appear particularly sensitive to residual astigmatism and to low contrast situations, including lower lighting.

Photic phenomena include glare, halos, and unique "ring" of light around point light sources, including car headlights, traffic lights, and street lights, among others. Many of these phenomena are a function of the MFIOL design, and all patients should be counseled that they will likely experience these symptoms to varying extent, especially in the early recovery period. For most patients the severity of photic phenomena diminishes over time; however, up to 5% of patients categorize their symptoms as severe and persistent. There may be a process of neuro-adaptation that occurs over time, considered more successful when both eyes have MFIOLs implanted, and with this neuro-adaptation these symptoms may diminish to unnoticeable or at least tolerable. When they do not, other measures must be taken to improve overall visual function.

Decision Tree for Evaluation and Management of Multifocal IOL Visual Disturbance

Case Figure 36-1 outlines a decision tree for evaluating and treating dissatisfaction after MFIOL implantation. Some patients have improvement in visual quality after YAG capsulotomy even with a relatively subtle PCO; however, it must be stressed that, until the prospect of IOL exchange is eliminated, YAG capsulotomy should not be performed. Once the posterior capsule is opened, IOL exchange becomes significantly more challenging and carries increased risks.

Many patient complaints may be addressed through correction of residual ametropia and maximizing the ocular surface through improving tear production and meibomian gland function. Topical cyclosporine and frequent lubricating drops will maximize tear production, while oral doxycycline or topical azithromycin improve meibomian gland function. Subtle IOL decentrations may be significant for MFIOLs, especially in patients with small pupils, and either topical cycloplegics to functionally uncover the IOL multifocality or argon laser iridoplasty to functionally center the pupil over the IOL optic may improve symptoms.

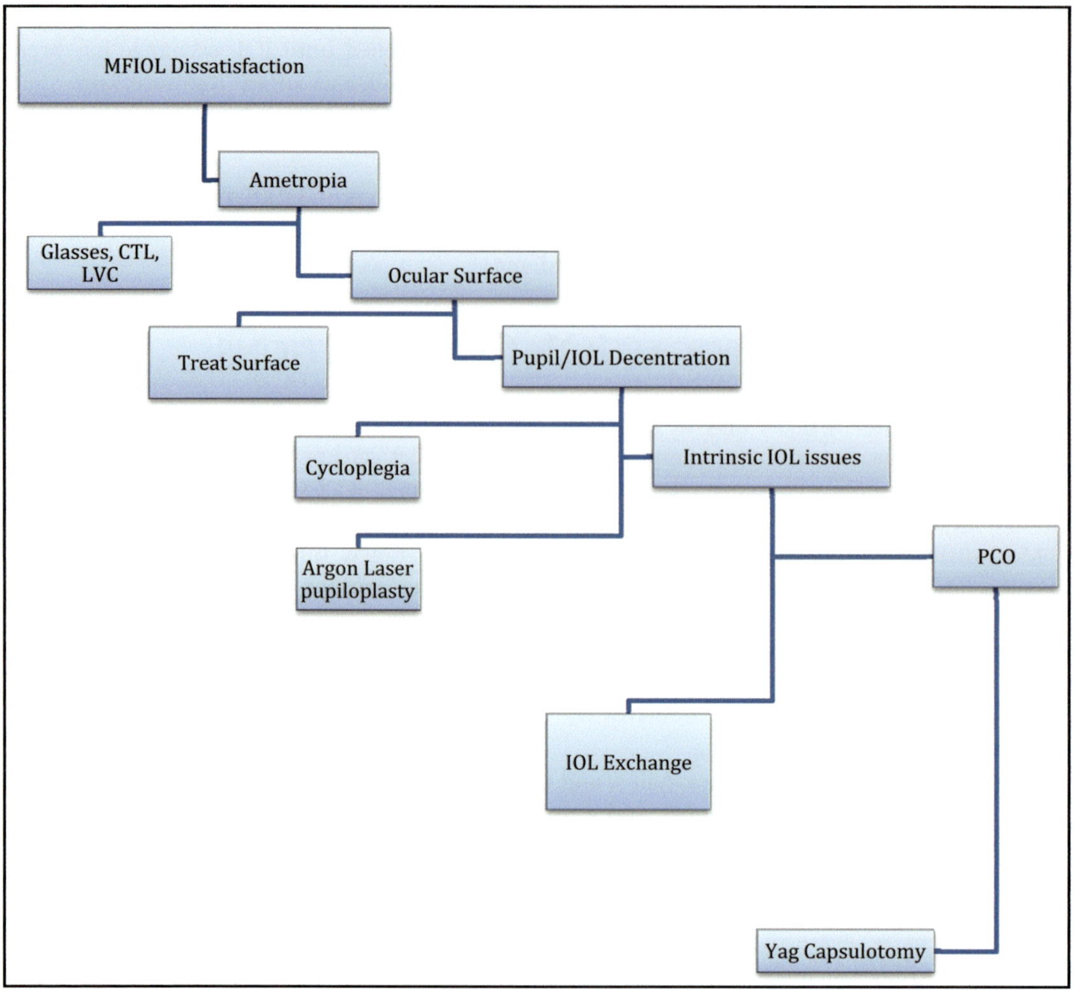

Case Figure 36-1. Decision tree for management of MFIOL dissatisfaction. In a case of MFIOL vision disturbance, residual ametropia and ocular surface issues should be evaluated and treated first. If symptoms persist, IOL decentration may be causing the issues, and a course of topical cycloplegic drops may temporarily alleviate the symptoms. If decentration is the major factor, argon laser iridoplasty may functionally center the pupil to correspond with the IOL optical center and visual axis. If none of these treatments or evaluations are effective, and if the issues have been present since surgery, then intrinsic MFIOL properties are likely the cause. If, after an appropriate time for adaptation, these symptoms persist and are disabling, then IOL exchange may be warranted. If patient symptoms were not present immediately after surgery but appear to be worsening over time, then PCO is a more likely source, and YAG capsulotomy may be warranted.

If the previously mentioned strategies are ineffective, intrinsic properties of MFIOLs are likely the cause of visual complaints. Once this has been established, some patients will opt to keep the MFIOL despite their symptoms due to the benefit at near and intermediate the lens provides; however, some patients will opt for IOL exchange.

In distinguishing between intrinsic MFIOL issues and other causes, especially PCO, determining onset of symptoms has significant value. Intrinsic IOL properties should be present immediately after surgery and are unlikely to change significantly for better or worse over time. Ocular surface issues will fluctuate during the recovery process and may worsen if dry eye and blepharitis are not addressed. Posterior capsule opacification will not be symptomatic immediately after surgery but should worsen over time if it is the source of visual complaints.

Retreatment Options and Bioptics

Patients with MFIOL implants are often intolerant to relatively small amounts of ametropia, especially astigmatism. Most studies have demonstrated significant subjective blur when residual astigmatism exceeds 0.5 D. Therefore, all patients considering MFIOL implants should have a full evaluation for LVC, including corneal topography and corneal thickness evaluation. Both LASIK and surface ablation appear equally effective after MFIOLs, but timing of the corneal procedure may dictate procedure choice. If surgery is planned before 3 months after RLE, it may be better to proceed with surface ablation rather than LASIK due to the potential for wound gape from the suction pressure applied during flap creation.

Bibliography

Alfonso JF, Fernández-Vega L, Baamonde MB, Montés-Micó R. Correlation of pupil size with visual acuity and contrast sensitivity after implantation of an apodized diffractive intraocular lens. *J Cataract Refract Surg.* 2007;33(3):430-438.

Barsam A, Voldman A, Holladay J, Bhogal M, Perry HD, Donnenfeld ED. Argon laser iridoplasty to improve visual function following multifocal intraocular lens implantation. *J Refract Surg.* 2012;15:281-283.

Blaylock JF, Si Z, Vickers C. Visual and refractive status at different focal distances after implantation of the ReSTOR multifocal intraocular lens. *J Cataract Refract Surg.* 2006;32(9):1464-1473.

Chiam PJ, Chan JH, Agarwal RK, Kasaby S. ReSTOR intraocular lens implantation in cataract surgery: quality of vision. *J Cataract Refract Surg.* 2006;32(9):1459-1463.

de Vries NE, Webers CA, Montés-Micó R, Ferrer-Blasco T, Nuijts RM. Visual outcomes after cataract surgery with implantation of a +3.00 D or +4.00 D aspheric diffractive multifocal intraocular lens: Comparative study. *J Cataract Refract Surg.* 2010;36(8):1316-1322.

de Vries NE, Webers CA, Touwslager WR, Bauer NJ, de Brabander J, Berendschot TT, Nuijts RM. Dissatisfaction after implantation of multifocal intraocular lenses. *J Cataract Refract Surg.* 2011;37(5):859-865.

Gil MA, Varon C, Rosello N, Cardona G, Buil JA. Visual acuity, contrast sensitivity, subjective quality of vision, and quality of life with 4 different multifocal IOLs. *Eur J Ophthalmol.* 2012;(2):175-187.

Jendritza BB, Knorz MC, Morton S. Wavefront-guided excimer laser vision correction after multifocal IOL implantation. *J Refract Surg.* 2008;24(3):274-279.

Mester U, Hunold W, Wesendahl T, Kaymak H. Functional outcomes after implantation of Tecnis ZM900 and Array SA40 multifocal intraocular lenses. *J Cataract Refract Surg.* 2007;33(6):1033-1040.

Salati C, Salvetat ML, Zeppieri M, Brusini P. Pupil size influence on the intraocular performance of the multifocal AMO-Array intraocular lens in elderly patients. *Eur J Ophthalmol.* 2007;17(4):571-578.

Shimizu K, Ito M. Dissatisfaction after bilateral multifocal intraocular lens implantation: an electrophysiology study. *J Refract Surg.* 2011;27(4):309-312.

Woodward MA, Randleman JB, Stulting RD. Dissatisfaction after multifocal intraocular lens implantation. *J Cataract Refract Surg.* 2009;35(6):992-997.

Please visit www.routledge.com/ 9781617110368
to access additional material.

Appendix
Case Index

Index

For Product Safety Concerns and Information please contact our
EU representative GPSR@taylorandfrancis.com Taylor & Francis
Verlag GmbH, Kaufingerstraße 24, 80331 München, Germany